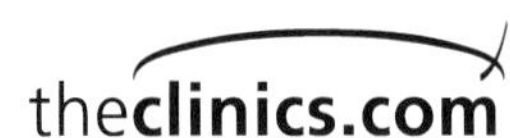

ENDOCRINOLOGY AND METABOLISM CLINICS OF NORTH AMERICA

Acute Endocrinology

GUEST EDITOR
Greet Van den Berghe, MD, PhD

CONSULTING EDITOR
Derek LeRoith, MD, PhD

December 2006 • Volume 35 • Number 4

SAUNDERS

An Imprint of Elsevier, Inc.
PHILADELPHIA LONDON TORONTO MONTREAL SYDNEY TOKYO

W.B. SAUNDERS COMPANY
A Division of Elsevier Inc.

1600 John F. Kennedy Boulevard • Suite 1800 • Philadelphia, Pennsylvania 19103-2899

http://www.theclinics.com

ENDOCRINOLOGY AND METABOLISM CLINICS OF NORTH AMERICA
December 2006
Editor: Rachel Glover

Volume 35, Number 4
ISSN 0889-8529
ISBN 1-4160-4308-X

Endocrinology and Metabolism Clinics of North America (ISSN 0889-8529) is published quarterly by Elsevier Inc., 360 Park Avenue South, New York, NY 10010-1710. Months of publication are March, June, September, and December. Business and editorial offices: 1600 John F. Kennedy Boulevard, Suite 1800, Philadelphia, PA 19103-2899. Customer Service Office: 6277 Sea Harbor Drive, Orlando, FL 32887-4800. Periodicals postage paid at New York, NY and additional mailing offices. Subscription prices are USD 193 per year for US individuals, USD 319 per year for US institutions, USD 99 per year for US students and residents, USD 242 per year for Canadian individuals, USD 383 per year for Canadian institutions, USD 264 per year for international individuals, USD 383 per year for international institutions and USD 138 per year for Canadian and foreign students/residents. To receive student/resident rate, orders must be accompained by name of affiliated institution, date of term, and the *signature* of program/residency coordinator on institution letterhead. Orders will be billed at individual rate until proof of status is received. Foreign air speed delivery is included in all *Clinics* subscription prices. All prices are subject to change without notice. POSTMASTER: Send address changes to *Endocrinology and Metabolism Clinics of North America*, Elsevier Periodicals Customer Service, 6277 Sea Harbor Drive, Orlando, FL 32887-4800. **Customer Service: (+1) 800-654-2452 (US). From outside of the US, call (+1) 407-345-4000; e-mail: hhspcs@harcourt.com.**

Reprints. For copies of 100 or more, of articles in this publication, please contact the Commercial Rights Department, Elsevier Inc., 360 Park Avenue South, New York, NY 10010-1710; phone: (+1) 212-633-3813; fax: (+1) 212-462-1935; e-mail: reprints@elsevier.com.

Endocrinology and Metabolism Clinics of North America is covered in *Index Medicus, EMBASE/Excerpta Medica, Current Contents/Clinical Medicine, Current Contents/Life Sciences, Science Citation Index, ISI/BIOMED, BIOSIS, and Chemical Abstracts.*

Printed in the United States of America.

CONSULTING EDITOR

DEREK LeROITH, MD, PhD, Chief, Division of Endocrinology, Metabolism, and Bone Diseases, Mount Sinai School of Medicine, New York, New York

GUEST EDITOR

GREET VAN DEN BERGHE, MD, PhD, Professor of Medicine, Department of Intensive Care Medicine, Katholieke Universiteit Leuven, Leuven, Belgium

CONTRIBUTORS

GABRIELE BASSI, MD, Resident Fellow, Istituto di Anestesiologia e Rianimazione dell'Università degli Studi di Milano, Azienda Ospedaliera, Polo Universitario San Paolo, Milano, Italy

ROGER BOUILLON, MD, PhD, FRCP, Clinic and Laboratory of Endocrinology, University Hospital Gasthuisberg, Leuven, Belgium

FREDERIEKE M. BROUWERS, MD, Visiting Fellow, Section on Medical Neuroendocrinology, Reproductive Biology and Medicine Branch, National Institute of Child Health and Human Development, Bethesda, Maryland

KENNETH BURMAN, MD, Chief, Endocrine Section, Washington Hospital Center, Washington, DC; Program Director, Endocrine Fellowship Program, Georgetown University and the Washington Hospital Center, Washington; and Professor, Department of Medicine, Georgetown University, Washington, District of Columbia

ENRICO CALZIA, MD, Associated Professor of Anesthesiology, Sektion Anästhesiologische Pathophysiologie und Verfahrensentwicklung, Universitätsklinikum, Ulm, Germany

YVES DEBAVEYE, MD, Department of Intensive Care, Catholic University of Leuven, Leuven, Belgium

GRAEME EISENHOFER, PhD, Staff Scientist, Clinical Neurocardiology Section, National Institute of Neurological Disorders and Stroke, National Institutes of Health, Bethesda, Maryland

PHILLIP GORDEN, MD, Investigator, Molecular and Cellular Physiology Section, National Institute of Diabetes and Digestive and Kidney Disease, National Institutes of Health, Bethesda, Maryland

JEAN-MARC GUETTIER, MD, Clinical Fellow, Inter-Institute Endocrine Training Program, National Institute of Diabetes and Digestive and Kidney Disease, National Institutes of Health, Bethesda, Maryland

ABBAS E. KITABCHI, PhD, MD, Professor of Medicine and Molecular Sciences; and Director, Division of Endocrinology, Diabetes and Metabolism, University of Tennessee Health Science Center, Memphis, Tennessee

LIES LANGOUCHE, PhD, Department of Intensive Care Medicine, Katholieke Universiteit Leuven, Leuven, Belgium

JACQUES W.M. LENDERS, MD, PhD, Professor, Department of Internal Medicine, Division of General Internal Medicine, Radboud University Nijmegen Medical Centre, Nijmegen, the Netherlands

LIESE MEBIS, MSC, Department of Intensive Care, Catholic University of Leuven, Leuven, Belgium

DIETER MESOTTEN, MD, PhD, Resident, Department of Intensive Care Medicine, University Hospital Gasthuisberg, Catholic University Leuven, Belgium

BEAT MÜLLER, MD, Professor of Internal Medicine and Endocrinology, Clinic of Endocrinology, Diabetes and Clinical Nutrition, Department of Internal Medicine, University Hospital Basel, Basel, Switzerland

SUZANNE MYERS ADLER, MD, Fellow, Division of Endocrinology and Metabolism, Georgetown University School of Medicine, Washington, District of Columbia

BINDU NAYAK, MD, Endocrine Fellow, Combined Endocrine Program, Georgetown University and the Washington Hospital Center, Washington, District of Columbia

EBENEZER A. NYENWE, MD, Senior Fellow in Endocrinology, Division of Endocrinology, Diabetes and Metabolism, University of Tennessee Health Science Center, Memphis, Tennessee

KAREL PACAK, MD, PhD, DSc, Chief, Section on Medical Neuroendocrinology, Reproductive Biology and Medicine Branch, National Institute of Child Health and Human Development, Bethesda, Maryland

PETER RADERMACHER, MD, Professor of Anesthesiology, Sektion Anästhesiologische Pathophysiologie und Verfahrensentwicklung, Universitätsklinikum, Ulm, Germany

PHILIPP SCHUETZ, MD, Resident in Internal Medicine and Endocrinology, Clinic of Endocrinology, Diabetes and Clinical Nutrition, Department of Internal Medicine, University Hospital Basel, Basel, Switzerland

GREET VAN DEN BERGHE, MD, PhD, Professor of Medicine, Department of Intensive Care Medicine, Katholieke Universiteit Leuven, Leuven, Belgium

ILSE VANHOREBEEK, PhD, Postdoctoral Fellow, Department of Intensive Care Medicine, Katholieke Universiteit Leuven, Leuven, Belgium

JOSEPH G. VERBALIS, MD, Professor of Medicine and Physiology; Chair, Department of Medicine, Georgetown University School of Medicine, Washington, District of Columbia

THEO J. VISSER, PhD, Professor of Medicine, Department of Internal Medicine, Erasmus University Medical Center, Rotterdam, the Netherlands

LEONARD WARTOFSKY, MD, Chairman, Department of Medicine, Washington Hospital Center, Washington, District of Columbia; Professor of Medicine, Physiology, Anatomy, and Genetics, Uniformed Services University of the Health Sciences, Bethesda, Maryland; and Professor of Medicine, Georgetown University School of Medicine, Washington, District of Columbia

CONTENTS

Thyroid storm represents the extreme manifestation of thyrotoxicosis as a true endocrine emergency. Although Graves' disease is the most common underlying disorder in thyroid storm, there is usually a precipitating event or condition that transforms the patient into life-threatening thyrotoxicosis. Treatment of thyroid storm involves decreasing new hormone synthesis, inhibiting the release of thyroid hormone, and blocking the peripheral effects of thyroid hormone. This multidrug, therapeutic approach uses thionamides, iodine, beta-adrenergic receptor antagonists, corticosteroids in certain circumstances, and supportive therapy. Certain conditions may warrant the use of alternative therapy with cholestyramine, lithium carbonate, or potassium perchlorate. After the critical illness of thyroid storm subsides, definitive treatment of the underlying thyrotoxicosis can be planned.

Myxedema coma is the term given to the most severe presentation of profound hypothyroidism and is often fatal in spite of therapy. Decompensation of the hypothyroid patient into a coma may be precipitated by a number of drugs, systemic illnesses (eg, pneumonia), and other causes. It typically presents in older women in the winter months and is associated with signs of hypothyroidism, hypothermia, hyponatremia, hypercarbia, and hypoxemia. Treatment must be initiated promptly in an intensive care unit setting.

implemented. In most cases, this systemic approach to diagnosis and therapy is rewarded with a good outcome for the patient.

Acute Adrenal Insufficiency **767**
Roger Bouillon

Adrenal insufficiency is a rare disorder, usually with gradually evolving clinical symptoms and signs. Occasionally, an acute adrenal insufficiency crisis can become a life-threatening condition because of acute interruption of a normal or hyperfunctioning adrenal or pituitary gland or sudden interruption of adrenal replacement therapy. Acute stress situations can aggravate the symptomatology. A simple strategy of diagnostic screening and early intervention with sodium chloride–containing fluids and hydrocortisone should be widely implemented for cases with suspicion of an acute Addison disease crisis. In contrast, the chronic replacement dosage for patients with adrenal insufficiency should be as low as possible with clear instructions for dosage adjustments in case of stress or acute emergencies.

The Dynamic Neuroendocrine Response to Critical Illness **777**
Lies Langouche and Greet Van den Berghe

The severity of striking alterations in the hypothalamic–anterior pituitary–peripheral hormone axes, which are the hallmark of severity of critical illness, is associated with a high risk for morbidity and mortality. Most attempts to correct the hormone balance are ineffective or harmful because of lack of pathophysiologic understanding. Extensive research has provided more insight in the biphasic neuroendocrine response to critical illness: the acute phase is characterized by an actively secreting pituitary but low peripheral effector hormone levels. In contrast, in prolonged critical illness, uniform suppression of the neuroendocrine axes, predominantly of hypothalamic origin, contributes to low serum levels of the respective target-organ hormones.

Changes Within the Growth Hormone/Insulin-like Growth Factor I/IGF Binding Protein Axis During Critical Illness **793**
Dieter Mesotten and Greet Van den Berghe

Interest in the somatotropic axis, with its complex network of interactions, during critical illness arose only a few decades ago. The distinguishing neuroendocrine features of prolonged critical illness were not differentiated from those during the acute phase until the early 1990s. This incomplete understanding of the somatotropic axis contributed to some disastrous results, such as the multicenter growth hormone trial. The goal of stimulating the somatotropic axis without a proper preceding neuroendocrine diagnosis should be held obsolete. Moreover, the fascinating link between regulators of carbohydrate metabolism, such as insulin and insulin-like

FORTHCOMING ISSUES

March 2007

Growth Hormone
Ken K.Y. Ho, MD, *Guest Editor*

June 2007

Andrology
Ronald Tamler, MD, *Guest Editor*

September 2007

Transplant Medicine
Tracy L. Breen, MD, *Guest Editor*

RECENT ISSUES

September 2006

Impaired Glucose Tolerance and Cardiovascular Disease
Willa A. Hseuh, MD, Preethi Srikanthan, MD, and Christopher J. Lyon, PhD, *Guest Editors*

June 2006

Molecular Basis of Inherited Pancreatic Disorders
Markus M. Lerch, MD, FRCP,
Thomas Griesbacher, MD,
David C. Whitcomb, MD, PhD, *Guest Editors*

March 2006

Endocrine Disorders During Pregnancy
Susan J. Mandel, MD, MPH
Guest Editor

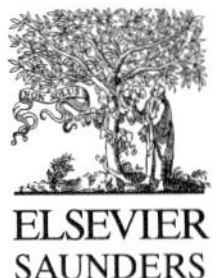

ELSEVIER
SAUNDERS

Endocrinol Metab Clin N Am
35 (2006) xiii–xv

ENDOCRINOLOGY
AND METABOLISM
CLINICS
OF NORTH AMERICA

Foreword

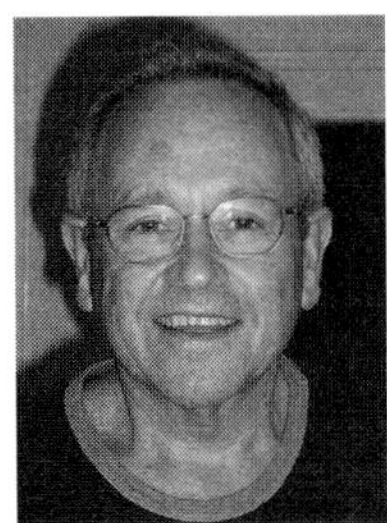

Derek LeRoith, MD, PhD
Consulting Editor

Once again, the *Endocrinology and Metabolism Clinics of North America* has assembled a cadre of world experts to review a number of very important aspects of acute endocrinology. Dr. Greet Van den Berghe, a world-renowned expert in critical care medicine has compiled this extremely topical issue.

The opening presentations cover thyroid storm and myxoedema coma, two classic endocrine emergencies. Nayak and Burman describe the normal physiology of thyroid hormone metabolism and the etiology of thyroid storm, which usually occurs in cases of Graves' disease. As they outline in their very practical review, signs and symptoms affect many organ systems of the body, and once the diagnosis is made, there are a number of therapeutic choices. Most cases will respond to medications, but occasionally, emergency surgery is required. The review by Wartofsky describes the fortunately uncommon occurrence of myxoedema coma, although patients with severe undiagnosed myxoedema are probably more common than thought, and myxoedema should always be considered in severely ill patients. Once again, multiple systems are affected, and signs and symptoms maybe quite subtle, especially in the elderly. Serum thyroid-stimulating hormone measurements are easily obtainable and are the mainstay for screening. As Wartofsky points out, because hypothyroidism may be secondary to hypopituitarism, corticosteroids should be used simultaneously to starting treatment for myxoedema, to avoid an adrenal crisis.

Pheochromocytomas are not very common and are often difficult to detect, although these should always be thought of when presenting symptoms are unusual. Paroxysmal hypertension, sweating, palpitations, and headaches

doi:10.1016/j.ecl.2006.10.001

are the classic symptoms, yet are absent in over half of the cases. In cases of pheochromocytoma emergencies, multi-system failure can be seen, particularly with hypertensive encephalopathy, arrythmias, and shock. Both alpha and beta adrenergic blockades are necessary; in the review by Brouwers and colleagues, there is a very explicit description of the management of such life-threatening conditions.

Both hyperglycemia and hypoglycemia may become critical conditions. Kitabchi describes the events occurring in hyperglycemic ketoacidosis, primarily, although not exclusively, an event seen in Type 1 diabetics, and non-ketotic hyperosmolar coma, seen more commonly in Type 2 diabetics. Despite our understanding of these conditions and of the appropriate management required, both are still relatively common, and may reflect poor management of patients with diabetes; thus, this review is timely and appropriate. The article on hypoglycemia by Guettier and Gorden, on the other hand, describes the classic causes and evaluation of patients with hypoglycemia and the management of the primary cause. Drug-induced hypoglycemia remains the most common type of hypoglycemia, particularly in patients with diabetes, and should be treated rapidly and effectively, because it often presents as an emergency condition.

Adrenal insufficiency may be primary or secondary to hypothalamic–pituitary disorders and requires immediate diagnosis and replacement therapy. The article by Bouillon is a practical approach that suggests that during the diagnosis, it may be necessary to institute therapy immediately to avoid a deterioration of the patient's condition.

The article by Langouche and Van den Berghe describes an interesting summary of studies that outline the hormonal deficiencies seen in acute and chronic illness. In both circumstances, peripheral hormone deficiency occurs. In acute illness, this is despite increased secretion of hypothalamic–pituitary hormones and suggests a degree of peripheral hormone resistance. In contrast, in chronic illness, there is an overall reduction in central hormone secretion. The concept is based on numerous studies and has a powerful message for the academic.

Mesotten and Van den Berghe then address the question of the growth hormone (GH)/insulin-like growth factor (IGF) in critical illness. There is a good although incomplete understanding of the effects of critical illness on this axis. On the other hand, use of rhGH or rhIGF-1 in these patients remains essentially a research opportunity. Both hormones have numerous effects in addition to protein anabolism, and these negative effects on metabolism may preclude their use; indeed, one study using GH in intensive care patients was associated with increased mortality.

Mebis and colleagues describe the alterations in the hypothalamic–pituitary–thyroid axis in critical illness, known to most clinicians as the "euthyroid sick syndrome." They also discuss the question of replacement of triiodothyronine (thyroxine is ineffective) under these circumstances, and although they don't give a clear answer to this question (because there isn't one), they correctly suggest that thyrotropin-releasing hormone replacement maybe more appropriate and safer.

Similarly, in the excellent article by Müller, there is a discussion, backed by studies, which suggests that a degree of "relative adrenal insufficiency" exists in cases of critical illness. However, as the author points out, the uncontrolled use of glucocorticoids under these circumstances may sometimes be more harmful than helpful. Judicious use is, therefore, suggested as we await the outcome of large controlled studies on this topic.

Catecholamines are widely used in maintaining tissue perfusion in patients with critical illnesses, although some of the side effects are quite serious and include increased oxygen consumption and enhanced gluconeogenesis. Dopamine, on the other hand, may suppress release of certain hormones and interfere with the body's immune response. Vasopressin has become the new wonder drug in maintaining cardiovascular stability, although its side effect profile is as yet undefined. All of these issues are covered in a very scholarly article by Bassi, Radermacher, and Calzia.

In their classic studies on intensive insulin therapy in medical and surgical intensive care patients, Van den Berghe and coworkers showed phenomenal improvements in outcomes. Vanhorebeek and Van den Berghe describe many studies of their own and by others on the mechanisms that may play a role in the success of an intensive insulin therapy program. In addition to blood glucose control, it is apparent that insulin therapy has effects on other metabolic parameters, such as lipids, and on tissue mitochondrial health. Insulin may also have nonmetabolic effects, such as on proinflammatory mediators, that may help explain the results.

Sodium and water imbalances are critical issues in patients with severe illnesses and are very commonly encountered. These conditions are divided into hypoosmolar disorders (excess water relative to solute) and hyperosmolar disorders (excess solute relative to water), making appropriate evaluation and management extremely important. A very practical expose is discussed by Verbalis.

In summary, this issue is a must read for endocrinologists, internists, and intensivists, contributing greatly to the understanding of important endocrinological disorders and providing practical guidelines to their treatment.

Derek LeRoith, MD, PhD
Division of Endocrinology, Metabolism, and Bone Diseases
Mount Sinai School of Medicine
One Gustave L. Levy Place, Box 1055
Atran 4-36
New York, NY 10029-6574, USA

E-mail address: derek.leroith@mssm.edu

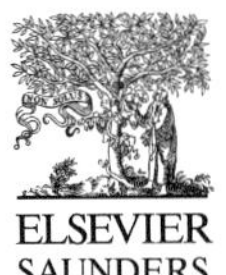

ELSEVIER
SAUNDERS

Endocrinol Metab Clin N Am
35 (2006) xvii–xviii

ENDOCRINOLOGY
AND METABOLISM
CLINICS
OF NORTH AMERICA

Preface

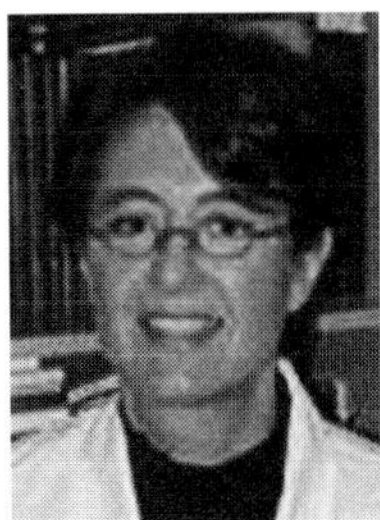

Greet Van den Berghe, MD, PhD
Guest Editor

Until recently, there were no other specialties in medicine so uncomfortable with each other, and hence so isolated, than endocrinology and critical care medicine. Fortunately, the two "alien" disciplines have recently joined forces in successful attempts to perform high-quality research to clarify the unknown. By integrating endocrinology in critical care medicine (or perhaps I should say vice versa), new experimental and clinical data on the complex endocrine and metabolic derangements accompanying nonendocrine severe illnesses became available, which generated important novel insights with relevant clinical implications. In addition, the state-of-the-art diagnosis and management of primary endocrine diseases that represent life-threatening situations leading to intensive care unit (ICU) admission have been updated. This issue aims at compiling all these new findings into one volume, thereby attempting to become the first compilation of interest to both disciplines, endocrinology and critical care medicine. It indeed covers both areas of "acute endocrinology" that are often taken care of at distant sites within hospitals. The first part deals with the classic life-threatening illnesses caused by primary endocrine diseases, such as thyrotoxicosis, hypothyroidism, pheochromocytoma, severe hyperglycemia and hypoglycemia, and acute adrenal crises. The second part of the issue looks at endocrinology from the ICU side, starting with a general overview of the dynamic neuroendocrine and metabolic stress responses in the condition of intensive care-dependent nonendocrine critical illness. Alterations within several of the endocrine axes briefly touched on in the overview article are then further discussed in detail in the following articles: critical illness–induced alterations within the

0889-8529/06/$ - see front matter
doi:10.1016/j.ecl.2006.09.001

growth hormone axis, the thyroid axis, and the pituitary adrenal axis; changes in catecholamines; glucose control; and salt and water metabolism. The last article on salt and water disturbances bridges the endocrine and nonendocrine causes and their specific approaches.

I sincerely hope that this volume provides a unique and up-to-date overview of the state-of-the-art knowledge of interest to the most alien of disciplines in medicine and stimulates further interdisciplinary research in this important and exciting field.

Greet Van den Berghe, MD, PhD
Department of Intensive Care Medicine
University Hospital Gasthuisberg
Herestraat 49
B-3000 Leuven, Belgium

E-mail address: greta.vandenberghe@med.kuleuven.be

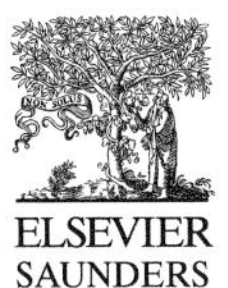
ELSEVIER
SAUNDERS

Endocrinol Metab Clin N Am
35 (2006) 663–686

ENDOCRINOLOGY
AND METABOLISM
CLINICS
OF NORTH AMERICA

Thyrotoxicosis and Thyroid Storm

Bindu Nayak, MD[a], Kenneth Burman, MD[a,b,c,*]

[a]*Department of Endocrinology, Georgetown University Hospital, 4000 Reservoir Road NW, Building D, Suite 232, Washington, DC 20007, USA*

[b]*Department of Endocrinology, Washington Hospital Center, 110 Irving Street NW, Room 2A-72, Washington DC 20010-2975, USA*

[c]*Department of Medicine, Georgetown University, 110 Irving Street NW, Room 2A-72, Washington DC 20010, USA*

In the spectrum of endocrine emergencies, thyroid storm ranks as one of the most critical illnesses. Recognition and appropriate management of life-threatening thyrotoxicosis is vital to prevent the high morbidity and mortality that may accompany this disorder. The incidence of thyroid storm has been noted to be less than 10% of patients hospitalized for thyrotoxicosis; however, the mortality rate due to thyroid storm ranges from 20 to 30% [1,2].

In common parlance, whereas hyperthyroidism refers to disorders that result from overproduction of hormone from the thyroid gland, thyrotoxicosis refers to any cause of excessive thyroid hormone concentration. Thyroid storm represents the extreme manifestation of thyrotoxicosis [3]. The point at which thyrotoxicosis transforms to thyroid storm is controversial, and is, to some degree, subjective. In an effort to standardize and objectify thyroid storm somewhat, as compared with severe thyrotoxicosis, Burch and Wartofsky [4] have delineated a point system assessing degrees of dysfunction in various systems (thermoregulatory, central nervous, gastrointestinal, and cardiovascular), as shown in Table 1. However, clinically, it is prudent to assume that someone with severe thyrotoxicosis has impending thyroid storm, and to treat them aggressively, rather than focus on specific definitions.

Etiology

The most common underlying cause of thyrotoxicosis in cases of thyroid storm is Graves' disease. Graves' disease is mediated by the thyrotropin

* Corresponding author. Department of Endocrinology, Washington Hospital Center, 110 Irving Street NW, Room 2A-72, Washington DC 20010-2975.

E-mail address: Kenneth.burman@medstar.net (K. Burman).

doi:10.1016/j.ecl.2006.09.008 ***endo.theclinics.com***

Table 1
Diagnostic criteria for thyroid storm

Diagnostic parameters	Scoring points
Thermoregulatory dysfunction	
Temperature	
99–99.9	5
100–100.9	10
101–101.9	15
102–102.9	20
103–103.9	25
≥104.0	30
Central nervous system effects	
Absent	0
Mild (agitation)	10
Moderate (delirium, psychosis, extreme lethargy	20
Severe (seizures, coma)	30
Gastrointestinal-hepatic dysfunction	
Absent	0
Moderate (diarrhea, nausea/vomiting, abdominal pain)	10
Severe (unexplained jaundice)	20
Cardiovascular dysfunction	
Tachycardia (beats/minute)	
90–109	5
110–119	10
120–129	15
≥140	25
Congestive heart failure	
Absent	0
Mild (pedal edema)	5
Moderate (bibasilar rales)	10
Severe (pulmonary edema)	15
Atrial fibrillation	
Absent	0
Present	10
Precipitating event	
Absent	0
Present	10

Scoring system: A score of 45 or greater is highly suggestive of thyroid storm; a score of 25–44 is suggestive of impending storm, and a score below 25 is unlikely to represent thyroid storm.

Adapted from Burch HB, Wartofsky L. Life-threatening thyrotoxicosis. Thyroid storm. Endocrinol Metab Clin North Am 1993;22(2):263–77.

receptor antibodies that stimulate excess and uncontrolled thyroidal synthesis and secretion of thyroid hormones (thyroxine [T_4] or triiodothyronine [T_3]). It occurs most frequently in young women, but can occur in either sex and any age group. However, thyroid storm can also occur with a solitary toxic adenoma or toxic multinodular goiter. Rare causes of thyrotoxicosis leading to thyroid storm would include hypersecretory thyroid carcinoma, thyrotropin-secreting pituitary adenoma, struma ovarii/teratoma, and human chorionic gonadotropia–secreting hydatidiform mole. Other causes include interferon alpha and interleukin-2–induced thyrotoxicosis during treatment for other diseases, such as viral hepatitis and HIV infection [5–8]. Particularly relevant is hyperthyroidism aggravated by iodine exposure, which can occur, for example, following the intravenous administration of radiocontrast dye, or during or after amiodarone administration.

Given the background of hyperthyroidism due to the above causes, a precipitating event usually ignites the transition from thyrotoxicosis to thyroid storm. Thyroid storm can be precipitated by systemic insults such as surgery, trauma, myocardial infarction, pulmonary thromboembolism, diabetic ketoacidosis, parturition, or severe infection [5]. Thyroid storm has also been reported to be precipitated by the discontinuation of antithyroid drugs, excessive ingestion or intravenous administration of iodine (eg, radiocontrast dyes, amiodarone), radioiodine therapy, and even pseudoephedrine and salicylate use. Salicylates may increase free thyroid hormone levels disproportionately [9]. In the past, thyroid surgery in patients who had uncontrolled hyperthyroidism was the most common cause of thyroid storm. However, appropriate recognition and preparation before thyroid surgery has decreased, but not eliminated, the perioperative incidence of thyroid storm. The most common precipitating cause of thyroid storm currently seems to be infection, although it is difficult to know if published reports mirror actual frequencies [10].

To appreciate the pathogenesis of thyroid storm, one must first consider the mechanism of action of thyroid hormone at the nuclear level. Circulating, or free, T_4 and T_3 are taken into the cytoplasm of cells. T_4 is converted to its active form, T_3, by 5′-deiodinase enzyme(s). Conversion of T_4 to T_3 is accomplished by deiodination in the outer ring of the T_4 molecule. The three deiodinase proteins are D1, D2, and D3. Type I deiodinase (D1) and Type II deiodinase (D2) facilitate outer ring deiodination of T_4 to T_3. Normally, deiodination of T_4 to T_3 provides only 20% to 30% of T_3 (with the remaining emanating from direct thyroid secretion); however, it may provide more than 50% of T_3 in the thyrotoxic state. D1 is sensitive to inhibition by propylthiouracil, and D2 is insensitive to it. D1 activity has been noted in the liver, kidney, thyroid, and pituitary. D2 is responsible for most of the T_3 production in the euthyroid state. D2 mRNA is expressed in vascular smooth muscle, thyroid, heart, brain, spinal cord, skeletal muscle, and placenta. Type 3 deiodinase (D3) catalyzes the conversion of T_4 to reverse T_3 and to 3,3′–diiodothyronine (T2) which are both inactive. D3 is mainly present in the central nervous system, skin, and placenta [11].

After T_4 is deiodinated to T_3, it can then exert its effect by passing into the nucleus and binding to thyroid hormone receptors or thyroid hormone–responsive elements, to induce gene activation and transcription [4,12]. Thyroid hormone exerts its influence through nongenomic and genomic or nuclear effects. Nongenomic effects (eg, mitochondrial) usually occur rapidly, whereas genomic effects require at least several hours to cause a modification of gene transcription. Thyroid hormone has specific effects in different tissues of the body. In the pituitary gland, T_3 exerts negative regulation on the transcription of the genes for the beta subunit and the common alpha subunit of thyrotropin, resulting in a suppressed thyrotropin in the context of thyrotoxicosis. Thyroid hormone also stimulates lipogenesis and lipolysis by inducing enzymes important early in the lipogenic pathway, including malic enzyme, glucose-6-phosphate dehydrogenase, and fatty acid synthetase. T_3 also accelerates the transcription of 3-hydroxy-3-methylglutaryl coenzyme A reductase. Although cholesterol production is increased, excretion of cholesterol in the bile is also accelerated, generally resulting in a decrease in total cholesterol. Thyroid hormone exerts its effect on bone by stimulating both osteogenesis and osteolysis, resulting in faster bone remodeling [12]. Thyroid hormone effects on the heart and cardiovascular system are many, resulting in decreased systemic vascular resistance, increased blood volume, increased contractility, and increased cardiac output [13].

One hypothesis to explain the cause of thyroid storm is an increase in the amount of free thyroid hormones. Of course, the elevated serum and intracellular levels of T_4/T_3 suppress thyrotropin, so that serum thyrotropin should be undetectable, except in very unusual cases (eg, pituitary thyrotropin-secreting adenoma). In one study comparing 6 subjects with thyroid storm to 15 subjects with more typical thyrotoxicosis, Brooks and colleagues [14] found that the mean free T_4 concentration was higher in subjects with thyroid storm, whereas the total T_4 concentration was similar in both groups. Another theory that may explain the pathogenesis of thyroid storm is a possible increase in target cell beta-adrenergic receptor density or postreceptor modifications in signaling pathways [4,15,16].

The important clinical point is that it is best to consider severe thyrotoxicosis or thyroid storm in ill patients and to approach and treat them in an active, preemptory fashion when possible. The distinction between severe thyrotoxicosis and life-threatening thyrotoxicosis, or thyroid storm, is a matter of clinical judgment. Although objective means such as the point scale by Burch and Wartofsky can, and perhaps should, be used, it is most prudent to treat a patient aggressively for his/her hyperthyroidism, rather than excessively contemplate whether this case really meets the criteria for thyroid storm. Close clinical monitoring is also required, usually in an intensive care unit. There is no arbitrary serum T_4 or T_3 cutoff that discriminates severe thyrotoxicosis from thyroid storm. Also, systemically ill patients have decreased ability to convert T_4 to T_3. Therefore, a minimally elevated T_3 or even a "normal" T_3 may be considered inappropriately elevated in the context of systemic illness.

Clinical presentation

The signs and symptoms of thyrotoxicosis are outlined in Table 2.

Table 2
Signs and symptoms of thyrotoxicosis

Organ system	Symptoms	Signs
Neuropsychiatric/Neuromuscular	Emotional lability	Muscle wasting
	Anxiety	Hyperreflexia
	Confusion	Fine tremor
	Coma	Periodic paralysis
Gastrointestinal	Hyperdefecation	
	Diarrhea	
Reproductive	Oligomenorrhea	Gynecomastia
	Decreased libido	Spider angiomas
Thyroid gland	Neck fullness	Diffuse enlargement
	Tenderness	Bruit
Cardiorespiratory	Palpitations	Atrial fibrillation
	Dyspnea	Sinus tachycardia
	Chest pain	Hyperdynamic precordium
		Congestive heart failure
Dermatologic	Hair loss	Pretibial myxedema
		Warm, moist skin
		Palmar erythema
Ophthalmologic	Diplopia	Exophthalmos
	Eye irritation	Ophthalmoplegia
		Conjunctival injection

Constitutional

One of the common findings in thyrotoxicosis is weight loss, despite having the same or greater caloric intake. The hypermetabolic state results in an imbalance of greater energy production compared with energy use, resulting in increased heat production and elimination. The thermogenesis leads to increased perspiration and heat intolerance. Other constitutional symptoms reported are generalized weakness and fatigue [17].

Neuropsychiatric

Neuropsychiatric manifestations of thyrotoxicosis include emotional lability, restlessness, anxiety, agitation, confusion, psychosis, and even coma [18]. In fact, behavioral studies reveal poor performance in memory and concentration testing proportional to the degree of thyrotoxicosis [17].

Gastrointestinal

Gastrointestinal symptoms include increased frequency of bowel movements due to increased motor contraction in the small bowel, leading to more rapid movement of intestinal contents.

Reproductive symptoms

Reproductive symptoms include changes in the menstrual cycle, including oligomenorrhea and anovulation. In men, symptoms can include decreased libido, gynecomastia, and development of spider angiomas, perhaps related to an increase in sex hormone-binding globulin and a subsequent increase in estrogen activity [17].

Cardiorespiratory

Cardiorespiratory symptoms of thyrotoxicosis include palpitations and dyspnea on exertion. The shortness of breath can be multifactorial in origin because of decreased lung compliance, engorged pulmonary capillary bed, or left ventricular failure. Thyrotoxic patients may also experience chest pain similar to angina pectoris, owing to increased myocardial oxygen demand and coronary artery spasm, although coronary artery disease should be excluded as appropriate. Physical findings with thyroid storm can include a hyperdynamic precordium with tachycardia, increased pulse pressure, and a strong apical impulse. A pleuropericardial rub may also be heard occasionally, and there may be evidence of heart failure [17].

Thyroid

Thyroid gland findings can vary, depending on the cause of the thyrotoxicosis. With Graves' disease, diffuse enlargement of the gland, and possibly a bruit, can be appreciated, caused by increased vascularity and blood flow. Other potential accompanying signs in Graves' disease include inflammatory ophthalmopathy and, possibly, localized dermal myxedema. The myxedema associated with Graves' disease tends to occur in the pretibial areas and can appear as asymmetric, raised, firm, pink-to-purple brown plaques of nonpitting edema. With a toxic multinodular goiter, physical findings of the thyroid gland may include one or more nodules. With subacute thyroiditis, a tender thyroid gland could be found, and may be accompanied by constitutional complaints of fever and malaise [17,19].

In older individuals, typical symptoms of thyrotoxicosis may not be apparent. Older patients may present with "apathetic" thyrotoxicosis, with some atypical symptoms including weight loss, palpitations, weakness, dizziness, syncope, or memory loss, and physical findings of sinus tachycardia or atrial fibrillation [17].

Diagnosis

In thyroid storm, the pattern of elevated free T_4 and free T_3 with a depressed thyrotropin (less than 0.05 μU/mL) can be comparable to the levels seen in thyrotoxicosis. After synthesis of thyroid hormone, the thyroid gland secretes mainly T_4. Approximately 80% of circulating T_3 is derived from monodeiodination of T_4 in peripheral tissues, whereas only about 20% emanates from direct thyroidal secretion. Both T_4 and T_3 are then bound to proteins: thyroxine-binding globulin, transthyretin, and albumin. Only a small fraction of the hormones, 0.025% of T_4 and 0.35% of T_3, are free and unbound [17,19]. Because the laboratory measurement of total T_3 and total T_4 measures mainly protein-bound hormone concentrations, results may be affected by conditions that affect protein binding. Thyroxine-binding globulin is elevated in infectious hepatitis and pregnancy, and in patients taking estrogens or opiates. In addition, many drugs interfere with protein binding, including heparin, furosemide, phenytoin, carbamazepine, diazepam, salicylates, and nonsteroidal anti-inflammatory drugs. Because of this interference with total thyroid hormone levels, free hormone concentrations are preferable in the diagnosis of thyrotoxicosis [9].

Serum total and free T_3 concentrations are elevated in most patients who have thyrotoxicosis because of increased thyroidal T_3 production and more rapid extrathyroidal conversion of T_4 to T_3. In less than 5% of patients who have thyrotoxicosis in North America, there can be an increase in serum-free T_3 while having a "normal" free T_4, referred to as "T_3 toxicosis" [17,19]. With Graves' disease and toxic nodular goiter, there tends to be a higher proportion of T_3, with a T_3/ T_4 ratio of greater than 20. With thyrotoxicosis caused by thyroiditis, iodine exposure, or exogenous levothyroxine intake, there is generally a greater proportion of T_4, with a T_3/ T_4 ratio of less than 15 [19].

Other possible laboratory findings associated with thyrotoxicosis include hyperglycemia, hypercalcemia, elevated alkaline phosphatase, leukocytosis, and elevated liver enzymes. The hyperglycemia tends to occur because of a catecholamine-induced inhibition of insulin release, and increased glycogenolysis. Mild hypercalcemia and elevated alkaline phosphatase can occur because of hemoconcentration and enhanced thyroid hormone–stimulated bone resorption [9,15,18,20].

Adrenocortical function is also affected by thyrotoxicosis. Thyrotoxicosis accelerates the metabolism of endogenous or exogenous cortisol by stimulating the rate-limiting step in the degradation of glucocorticoids, which is accomplished by the hepatic enzymes, $\Delta 4,5$ steroid reductases. Therefore, cortisol and other steroids, including corticosterone, deoxycorticosterone, and aldosterone are metabolized at an accelerated rate [21]. However, with thyrotoxicosis, both degradation and production of cortisol should be accelerated, resulting in a normal to increased circulating cortisol level. Given the stressful condition of thyroid storm, a normal cortisol level may be interpreted as an indication of some degree of adrenal insufficiency. Objectively, basal serum cortisol and cortisol responses to a corticotropin stimulation test should be normal. However, it has been found that adrenocortical reserve in long-standing, severe thyrotoxicosis can be diminished [21]. Tsatsoulis and colleagues [22] assessed adrenocortical reserve in 10 subjects with severe, long-standing (4–6 months) thyrotoxicosis with a low-dose corticotropin stimulation test following dexamethasone pretreatment. The subjects were tested while they were thyrotoxic before treatment, and again after treatment, once they had become euthyroid. The cortisol response to the corticotropin stimulation test decreased significantly when subjects were thyrotoxic, compared with the cortisol response in the euthyroid state, perhaps indicating a relative adrenal insufficiency [10,22]. Interpretation of corticotropin stimulation tests in the context of serious illnesses is an important issue, but beyond the scope of this article.

Radiologic imaging is not required to make the diagnosis of thyrotoxicosis or thyroid storm. However, in the evaluation of thyroid storm, a chest radiograph (or chest CT without contrast when appropriate) would be helpful to seek a possible infectious source as a precipitant. Although not always indicated for diagnosis, given the urgency and clinical context, nuclear medicine imaging with radioactive iodine uptake and scanning would reveal a greatly increased uptake of radioiodine as early as 1 or 2 hours after administration of the isotope, indicating rapid intraglandular turnover of iodine [15]. It is frequently helpful, and generally easier in the setting of an intensive care unit, to obtain a thyroid sonogram with Doppler flow to assess thyroid gland size, vascularity, and the presence of nodules that may require further attention. Typically, a thyroid gland secreting excessive hormones would be enlarged and have enhanced Doppler flow. On the other hand, in the setting of subacute, postpartum, or silent thyroiditis, or exogenous causes of hyperthyroidism, the thyroid gland would be expected to be small, with decreased Doppler flow.

Electrocardiogram manifestations of thyrotoxicosis most commonly include sinus tachycardia and atrial fibrillation. Sinus tachycardia occurs in approximately 40% of cases, whereas atrial fibrillation occurs in 10% to 20% of patients who have thyrotoxicosis, with a tendency to occur more commonly in patients older than 60, who are more likely to have underlying structural heart disease [23]. The extent of evaluation before therapy depends on the urgency of the clinical condition, and additional studies can be obtained once antithyroid therapy is initiated.

Management

The medical management of thyroid storm consists of an array of medications that act to halt the synthesis, release, and peripheral effects of thyroid hormone. Management of thyroid storm is outlined in Table 3. This multidrug approach has proven to be vitally important in the expeditious control of life-threatening thyrotoxicosis. This therapeutic armamentarium has multiple targets: stopping synthesis of new hormone within the thyroid gland; halting the release of stored thyroid hormone from the thyroid gland; preventing conversion of T_4 to T_3; controlling the adrenergic symptoms associated with thyrotoxicosis; and controlling systemic decompensation with supportive therapy [5,18].

The order of therapy in treating thyroid storm is very important, with regard to use of thionamide therapy and iodine therapy. In most patients, inhibition of thyroid gland synthesis of new thyroid hormone with a thionamide should be initiated before iodine therapy, to prevent the

Table 3
Management of thyroid storm

Medication	Dosage	Mechanism of action	Conditions of use
I. Inhibition of new hormone production			
Propylthiouracil	200–400 mg po q 6–8 h[a]	Inhibits new hormone synthesis; decreases T4-to-T3 conversion	First-line therapy
or			
Methimazole	20–25 mg po q 6 h[a]	Inhibits new hormone synthesis	First-line therapy
II. Inhibition of thyroid hormone release			
Potassium iodide[b] SSKI	5 drops po q 6 h	Blocks release of hormone from gland	Administer at least 1 hr after thionamide
Lugol's solution[b]	4–8 drops po q 6–8 h	Blocks release of hormone from gland	Administer at least 1 hr after thionamide
Sodium ipodate[c] (308 mg iodine/500 mg tab)	1–3 g po qd	Blocks release of hormone from gland; inhibits T4-to-T3 conversion	Administer at least 1 h after thionamide
Iopanoic acid[c]	1 g po q 8 h for 24 h, then 500 mg po q 12 h	Blocks release of hormone from gland; inhibits T4-to-T3 conversion	Administer at least 1 h after thionamide
III. Beta-adrenergic blockade			
Propranolol	60–80 mg po q 4 h or 80–120 mg q 6 h	Beta-adrenergic blockade; decreases T4-to-T3 conversion	
Cardioselective agents:			
Atenolol	50–200 mg po qd	Beta-adrenergic blockade	Use when cardioselective agents preferred
Metoprolol	100–200 mg po qd		
Nadolol	40–80 mg po qd		
Intravenous agent:			
Esmolol	50–100 µg/kg/min	Beta-adrenergic blockade	Use when oral agents contraindicated; Consider use in heart failure

(*continued on next page*)

Table 3 (*continued*)

Medication	Dosage	Mechanism of action	Conditions of use
IV. Supportive treatment			
Acetaminophen	325–650 po/pr q 4–6 h as needed	Treatment of hyperthermia	Preferred treatment over salicylates
Hydrocortisone	100 mg IV q 8 h	Decreases T4-to-T3 conversion; vasomotor stability	Use when patient hypotensive to treat possible concomitant adrenal insufficiency
V. Alternative Therapies			
Lithium carbonate	300 mg po q 8 h[d]	Blocks release of hormone from gland; inhibits new hormone synthesis	Used when thionamide or iodide therapy is contraindicated; lithium levels should be checked regularly
Potassium perchlorate	1 g po qd	Inhibits iodide uptake by thyroid gland	Used in combination with thionamide in treatment of Type II amiodarone-induced thyrotoxicosis
Cholestyramine	4 g po qid	Decreases reabsorption of thyroid hormone from enterohepatic circulation	Used in combination with thionamide therapy

[a] Rectal formulations are described in article.

[b] SSKI (1 g/mL) contains 76.4% iodine. Five drops four times a day (assuming 20 drops/mL) contain about 764 mg iodine. Lugol's solution (125 mg/mL of total iodine) contains, in each 100 mL, 5 g of iodine and 10 g of potassium iodide. Four drops four times a day contain about 134 mg of iodine [40].

[c] These agents are no longer commercially available.

[d] Lithium dose should be adjusted to achieve serum concentration of 0.6–1.0 meq/L.

stimulation of new thyroid hormone synthesis that can occur if iodine is given initially [4,5,18]. However, the time delay between antithyroid agents administration and iodine administration is a matter of controversy, and can be only 30 to 60 minutes, depending on the clinical urgency.

Antithyroid drug therapy with thionamides has been used for treatment of thyrotoxicosis since the introduction of this class of medicine in 1943. The two specific antithyroid agent classes are thiouracils and imidazoles. Propylthiouracil is a thiouracil, whereas methimazole and carbimazole are imidazoles. Although propylthiouracil and methimazole are used widely in the United States, carbimazole is not available in the United States, and is more commonly used in Europe. Carbimazole is metabolized rapidly to methimazole [24,25].

Within the thyroid gland, the thionamides interfere with the thyroperoxidase-catalyzed coupling process by which iodotyrosine residues are combined to form T_4 and T_3. Thionamides may also have an inhibitory effect on thyroid follicular cell function and growth [24]. Outside the thyroid gland, propylthiouracil, but not methimazole, inhibits conversion of T_4 to T_3. Thionamides may also have clinically important immunosuppressive effects, including decreasing antithyrotropin-receptor antibodies over time, and decreasing other immunologically important molecules, such as intracellular adhesion molecule 1 and soluble interleukin-2. Antithyroid drugs may also induce apoptosis of intrathyroidal lymphocytes and decrease HLA antigen class II expression [26].

Methimazole has a longer half-life than propylthiouracil, permitting less frequent dosing [27]. Although methimazole is free in the serum, 80%–90% of propylthiouracil is bound to albumin [24,26]. Either agent may be used to treat thyroid storm. Propylthiouracil has the additional theoretical advantage of inhibiting peripheral conversion of T_4 to T_3. On the other hand, the duration of action of methimazole is longer, such that it can be administered less frequently, as compared with three to four times daily for propylthiouracil (PTU). The authors recommend that the dosing in thyroid storm for propylthiouracil be 800 to 1200 mg daily in divided doses of 200 mg or 300 mg every 6 hours. The dosing for methimazole is 80 to 100 mg daily in divided doses of 20 to 25 mg every 6 hours (although once stable, the frequency of dosing can be decreased to once or twice daily) [18]. Typically, administration has been by mouth; however, both methimazole and propylthiouracil can be administered rectally [28–31]. Given that methimazole was shown to have similar pharmacokinetics for both oral and intravenous use in normal subjects and in subjects with hyperthyroidism, the parenteral route for methimazole should also be considered [32]. Although there are no commercially available parenteral formulations of the thionamides, there are case reports of methimazole being administered intravenously in circumstances where the oral and rectal route of administration could not be used [33,34].

The rectal formulations of the antithyroid drugs have been either as enemas or suppositories. Nabil and colleagues [28] used a suppository formulation of methimazole, in which 1200 mg of methimazole was dissolved in 12 mL of water with two drops of Span 80, mixed with 52 mL of cocoa butter. Yeung and colleagues [29] used an enema preparation of propylthiouracil, in which 12 50 mg tablets of propylthiouracil were dissolved in 90 mL of sterile water and administered by foley catheter inserted into the rectum, with the balloon inflated to prevent leakage. Walter and colleagues [30] used an enema formulation of propylthiouracil, composed of eight 50 mg tablets dissolved in 60 mL of Fleet's mineral oil or in 60 mL of Fleet's phospho soda. Jongjaroenprasert and colleagues [31] compared the use of an enema preparation of propylthiouracil with a suppository preparation, assessing bioavailability and effectiveness. For the enema preparation, eight 50 mg tablets of propylthiouracil were dissolved in 90 mL of sterile water. For the suppository formulation, 200 mg of propylthiouracil were dissolved in a polyethylene glycol base and put into suppository tablets. The enema form provided better bioavailability than the suppository form. However, both preparations proved to have comparable therapeutic effect. Hodak and colleagues [33] prepared the intravenous preparation of methimazole by reconstituting 500 mg of methimazole powder with 0.9% sodium chloride solution to a final volume of 50 mL. The solution of 10 mg/mL was then filtered through a 0.22-μm filter and subsequently administered as a slow, intravenous push over 2 minutes, followed by a saline flush. Routine pharmacologic sterility tests need to be performed as indicated by local regulations.

Common adverse side effects of the antithyroid drugs include an abnormal sense of taste, pruritus, urticaria, fever, and arthralgias. More rare and serious side effects are agranulocytosis, hepatotoxicity, and vasculitis. With a criterion of absolute granulocyte count of less than 500 per cubic millimeter, 0.37% of subjects receiving propylthiouracil and 0.35% of subjects receiving methimazole developed agranulocytosis, in a large case series [35]. Most cases of agranulocytosis occur within the first 3 months of treatment, but can occur anytime after starting therapy. With methimazole, agranulocytosis tends to be dose-related, with occurrence being rare at doses of less than 40 mg daily. However, agranulocytosis does not appear to be dose-related with propylthiouracil use [25,26]. Nonetheless, agranulocytosis can occur at any time with either medication, and close monitoring is mandatory.

The use of granulocyte colony-stimulating factor (G-CSF) for treatment of agranulocytosis induced by antithyroid medications has been studied in a large retrospective study and a prospective controlled study. In the prospective study, Fukata and colleagues [36] showed that the use of G-CSF did not shorten recovery time in the treated, compared with the untreated, groups with moderate or severe agranulocytosis. In the retrospective study, Tajiri and colleagues [37,38] showed that G-CSF therapy did shorten recovery time in patients with antithyroid drug–induced agranulocytosis, as long as the absolute granulocyte count was above $0.1 \times 10(9)/L$. Therefore, the use of G-CSF can be recommended for treatment of antithyroid drug–induced agranulocytosis, with consideration of the individual context [26].

Hepatotoxicity can also occur in 0.1% to 0.2% of patients using antithyroid drugs. Hepatotoxicity related to propylthiouracil tends to be an allergic hepatitis with evidence of hepatocellular injury, whereas hepatotoxicity related to methimazole tends to result in hepatic abnormalities typical of a cholestatic process [26]. Vasculitis may also occur with antithyroid drug use, associated more commonly with propylthiouracil than with methimazole. This toxic antithyroid drug reaction is associated with some serologic markers: most patients have perinuclear antineutrophil cytoplasmic antibodies and antimyeloperoxidase antineutrophil cytoplasmic antibodies.

Some patients develop antineutrophil cytoplasmic antibody–positivity, which is associated with acute renal insufficiency, arthritis, skin ulcerations, vasculitic rash, and possibly sinusitis or hemoptysis [26].

In the setting of thyroid storm, iodine therapy complements the effects of thionamide therapy. Thionamide therapy decreases the synthesis of new hormone production; iodine therapy blocks the release of prestored hormone, and decreases iodide transport and oxidation in follicular cells. This decrease in organification due to increasing doses of inorganic iodide is known as the "Wolff-Chaikoff" effect. Small increments in available iodide cause increased formation of thyroid hormone; however, large amounts of exogenous iodide actually inhibit hormone formation. At iodide concentrations greater than 1 μmol/L, iodination is inhibited. However, despite maintenance of high doses of iodide, the thyroid gland eventually escapes this inhibition after approximately 48 hours. This escape occurs as the iodide transport system adapts to the higher concentration of iodide by modulating the activity of the sodium-iodide symporter [39]. Although iodide is effective at rapidly reducing serum thyroid hormone levels, usually within 7 to 14 days, most patients escape the inhibition and return to hyperthyroidism within 2 to 3 weeks, if no other treatment is given. Therefore, the use of iodide to treat thyrotoxicosis is of limited use, and thus is used only in severe thyrotoxicosis or thyroid storm in combination with thionamide therapy [40].

Administering iodine therapy before thionamide therapy affects short-term and longer-term treatment options for thyrotoxicosis. In the acute setting, if iodine therapy is given before thionamide therapy, new hormone synthesis can be stimulated. When planning definitive therapy for thyrotoxicosis after the acute phase of thyroid storm, use of exogenous iodine at any time can predispose a patient to increased surgical risk because of the enrichment of thyroid hormone stores, and can cause postponement of radioiodine ablation until an adequate clearance of the iodine load occurs [4]. Initial blockade of iodine organification begins within 1 hour of treatment with thionamide therapy. Therefore, to block the release of preformed thyroid hormone safely, iodine therapy should be administered no sooner than 30 to 60 minutes after thionamide therapy [5]. The biphasic effects of iodine are important and can be summarized. Over a short term of 1 to 3 weeks, iodine inhibits thyroid hormone synthesis and can be used as an effective antithyroid agent, especially in conjunction with propylthiouracil or methimazole. In all patients, but especially in those who are not also receiving propylthiouracil or methimazole, there may be escape from the Wolff-Chaikoff effect after 2 to 3 weeks of iodine administration, and exacerbation of hyperthyroidism may ensue. The chance of this latter hyperthyroid phase occurring is decreased, but not eliminated, by the adjunctive administration of propylthiouracil or methimazole.

Oral formulations of inorganic iodine include Lugol's solution and saturated solution of potassium iodide. The dosing for these preparations in thyroid storm is 0.2 to 2 g daily, with four to eight drops of Lugol's solution (assuming 20 drops/mL, 8 mg iodine/drop) every 6 to 8 hours and five drops of saturation solution of potassium iodide (with 20 drops/mL, 38 mg iodide/drop) every 6 hours [4,40]. Parenteral sources of iodine, including sodium iodide, are no longer available in the United States. The oral iodinated contrast agents, iopanoic acid and sodium ipodate, have multiple effects on thyroid hormone in the periphery and within the thyroid gland. These iodinated contrast agents competitively inhibit Types 1 and 2 5′-monodeiodinase in the liver, brain, and thyroid, blocking conversion of T_4 to T_3, resulting in a rapid decrease in T_3 and an increase in reverse T_3. These iodinated contrast agents have also been found to inhibit binding of T_3 and T_4 to cellular receptors [10,18]. In thyroid storm, sodium ipodate (308 mg iodine/500mg capsule) is dosed at 1 to 3 g daily. Usually, iopanoic acid is dosed at 1g every 8 hours for the first 24 hours, followed by 500 mg twice daily [4,41]. Unfortunately, however, these very effective antithyroid agents are no longer marketed commercially or available.

Controlling the cardiovascular manifestations of thyrotoxicosis is a vital part of management. The cardiovascular changes seen with thyrotoxicosis occur because of the different effects of thyroid hormone on the heart and on systemic vasculature. Thyroid hormone decreases systemic vascular resistance by a direct vasodilatory action on smooth muscle and by endothelial release of nitric oxide or other endothelial-derived vasodilators. In response to thyroid hormone administration in hypothyroid patients, systemic vascular resistance may decrease by as much as 50% to 70% [42]. The decreased systemic vascular resistance leads to increased blood flow to the heart and other organs.

The effect of thyroid hormone on the heart is mediated partly by the genomic effects of T_3 binding to specific nuclear receptors. This binding activates thyroid hormone response elements within promoter enhancer regions of certain genes, which are partly responsible for modulating cardiac structure and contractility. Specifically, T_3 activates transcription of the α-myosin heavy chain (MHC-α) and represses transcription of the β-myosin heavy chain (MHC-β). Myofibrillar proteins, which compose the thick filaments of the cardiac myocyte, are made up of MHC-αs or MHC-βs. Three myosin isoforms have been identified in ventricular muscle: V1, made of MHC-α/α; V2, made of MHC-α/β; and V3, made of MHC-β/β. Thyroid hormone increases the synthesis of V1 and decreases the synthesis of V2, resulting in an increase in the velocity of muscle fiber shortening, because V1 has higher ATPase enzymatic activity [43].

T_3 also regulates production of the sarcoplasmic reticulum proteins, calcium-activated ATPase, phospholamban, and various plasma-membrane ion transporters through transcriptional and posttranscriptional effects. In addition to these genomic effects of T_3 in the heart, thyroid hormone also has nongenomic actions, directly altering the performance of sodium, potassium, and calcium channels [13,42].

Beta-blockade is essential in controlling the peripheral actions of thyroid hormone. The use of a beta-adrenergic receptor antagonist in the management of thyrotoxic crisis was first reported in 1966 with the agent pronethalol [44]. Soon thereafter, propranolol became the most commonly used beta-blocker in the United States [18]. In thyroid storm, propranolol is dosed at 60 to 80 mg every 4 hours, or 80 to 120 mg every 4 hours. The onset of action after oral dosing takes place within 1 hour. For a more rapid effect, propranolol can also be administered parenterally, with a bolus of 0.5 to 1 mg over 10 minutes followed by 1 to 3 mg over 10 minutes, every few hours, depending on the clinical context [15,41]. Esmolol can also be administered parenterally at a dose of 50 to 100 μg/kg/min [24]. Relatively large doses of propranolol are required in the setting of thyrotoxicosis because of the faster metabolism of the drug, and possibly because of a greater quantity of cardiac beta-adrenergic receptors [42].

Intravenous administration of beta-blockers should be performed in a monitored setting. In addition to its effect on beta-adrenergic receptors, propranolol in large doses (greater than 160 mg daily) can decrease T_3 levels by as much as 30%. This effect, mediated by the inhibition of 5′monodeiodinase, is mediated slowly over 7 to 10 days. Because propranolol has a short half-life and an increased requirement during thyrotoxicosis, multiple large daily doses are required. Longer-acting cardioselective beta-adrenergic receptor antagonists may be used also, and would require less frequent dosing. Atenolol can be used in thyrotoxicosis, with doses ranging from 50 to 200 mg daily, but may require twice daily dosing to achieve adequate control [25]. Other oral agents that can be used include metoprolol at 100 to 200 mg daily and nadolol at 40 to 80 mg daily [24]. The actual administered dose is determined by the clinical context, and modified as the clinical situation changes. Cardiovascular manifestations and responses should be monitored closely, with subsequent modulation of the dose of medication as appropriate.

Relative contraindications to beta-adrenergic receptor antagonist use include a history of moderate to severe heart failure or the presence of reactive airway disease. With the latter, beta-1 selective receptor antagonists, such as metoprolol or atenolol, would be recommended but, again, the individual clinical context must be considered carefully [25]. Beta-blockade may result in hypotension in some patients who have heart failure and are being treated for thyrotoxicosis. Because the use of beta-adrenergic receptor antagonists can be beneficial in the treatment of thyrotoxicosis, careful consideration is required. If the cause of the heart failure were likely to be underlying tachycardia, beta-blockade would be particularly useful. However, in situations in which the cause of the heart failure cannot be ascertained easily, beta-blockade should only be administered with a short-acting drug, under close hemodynamic monitoring [42].

One of the significant cardiovascular complications of thyrotoxicosis is atrial fibrillation, occurring in 10% to 35% of cases [45]. The issue of anticoagulation in atrial fibrillation in the setting of thyrotoxicosis has been controversial. Studies assessing the incidence of embolic events in thyrotoxic patients who have atrial fibrillation have yielded conflicting information regarding the incidence of embolism [46,47]. In the largest retrospective study, it appears that thyrotoxic patients who have atrial fibrillation are not at greater risk for embolic events, compared with age-matched patients who have atrial fibrillation due to other causes [47]. The standard risk factors for embolic events in atrial fibrillation, including increased age and underlying heart disease, apply to thyrotoxic patients. The Seventh American College of Chest Physicians Conference on Antithrombotic and Thrombolytic Therapy recommends that, in thyrotoxic patients who have atrial fibrillation, antithrombotic therapies should be selected based on the presence of stroke risk factors [48]. Therefore, standard therapy with warfarin or aspirin would be indicated, according to these guidelines. Thyrotoxic patients may require a lower maintenance dose of warfarin than euthyroid patients because of increased clearance of vitamin K–dependent clotting factors [43].

Glucocorticoids, including dexamethasone and hydrocortisone, have also been used in the treatment of thyroid storm because they have an inhibitory effect on peripheral conversion of T_4 to T_3. Therefore, glucocorticoids can be effective in reducing T_3 levels as adjunctive therapy. The clinical relevance of this minor effect is unknown. Also, glucocorticoids are used in thyroid storm to treat possible relative adrenal insufficiency. One study found inappropriately normal levels of serum cortisol in a series of subjects with thyroid storm. This study found improved survival in those subjects treated with glucorticoids [4,49]. In patients who have severe thyrotoxicosis, especially in conjunction with hypotension, treatment with glucocorticoids has become standard practice because of the possibility of relative adrenal insufficiency, or the possibility of undiagnosed Addison's disease or adrenal insufficiency [21]. Dosing of glucorticoids in thyroid storm can be with hydrocortisone 100 mg intravenously every 8 hours, with tapering as the signs of thyroid storm improve.

Alternative therapies

Several therapeutic agents used in the treatment of thyrotoxicosis are only considered when the first-line therapies of thionamides, iodide, beta-blockers, and glucocorticoids fail or cannot be used owing to toxicity. When iodide therapy cannot be used, another agent that can be used to inhibit thyroid hormone release is lithium. Lithium can be used when thionamide therapy is contraindicated because of toxicity or adverse reactions; it can also be used in combination with PTU or methimazole [50]. In summary, lithium has several effects on the thyroid gland, including directly decreasing thyroid hormone secretion and thereby increasing intrathyroidal iodine content, and inhibiting coupling of iodotyrosine residues that form iodothyronines (T_4 and T_3) [51–53]. In thyroid storm, the dosing for lithium is 300 mg every 8 hours [24]. To avoid lithium toxicity, lithium level should be monitored regularly (perhaps even daily) to maintain a concentration of about 0.6–1.0 mEq/L [18,24]. Very frequent monitoring of serum lithium levels is mandatory, especially because the serum lithium concentrations may change as the patient is rendered more euthyroid.

Potassium perchlorate is another therapeutic agent used historically in the treatment of thyrotoxicosis. The perchlorate anion, ClO4-, is a competitive inhibitor of iodide transport [24]. However, its use fell out of favor for the treatment of thyrotoxicosis because of possible side effects of aplastic anemia and nephrotic syndrome. After thionamides became available, the risk of using potassium perchlorate outweighed its benefits. Recently, there has been a resurgence of interest in this agent, especially in selected patients who have amiodarone-induced thyrotoxicosis (AIT). For treatment of cardiac arrhythmias, amiodarone can cause hypothyroidism or hyperthyroidism. Hypothyroidism is more prevalent in high-iodine intake regions, and AIT is more prevalent in low-iodine intake areas. AIT has been classified into two categories: Type I and Type II. Type I AIT frequently occurs in individuals with underlying thyroid abnormalities, such as nodular goiter or latent autoimmunity. The pathogenesis of the thyrotoxicosis is presumed to be caused by iodine-induced accelerated thyroid hormone synthesis. Type II AIT is considered to be a form of destructive thyroiditis, induced by amiodarone. Glucocorticoids have been successful in treating Type II AIT, and the combination of potassium perchlorate and methimazole has been successful in the treatment of Type I AIT. The potassium perchlorate exerts its action by inhibiting iodide uptake by the thyroid gland while organification is inhibited by methimazole. The regimen of potassium perchlorate (1 g daily) and methimazole (30–50 mg daily) has been found to normalize thyroid hormone levels successfully, with an average duration of treatment of 4 weeks. With a limited treatment course of approximately 4 weeks, and a dose of potassium perchlorate that is no greater than 1 g daily, the adverse effects of aplastic anemia and nephrotic syndrome did not occur in several studies [54–56].

Before beta-adrenergic receptor antagonists were used to counteract the peripheral effects of thyroid hormone, the antiadrenergic agents, reserpine and guanethidine, were often used. Reserpine is an alkaloid agent that depletes catecholamine stores in sympathetic nerve terminals and the central nervous system. Guanethidine also inhibits the release of catecholamines. Side effects of these medications include hypotension and diarrhea. Reserpine can also have central nervous system depressant effects. Therefore, these agents would be indicated only in rare situations where beta-adrenergic receptor antagonists are contraindicated, and when there is no hypotension or evidence of central nervous system–associated mental status changes [4]. Dosing for guanethidine in thyroid storm is 30 to 40 mg orally every 6 hours, and for reserpine 2.5 to 5 mg intramuscularly every 4 hours [18].

Cholestyramine, an anion exchange resin, has also been used in the treatment of thyrotoxicosis, to help decrease reabsorption of thyroid hormone from the enterohepatic circulation [57]. Thyroid hormone is metabolized mainly in the liver, where it is conjugated to glucuronides and sulfates. These conjugation products are then excreted in the bile. Free hormones are released in the intestine and finally reabsorbed, completing the enterohepatic circulation of thyroid hormone. In states of thyrotoxicosis, there is increased enterohepatic circulation of thyroid hormone. Cholestyramine therapy has been studied in the treatment of thyrotoxicosis as an adjunctive therapy to thionamides, and has been found to decrease thyroid hormone levels rapidly. In several trials, cholestyramine therapy, in combination with methimazole or propylthiouracil, caused a more rapid decline in thyroid hormone levels than standard therapy with thionamides alone. Cholestyramine was also found to be useful in rapidly decreasing thyroid hormone levels in a case of iatrogenic hyperthyroidism. In these trials, cholestyramine was dosed at 4 g orally four times a day [57–60]. The effect of cholestyramine is generally minimal and it should not be administered at the exact same time as other medications because it may inhibit their absorption. On the other hand, cholestyramine is not expected to be associated with significant adverse effects.

When clinical deterioration occurs in thyroid storm, despite the use of all of these medications, removal of thyroid hormone from circulation would be a therapeutic consideration. Plasmapheresis, charcoal hemoperfusion, resin hemoperfusion, and plasma exchange have been found to be effective in rapidly reducing thyroid hormone levels in thyroid storm [61–63].

Supportive care/treatment of precipitating cause

Supportive care is an important part of the multisystem therapeutic approach to thyroid storm. Because fever is very common with severe thyrotoxicosis, antipyretics should be used; acetaminophen is the preferable choice. Salicylates should be avoided in thyrotoxicosis because salicylates can decrease thyroid protein binding, causing an increase in free thyroid hormone levels [18,41]. External cooling measures, such as alcohol sponging, ice packs, or a cooling blanket, can also be used. Fluid loss and dehydration are also common in severe thyrotoxicosis. The fluid losses could result from the combination of fever, diaphoresis, vomiting, and diarrhea. Intravenous fluids with dextrose (isotonic saline with 5% or 10% dextrose) should be given to replenish glycogen stores [41]. Patients should also receive multivitamins, particularly thiamine, to prevent Wernicke's encephalopathy, which could result from the administration of intravenous fluids with dextrose in the presence of thiamine deficiency [2].

Treating the precipitating cause of thyrotoxicosis is particularly important, considering that the most common precipitant is thought to be infection. If a precipitating factor were not readily apparent, a vigorous search for an infectious source would be warranted in the febrile thyrotoxic patient; this would be done with blood, urine, and sputum cultures, and a chest radiograph or noncontrast CT. Generally, however, empiric antibiotics are not recommended without an identified source of infection. In cases of thyroid storm precipitated by diabetic ketoacidosis, myocardial infarction, pulmonary embolism, or other acute processes, appropriate management of the specific underlying problem should proceed along with the treatment of the thyrotoxicosis [4].

Perioperative management

The history of thyroid surgery, or surgery in the setting of thyrotoxicosis, began in the late nineteenth century with dismal results and high mortality. Much of the mortality associated with thyroid surgery in the past was because of postoperative thyroid storm. Even in the early twentieth century, mortality ranged from 8% with very experienced surgeons, to 20% in less experienced medical centers. In 1923, with the start of inorganic iodine use preoperatively, mortality rates decreased to less than 1% with experienced surgeons. Then, in the 1940s, thionamides began to be used in preoperative preparation of thyrotoxic patients. Finally, in the 1960s, preoperative beta-adrenergic receptor blockade with propranolol emerged, with even better outcomes [25].

Preoperative management of the thyrotoxic patient can be subdivided into two categories: preparation for elective or nonurgent procedures and preparation for emergent procedures. When rapid control of thyrotoxicosis is not required, as would be the case for an elective or nonurgent procedure, the standard course of therapy would be to achieve euthyroidism before surgery. In this situation, thionamide therapy would be recommended and would facilitate euthyroidism within several weeks [25]. The use of iodine as a method of decreasing thyroid vascularity and friability before thyroid surgery has been debated. Since the early twentieth century, when the routine use of iodine for preoperative preparation for thyroidectomy in the treatment of thyrotoxicosis began, surgeons have believed that iodine decreases thyroid gland vascularity and friability [25]. Several studies have shown some evidence that iodine treatment does decrease blood flow to the thyroid gland [64,65]. However, one retrospective study comparing surgical outcomes in 42 hyperthyroid patients who underwent subtotal thyroidectomy with propranolol treatment alone, or propranolol and iodine treatment, revealed no benefit in terms of blood loss intraoperatively [66]. Therefore, in the preparation of thyrotoxic patients for a nonemergent procedure, iodine use may be indicated only if thionamides cannot be tolerated.

In the preoperative preparation of thyrotoxic patients for emergent procedures, time is of the essence. Rapid lowering of thyroid hormone levels, control of thyroid hormone release, and control of peripheral manifestations of thyroid hormone are needed. In this situation, several regimens have been tried with success, using the same therapeutic modalities that are used in the treatment of thyroid storm [25]. Management of rapid preparation of

Table 4
Rapid preparation of thyrotoxic patients for emergent surgery

Drug class	Recommended drug	Dosage	Mechanism of action	Continue postoperatively?
Beta-adrenergic Blockade	Propranolol	40–80 mg po tid-qid	Beta-adrenergic blockade; decreased T4-to-T3 conversion (high dose)	Yes
	or Esmolol	50–100 μg/kg/min	Beta-adrenergic blockade	Change to oral propranolol
Thionamide	Propylthiouracil	200 mg po q 4 h[a]	Inhibition of new thyroid hormone synthesis; decreased T4-to-T3 conversion	Stop immediately after near total thyroidectomy; continue after nonthyroidal surgery
	or Methimazole	20 mg po q 4 h[a]	Inhibition of new thyroid hormone synthesis	Stop immediately after near total thyroidectomy; continue after nonthyroidal surgery
Oral cholecysto-graphic agent	Iopanoic acid	500 mg po bid	Decreased release of thyroid hormone; decreased T4-to-T3 conversion	Stop immediately after surgery[b]
Corticosteroid	Hydrocortisone	100 mg po or IV q 8 h	Vasomotor stability; decreased T4-to-T3 conversion	Taper over first 72 h
	or Dexamethasone	2 mg po or IV q 6 h	Vasomotor stability; decreased T4-to-T3 conversion	Taper over first 72 h
	or Betamethasone	0.5 mg po q 6 h, IM or IV	Vasomotor stability; decreased T4-to-T3 conversion	Taper over first 72 h

[a] May be given per nasogastric tube or rectally.
[b] Not for prolonged use after nonthyroidal surgery in thionamide-intolerant patients.
From Langley RW, Burch HB. Perioperative management of the thyrotoxic patient. Endocrinol Metab Clin of North Am 2003;32:519–34; with permission.

thyrotoxic patients for emergent surgery is outlined in Table 4. One study used a 5-day course of betamethasone, iopanoic acid (no longer commercially available), and propranolol, with thyroidectomy performed on the sixth day in 14 hyperthyroid subjects. Rapid lowering of thyroid hormone levels occurred with good surgical outcomes [67].

Following thyroid surgery in hyperthyroid patients, therapy with beta-adrenergic receptor antagonists may still be required for a short period of time because the half-life of T_4 is 7 to 8 days. However, after thyroidectomy, thionamide therapy usually can be stopped postoperatively, assuming that there is little thyroid tissue remaining. The authors tend to stop the antithyroid agents on days 1 to 3 postoperatively, depending on the clinical context. Preoperative management of hyperthyroidism aims to drive thyroid hormone levels to a euthyroid status before surgery. With adequately prepared hyperthyroid patients, morbidity and mortality due to thyroid or non-thyroid surgery is low [25].

Definitive therapy

Definitive therapy of thyrotoxicosis must be considered after the life-threatening aspects of thyroid storm are treated. As the thyrotoxic patient shows clinical improvement with therapy, some of the treatment modalities can be modulated or withdrawn; iodine therapy can be discontinued and glucocorticoids can be tapered. Thionamide therapy, at gradually decreasing doses, usually is required for weeks to months after thyroid storm, to attain euthyroidism. Beta-adrenergic receptor blockade is also needed while the patient is still thyrotoxic. Definitive therapy with radioactive iodine ablation may not be able to be used for several weeks or months following treatment with iodine for thyroid storm. Following the resolution of thyroid storm, the thyrotoxic patient continues to require close follow-up and monitoring, with plans for definitive therapy to prevent a future recurrence of life-threatening thyrotoxicosis [4].

Summary

Thyrotoxicosis and thyroid storm pose a critical diagnostic and therapeutic challenge to the clinician. Recognition of life-threatening thyrotoxicosis and prompt use of the arsenal of medications aimed at halting the thyrotoxic process at every level is essential to successful management. With the array of therapeutic interventions, treatment aimed at stopping synthesis of new hormone within the thyroid gland, halting the release of stored thyroid hormone from the thyroid gland, preventing conversion of T_4 to T_3, and providing systemic support of the patient can transition the thyroid storm patient out of critical illness. Once this transition occurs, definitive therapy of thyrotoxicosis can be planned.

References

[1] Jameson L, Weetman A. Disorders of the thyroid gland. In: Braunwald E, Fauci A, Kasper D, et al, editors. Harrison's principles of internal medicine. 15th edition. New York: McGraw-Hill; 2001. p. 2060–84.
[2] Tietgens ST, Leinung MC. Thyroid storm. Med Clin North Am 1995;79:169–84.

[3] Larsen PR, Davies TF. Thyrotoxicosis. In: Larsen PR, Kronenberg HM, et al, editors. Williams textbook of endocrinology. 10th edition. Philadelphia: WB Saunders Co; 2002. p. 374–421.
[4] Burch HB, Wartofsky L. Life-threatening thyrotoxicosis. Thyroid storm. Endocrinol Metab Clin North Am 1993;22:263–77.
[5] Goldberg PA, Inzucchi SE. Critical issues in endocrinology. Clin Chest Med 2003;24: 583–606.
[6] Wong V, Xi-Li F, Geoge J, et al. Thyrotoxicosis induced by alpha-interferon therapy in chronic viral hepatitis. Clin Endocrinol (Oxf) 2002;56:793–8.
[7] Lin YQ, Wang X, Muthy MS, et al. Life-threatening thyrotoxicosis induced by combination therapy with peg-interferon and ribavirin in chronic hepatitis C. Endocr Pract 2005;11(2): 135–9.
[8] Jimenez C, Moran SA, Sereti I, et al. Graves' disease after Interleukin-2 therapy in a patient with Human Immunodeficiency Virus infection. Thyroid 2004;14(12):1097–101.
[9] Pimental L, Hansen K. Thyroid disease in the emergency department: a clinical and laboratory review. J Emerg Med 2005;28:201–9.
[10] Panzer C, Beazley R, Braverman L. Rapid preoperative preparation for severe hyperthyroid Graves' disease. J Clin Endocrinol Metab 2004;89:2142–4.
[11] Bianco AC, Larsen PR. Intracellular pathways of iodothyronine metabolism. In: Braverman LE, Utiger RD, editors. Werner's & Ingbar's The thyroid. 9th edition. Philadelphia: Lipincott, Williams & Wilkins; 2005. p. 109–33.
[12] Motomura K, Brent G. Mechanisms of thyroid hormone action. Endocrinol Metab Clin North Am 1998;27:1–23.
[13] Klein I, Ojama K. Thyroid hormone and the cardiovascular system. N Engl J Med 2001; 344(7):501–8.
[14] Brooks MH, Waldstein SS. Free thyroxine concentrations in thyroid storm. Ann Intern Med 1980;93(5):694–7.
[15] Sarlis NJ, Gourgiotis L. Thyroid emergencies. Rev Endocr Metab Disord 2003;4:129–36.
[16] Silva JE, Landsberg L. Catecholamines and the sympathoadrenal system in thyrotoxicosis. In: Braverman LE, Utiger RD, editors. Werner's and Ingbar's The thyroid. 6th edition. Philadelphia: Lipincott, Williams & Wilkins; 1991. p. 816–27.
[17] Dabon-Almirante CL, Surks M. Clinical and laboratory diagnosis of thyrotoxicosis. Endocrinol Metab Clin North Am 1998;27(1):25–35.
[18] Wartofsky L. Thyrotoxic storm. In: Braverman LE, Utiger RD, editors. Werner's & Ingbar's The thyroid. 9th edition. Philadelphia: Lipincott, Williams & Wilkins; 2005. p. 652–7.
[19] Ladenson P. Diagnosis of thyrotoxicosis. In: Braverman LE, Utiger RD, editors. Werner's & Ingbar's The thyroid. 9th edition. Philadelphia: Lipincott, Williams & Wilkins; 2005. p. 660–4.
[20] Burman KD, Monchik JM, Earll JM, et al. Ionized and total serum calcium and parathyroid hormone in hyperthyroidism. Ann Intern Med 1976;84:668–71.
[21] Dluhy RG. The adrenal cortex in thyrotoxicosis. In: Braverman LE, Utiger RD, editors. Werner's & Ingbar's The thyroid. 9th edition. Philadelphia: Lipincott, Williams & Wilkins; 2005. p. 602–3.
[22] Tsatsoulis A, Johnson EO, Kalogera CH, et al. The effect of thyrotoxicosis on adrenocortical reserve. Eur J Endocrinol 2000;142:231–5.
[23] Wald D. ECG manifestations of selected metabolic and endocrine disorders. Emerg Med Clin North Am 2006;24:145–57.
[24] Cooper D. Treatment of thyrotoxicosis. In: Braverman LE, Utiger RD, editors. Werner's & Ingbar's The thyroid. 9th edition. Philadelphia: Lipincott, Williams & Wilkins; 2005. p. 665–94.
[25] Langley RW, Burch HB. Perioperative management of the thyrotoxic patient. Endocrinol Metab Clin North Am 2003;32:519–34.
[26] Cooper DS. Antithyroid drugs. N Engl J Med 2005;352:905–17.

[27] Wartofsky L. A method for assessing the latency, potency, and duration of action of antithyroid agents in man. Verlag der Wiener Medizinischen Akademie 1974;121–35.

[28] Nabil N, Miner DJ, Amatruda JM. Methimazole: an alternative route of administration. J Clin Endocrinol Metab 1982;54(1):180–1.

[29] Yeung S, Go R, Balasubramanyam A, et al. Rectal administration of iodide and propylthiouracil in the treatment of thyroid storm. Thyroid 1995;5(5):403–5.

[30] Walter RM, Bartle WR. Rectal administration of propylthiouracil in the treatment of Graves' disease. Am J Med 1990;88:69–70.

[31] Jongjaroenprasert W, Akarawut W, Chantasart D, et al. Rectal administration of propylthiouracil in hyperthyroid patients: comparison of suspension enema and suppository form. Thyroid 2002;12(7):627–31.

[32] Okamura Y, Shigemusa C, Tatsuhara T. Pharmacokinetics of methimazole in normal subjects and hyperthyroid patients. Endocrinol Jpn 1986;33:605–15.

[33] Hodak SP, Huang C, et al. Intravenous methimazole in the treatment of refractory hyperthyroidism. Thyroid 2006; in press.

[34] Sowinski J, Junik R, Gembicki M. Effectiveness of intravenous administration of methimazole in patients with thyroid crisis. Endokrynol Pol 1988;39:67–73.

[35] Tajiri J, Noguchi S. Antithyroid drug-induced agranulocytosis: special reference to normal white blood cell count agranulocytosis. Thyroid 2004;14:459–62.

[36] Fukata S, Kuma K, Sugawara M. Granulocyte colony-stimulating factor (G-CSF) does not improve recovery from antithyroid drug-induced agranulocytosis. A prospective study. Thyroid 1999;9:29–31.

[37] Tajiri J, Noguchi S. Antithyroid drug-induced agranulocytosis: how has granulocyte colony-stimulating factor changed therapy? Thyroid 2005;15(3):292–7.

[38] Tajiri J, Noguchi S, Okamura S, et al. Granulocyte colony-stimulating factor treatment of antithyroid drug-induced granulocytopenia. Arch Intern Med 1993;153:509–14.

[39] Taurog A. Hormone synthesis: thyroid iodine metabolism. In: Braverman LE, Utiger RD, editors. Werner's & Ingbar's The thyroid. 6th edition. Philadelphia: Lipincott, Williams & Wilkins; 1991. p. 51–97.

[40] Burman K. Hyperthyroidism. In: Becker K, editor. Principles and practice of endocrinology and metabolism. 2nd edition. Philadelphia: J.B. Lipincott Company; 1995. p. 367–85.

[41] McKeown NJ, Tews MC, Gossain V, et al. Hyperthyroidism. Emerg Med Clin N Amer 2005;23:669–85.

[42] Klein I, Ojamaa K. Thyrotoxicosis and the heart. Endocrinol Metab Clin North Am 1998; 27(1):51–61.

[43] Fadel BM, Ellahham S, Ringel MD, et al. Hyperthyroid heart disease. Clin Cardiol 2000;23: 402–8.

[44] Hughes G. Management of thyrotoxic crisis with a beta-adrenergic blocking agent. Br J Clin Pract 1966;20:579.

[45] Presti CE, Hart RG. Thyrotoxicosis, atrial fibrillation, and embolism, revisited. Am Heart J 1989;117:976–7.

[46] Bar-Sela S, Ehrenfield M, Eliakim M. Arterial embolism in thyrotoxicosis with atrial fibrillation. Arch Intern Med 1981;141:1191.

[47] Peterson P, Hansen JM. Stroke in thyrotoxicosis with atrial fibrillation. Stroke 1988;19(1): 15–8.

[48] Singer DE, Albers GW, Dalen JE. Antithrombotic therapy in atrial fibrillation: the seventh ACCP conference on antithrombotic and thrombolytic therapy. Chest 2004;126: 429–56.

[49] Mazzaferri EL, Skillman TG. Thyroid storm. A review of 22 episodes with special emphasis on the use of guanethidine. Arch Intern Med 1969;124(6):684–90.

[50] Boehm TM, Burman KD, Barnes S, et al. Lithium and iodine combination therapy for thyrotoxicosis. Acta Endocrinol (Copenh) 1980;94:174–83.

[51] Berens SC, Bernstein RS, Robbins J, et al. Antithyroid effects of lithium. J Clin Invest 1970; 49(7):1357–67.
[52] Burrow GN, Burke WR, Himmelhoch JM, et al. Effect of lithium on thyroid function. J Clin Endocrinol Metab 1971;32(5):647–52.
[53] Spaulding SW, Burrow GN, Bermudez F, et al. The inhibitory effect of lithium on thyroid hormone release in both euthyroid and thyrotoxic patients. J Clin Endocrinol Metab 1972;35(6):905–11.
[54] Erdogan MF, Gulec S, Tutar E, et al. A stepwise approach to the treatment of amiodarone-induced thyrotoxicosis. Thyroid 2003;13(2):205–9.
[55] Bartalena L, Brogioni S, Grasso L, et al. Treatment of amiodarone-induced thyrotoxicosis, a difficult challenge: results of a prospective study. J Clin Endocrinol Metab 1996;81(8): 2930–3.
[56] Martino E, Aghini-Lombardi F, Mariotti S, et al. Treatment of amiodarone associated thyrotoxicosis by simultaneous administration of potassium perchlorate and methimazole. J Endocrinol Invest 1986;9:201–7.
[57] Solomon BL, Wartofsky L, Burman KD. Adjunctive cholestyramine therapy for thyrotoxicosis. Clin Endocrinol (Oxf) 1993;38:39–43.
[58] Shakir KM, Michaels RD, Hays JH, et al. The use of bile acid sequestrants to lower serum thyroid hormones in iatrogenic hyperthyroidism. Ann Intern Med 1993;118(2):112–3.
[59] Mercado M, Mendoza-Zubieta V, Bautista-Osorio R, et al. Treatment of hyperthyroidism with a combination of methimazole and cholestyramine. J Clin Endocrinol Metab 1996; 81(9):3191–3.
[60] Tsai WC, Pei D, Wang T, et al. The effect of combination therapy with propylthiouracil and cholestyramine in the treatment of Graves' hyperthyroidism. Clin Endocrinol (Oxf) 2005; 62(5):521–4.
[61] Burman KD, Yeager HC, Briggs WA, et al. Resin hemoperfusion: a method of removing circulating thyroid hormones. J Clin Endocrinol Metab 1976;42:70–8.
[62] Ashkar F, Katims RB, Smoak WM, et al. Thyroid storm treatment with blood exchange and plasmapheresis. JAMA 1970;214:1275–9.
[63] Tajiri J, Katsuya H, Kiyokawa T, et al. Successful treatment of thyrotoxic crisis with plasma exchange. Crit Care Med 1984;12(6):536–7.
[64] Marigold JH, Morgan AK, Earle DJ, et al. Lugol's iodine: its effect on thyroid blood flow in patients with thyrotoxicosis. Br J Surg 1985;72:45–7.
[65] Marmon L, Au FC. The preoperative use of iodine solution in thyrotoxic patients prepared with propranolol. Is it necessary? Am Surg 1989;55:629–31.
[66] Chang DC, Wheeler MH, Woodcock JP, et al. The effect of preoperative Lugol's iodine on thyroid blood flow in patients with Graves' hyperthyroidism. Surgery 1987;102:1055–61.
[67] Baeza A, Aguayo J, Barria M, et al. Rapid preoperative preparation in hyperthyroidism. Clin Endocrinol (Oxf) 1991;35(5):439–42.

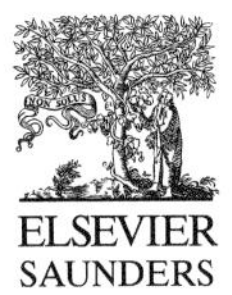

ELSEVIER
SAUNDERS

Endocrinol Metab Clin N Am
35 (2006) 687–698

ENDOCRINOLOGY
AND METABOLISM
CLINICS
OF NORTH AMERICA

Myxedema Coma

Leonard Wartofsky, MD[a,b,c,*]

[a]*Department of Medicine, Washington Hospital Center, Room 2A-62, 110 Irving Street NW, Washington, DC 20010–2975, USA*
[b]*Uniformed Services University of the Health Sciences, 4301 Jones Bridge Road, Bethesda, MD 20814, USA*
[c]*Georgetown University School of Medicine, 3900 Reservoir Road, Washington, DC 20007, USA*

Myxedema coma represents the most extreme form of hypothyroidism, so severe as to readily progress to death unless diagnosed promptly and treated vigorously. Two of the 12 patients first reported with hypothyroidism in 1879 likely died as a result of myxedema coma [1]. There are perhaps 300 cases reported in the literature; thus, although it is, fortunately, rare today, it is important to recognize because of the high associated mortality. A number of the case reports have been collated and reviewed over recent years [2–5].

Because hypothyroidism is some eightfold more common in women than in men, most patients who might present with myxedema coma are women. Because hypothyroidism is most common in the later decades of life, most of these women are elderly. It is important to maintain a high index of suspicion, especially if faced with an elderly female patient with signs and symptoms compatible with hypothyroidism who is beginning to manifest mental status changes and some of the typical findings described in this article. Like uncomplicated hypothyroidism, the diagnosis rests on a determination of serum thyroid-stimulating hormone (TSH). Most hospital and commercial laboratories can turn around a TSH result within hours, and once the diagnosis is made, therapy should be initiated immediately. Nevertheless, even with reasonably early diagnosis and customary therapy, the mortality rate approaches 50% to 60%.

Clinical presentation

Precipitating events

A review of the literature indicates that most patients with myxedema coma seem to present in winter and that a low body temperature

* Department of Medicine, Washington Hospital Center, Room 2A-62, 110 Irving Street NW, Washington, DC 20010-2975.
E-mail address: leonard.wartofsky@medstar.net

0889-8529/06/$ - see front matter
doi:10.1016/j.ecl.2006.09.003

(hypothermia) is usually present. Extremely cold weather actually seems to lower the threshold for vulnerability, with an otherwise stable hypothyroid individual slipping into a coma after cold exposure. The pathogenesis can be more complex, however, with other patients' clinical state evolving into a coma after development of pneumonia, sepsis from any cause, stroke, or cardiovascular compromise (Box 1).

Pneumonia may be a primary initiating event or may occur secondarily after a stroke or aspiration. Other clinical features that are typical of myxedema coma, such as carbon dioxide retention, hyponatremia, hypoglycemia, and hypoxemia, could potentially also contribute to the development of coma in a hypothyroid patient, particularly because they represent potential causes of coma in euthyroid subjects. Patients are likely to present with a slowly developing coma in the hospital setting after being admitted with some other event, such as a fracture. In such cases, the underlying diagnosis may not have been suspected; hence, the slower metabolism of drugs and higher attendant risk of adverse events are not appreciated. Thus, carbon dioxide retention leading to coma could be a feature of relative drug overdosage associated with suppression of respiratory drive, such as from sedatives, narcotic analgesics, antidepressants, hypnotics, and anesthetics. An association with amiodarone therapy has also been reported [6].

Box 1. Myxedema coma: exacerbating or precipitating factors

Hypothermia
Cerebrovascular accidents
Congestive heart failure
Infections
Drugs
Anesthetics
Sedatives
Tranquilizers
Narcotics
Amiodarone
Lithium carbonate
Gastrointestinal bleeding
Trauma
Metabolic disturbances exacerbating myxedema coma
Hypoglycemia
Hyponatremia
Acidosis
Hypercalcemia
Hypoxemia
Hypercapnia

Whatever the precipitating cause, the course is typically one of lethargy progressing to stupor and then coma, with respiratory failure and hypothermia, all of which may be hastened by the administration of the latter types of drugs that depress respiration and other brain functions. The characteristic features of severe hypothyroidism are present, such as dry skin, sparse hair, a hoarse voice, periorbital edema and nonpitting edema of the hands and feet, macroglossia, and delayed deep tendon reflexes, and moderate to profound hypothermia is common. In addition to hyponatremia and hypoglycemia, a routine laboratory evaluation may indicate anemia, hypercholesterolemia, and high serum lactate dehydrogenase and creatine kinase concentrations [7].

General description

If it is possible to obtain a past medical history of the patient, there could be a prior history of antecedent thyroid disease, radioiodine therapy or thyroidectomy, or thyroid hormone therapy that was inappropriately discontinued. Thus, physical examination may show a surgical scar on the neck and no palpable thyroid tissue, or there could be a goiter. Much more rarely, in perhaps 5% of cases of myxedema coma, the underlying cause is hypothalamic or pituitary disease rather than primary thyroid failure as the cause of hypothyroidism. One patient was reported who proved to have myxedema coma attributable to primary thyroid failure and pituitary insufficiency from Sheehan syndrome [7]. For a clinical profile, it is useful to examine the 24 patients (20 women and 4 men, mean age of 73 years) with myxedema coma reported from a hospital survey in Germany (although the authors reclassified 12 patients as having severe hypothyroidism but not coma) [8]. There was underlying primary hypothyroidism in 23 (previously recognized in 9) patients and central hypothyroidism in 1. Presenting findings included hypoxemia in 80%, hypercapnia in 54%, and hypothermia with a temperature less than 94°F in 88%. Six patients (25%) died in spite of treatment with thyroid hormone.

Neuropsychiatric manifestations

In patients with myxedema coma, there may be a history of lethargy, slowed mentation, poor memory, cognitive dysfunction, depression, or even psychosis, as can also be seen in patients with uncomplicated hypothyroidism. They do not complain of these symptoms, however, because of their impaired state of consciousness. Focal or generalized seizures may be seen in up to 25% of patients, possibly related to hyponatremia, hypoglycemia, or hypoxemia because of reduced cerebral blood flow [9].

Hypothermia

As noted previously [8], hypothermia is present in virtually all patients and may be quite profound (<80°F). In many of the reported cases, hypothermia was the first clinical clue to the diagnosis of myxedema coma. The ultimate response to therapy and survival has been shown to correlate with the degree of hypothermia, with the worst prognosis in patients with a core body temperature less than 90°F.

Cardiovascular manifestations

Typical cardiovascular findings in myxedema coma as well as in hypothyroid heart disease include nonspecific electrocardiographic abnormalities, cardiomegaly, bradycardia, and reduced cardiac contractility. One recent case report described a patient who presented with prolonged QT and polymorphic ventricular tachycardia (torsades de pointe) [10]. Low stroke volume and cardiac output occur as a result of the reduction in cardiac contractility, but frank congestive heart failure is rare. Cardiac enlargement may be real and attributable to ventricular dilatation or could represent a pericardial effusion. Hypotension may be present because of decreased intravascular volume and cardiovascular collapse, and shock may occur late in the course of the disease. In shock, the hypotension may be refractory to vasopressor therapy unless thyroid hormone is also being given.

Respiratory system

The reduced hypoxic respiratory drive and decreased ventilatory response to hypercapnia known to occur in hypothyroidism [11] are likely responsible for the respiratory depression commonly seen in myxedema coma, but impaired respiratory muscle function and obesity may exacerbate the hypoventilation [12–14]. The respiratory depression leads to alveolar hypoventilation and progressive hypoxemia and, ultimately, to carbon dioxide narcosis and coma. Although there are many contributing causes to the coma in these patients, the principal factor seems to be a depressed respiratory center response to carbon dioxide [15,16]. Mechanically assisted ventilation is required in most patients, irrespective of the cause of the respiratory depression and hypoventilation. Respiration may be impaired in these patients as well by the presence of pleural effusions or ascites, by reduced lung volume, and by macroglossia and edema (myxedema) of the nasopharynx and larynx, which serve to reduce the effective airway opening. Even after initiation of thyroid hormone therapy, assisted ventilation may have to be continued because of delayed recovery [17].

Gastrointestinal manifestations

Patients with myxedema coma may have anorexia, nausea, abdominal pain, and constipation with fecal retention. A distended quiet abdomen may be present, reduced intestinal motility is common, and paralytic ileus and megacolon may occur. A type of neurogenic oropharyngeal dysphagia has been described that is associated with delayed swallowing, aspiration, and risk of aspiration pneumonia [18]. Gastric atony, if present, may serve to reduce absorption of oral medications.

Infections

Because hypothermia is the rule in myxedema coma, the presence of a "normal" temperature should be a clue to underlying infection. Other signs of infection, such as diaphoresis and tachycardia, are also absent. Patients who fail to survive often have been shown to have had unrecognized infection and sepsis. The possibility of an underlying infection should always be considered while maintaining a low threshold for initiation of systemic antibiotic coverage [19]. The presence of pneumonia also worsens or even causes hypoventilation, and there is a heightened risk of pneumonitis attributable to aspiration caused by neurogenic dysphagia, semicoma, or seizures [9,18].

Renal and electrolyte manifestations

Patients may have bladder atony with urinary retention. Hyponatremia in any patient may cause lethargy and confusion, and hyponatremia and a reduced glomerular filtration rate are consistent findings in patients with myxedema coma. The hyponatremia results from an inability to excrete a water load, which is caused by decreased delivery of water to the distal nephron [20] and excess vasopressin secretion [21]. Urinary sodium excretion is normal or increased, and urinary osmolality is high relative to plasma osmolality.

Diagnosis

The probable diagnosis of myxedema coma should readily come to mind, given a patient with a history of or physical findings compatible with hypothyroidism in the presence of stupor, confusion, or coma, especially in the setting of hypothermia. Given a reasonable index of suspicion, therapy with thyroid hormone should be begun immediately, while awaiting the results of measurements of serum thyrotropin (TSH) and thyroxine (T4). In elderly patients, however, especially those with underlying cardiac disease, thyroid hormone therapy should be undertaken more cautiously because of the risks. Given the presence of the previously mentioned abnormalities that are characteristic of myxedema coma, such as hypothermia, hypoventilation, and hyponatremia in a lethargic, somnolent, or comatose patient, however, the diagnosis must be entertained, appropriate blood tests drawn and sent to the laboratory, and therapy initiated. Indeed, in many patients, the clinical features may be sufficiently clear to make measurements of serum TSH and T4 necessary only for confirmation of the diagnosis.

Today, in most hospitals, both hormones can be measured in several hours on a routine basis or, if necessary, should be so requested on an emergency basis. Although markedly elevated serum TSH would be expected, patients with severe nonthyroidal systemic illness may demonstrate a phenomenon parallel to the "euthyroid sick" syndrome [22], which can be called the "hypothyroid sick" syndrome. In such circumstances, pituitary TSH secretion is reduced and the blood levels may not be as high as one might otherwise expect [22,23]. As mentioned previously, approximately 5% of cases of myxedema coma are diagnosed on the basis of central hypothyroidism and could have normal or low serum TSH concentrations. Irrespective of whether the disease is primary or secondary thyroid failure, all patients with myxedema coma have low serum total and free T4 and triiodothyronine (T3) concentrations. In patients with the hypothyroid sick syndrome, serum T3 levels may be unusually low (<25 ng/mL).

Treatment

Therapy with thyroid hormone alone without addressing all the other metabolic derangements described previously would likely be inadequate for recovery. Because of the potentially high mortality without vigorous multifaceted therapy, all patients should be admitted to an intensive care unit to permit continuous close monitoring of their pulmonary and cardiac status. A central venous pressure line should be used to monitor volume repletion therapy, and a pulmonary artery catheter should be inserted in patients with cardiac disease.

Ventilatory support

Thorough attention to an evaluation of respiratory function should include assessment of pulmonary function (blood gas measurements) and physical examination and imaging to rule out pneumonia or airway obstruction attributable to macroglossia or myxedema of the larynx. Insertion of an endotracheal tube or performance of a tracheostomy may be required to achieve adequate oxygenation. Given that an open upper airway is ensured, mechanical ventilatory support is required to relieve or prevent hypoxemia and hypercapnia and antibiotic therapy should be considered. Mechanical ventilatory support is required typically for 24 to 48 hours, especially in patients whose hypoventilation and coma result from drug-induced respiratory depression, and some patients may require it for several weeks [17]. Frequent monitoring of arterial blood gases is warranted during the period of ventilatory support, and extubation should not be considered until the patient is fully conscious. On those rare occasions when a patient with myxedema coma might require emergency surgery, management should follow these same general principles [24].

Hypothermia

External warming of patients with hypothermia with an electric blanket is advisable but should be done cautiously because of the risk of hypotension caused by vasodilatation with a fall in peripheral vascular resistance. Therapy with thyroid hormone is absolutely essential for ultimate restoration of normal body temperature, but the amelioration of hypothermia by thyroid hormone may take several days.

Hypotension

Because external warming may worsen hypotension, it should be preceded and accompanied by careful intravenous volume repletion, initially with 5% to 10% glucose in half-normal saline or as isotonic sodium chloride if hyponatremia is present. Some patients require vasopressors to maintain their blood pressure until thyroid hormone action begins. Because of its nonspecific presumed effects on vascular stabilization, hydrocortisone (100 mg administered intravenously every 8 hours) is usually administered and is definitely warranted if pituitary disease or concomitant primary adrenal insufficiency is suspected.

Hyponatremia

A dilemma that may arise in these patients relates to the need to administer fluids for hypotension and the indication for fluid restriction for hyponatremia. A cautious approach would be to administer some saline (and glucose) intravenously to replace daily losses in the comatose patient but to limit the volume in those with only mild to moderate hyponatremia (serum sodium concentrations of 120–130 mEq/L) such that all water lost is not replaced. Conversely, if the serum sodium concentration is less than 120 mEq/L, it may be appropriate to administer a small amount of hypertonic saline (3% sodium chloride, 50–100 mL), followed by an intravenous bolus dose of furosemide (40–120 mg) to promote water diuresis [25]. Hyponatremia undoubtedly contributes to the mental status changes in patients with myxedema coma, especially in patients with serum sodium concentrations less than 120 mEq/L.

Glucocorticoid therapy

As mentioned previously, steroid therapy is indicated in those patients with myxedema coma attributable to pituitary or hypothalamic disease because they may have corticotropin deficiency as well as TSH deficiency. Primary adrenal insufficiency could be present in patients with primary hypothyroidism caused by Hashimoto disease on an autoimmune basis (Schmidt syndrome). There may be other clinical and laboratory clues to the coexistence of adrenal insufficiency in patients with myxedema coma, such as hypotension, hypoglycemia, hyponatremia, hyperkalemia, hypercalcemia, lymphocytosis, and azotemia. In most patients with myxedema coma, the serum cortisol concentrations are within the reference range.

It is generally deemed prudent to treat with hydrocortisone because of the possibility of coexistent primary or secondary adrenal insufficiency but also because of the possibility that thyroid hormone therapy may increase cortisol clearance and precipitate adrenal insufficiency. Hydrocortisone usually is given intravenously (50–100 mg every 6 to 8 hours for several days), after which it is tapered and discontinued on the basis of clinical response and plans for further diagnostic evaluation. Such short-term glucocorticoid therapy is safe and can be discontinued when the patient has improved and pituitary-adrenal function has been assessed to be adequate.

Myxedema coma and surgery

A brief consideration of operative intervention in the myxedematous patient may be of interest to some readers. Although elective surgery would be out of the question in a patient with myxedema coma, the situation might present on occasion because the diagnosis was made during the postoperative recovery period, as might often be the case in emergency surgery. Myxedema coma has also been described during obstetric labor [26]. The general perioperative management of patients with hypothyroidism has been reviewed [27], and some of the issues have been described in case reports [28]. Perhaps the most important postoperative issue is the maintenance of an open airway [29,30], and this must be closely monitored in the recovery room.

Thyroid hormone therapy

Patients with myxedema coma need thyroid hormone and die without it. Nevertheless, although the need to treat these patients with thyroid hormone is so patently obvious, the regimen by which to conduct this treatment remains somewhat controversial. The question is how to restore the low serum and tissue thyroid hormone concentrations to normal safely, and the controversy, simply put, relates to whether to administer T4 or T3. On the basis of provision of the organism's need for T3, based on the physiologic monodeiodination of T4 and its conversion to T3, we universally aver that therapy of "garden variety" hypothyroidism is best done with T4 alone. An important potential drawback to total reliance on the generation of T3 from T4 is that the rate of extrathyroidal conversion of T4 to T3 is reduced in the sick hypothyroid patient [22]. Perhaps in favor of T3 therapy is the fact that its onset of action is considerably more rapid than that of T4, which could increase chances for survival [25]. An earlier beneficial effect on neuropsychiatric symptoms may be inferred from studies in baboons showing that T3 crosses the blood-brain barrier more readily than does T4 [31].

Whether one is administering T4 or T3, additional concerns relate to the dosage, frequency, and route of administration. We need to choose an approach to thyroid hormone therapy that balances concern for the high mortality of untreated myxedema coma against the risks of high-dose thyroid hormone therapy, which may include atrial tachyarrhythmias or myocardial infarction. Given the high mortality, we believe that there is a benefit to achieving effective tissue levels of the thyroid hormones as quickly as possible. No one really knows what constitutes the optimal therapeutic approach, however, and recommendations tend to be empiric at best. One argument for using T4 is that serum levels are easier to measure than are those for serum T3, but this is really not the case any longer in modern laboratories. Serum T4 measurements may be easier to interpret, however, because the values do not vary as much between doses as would serum T3 values. T4 therapy may also provide a steadier and smoother, albeit slower, onset of action with a lower risk of adverse effects. Conversely, the onset of action of T3 is quicker, and its serum (and probably tissue) concentrations fluctuate more between doses. In either case, monitoring serum TSH values can provide the information necessary to adjust dosage to achieve the desired impact of treatment at the tissue level. In the comatose patient, it is necessary to give the thyroid hormone by nasogastric (NG) tube or by parenteral injection. Risks of aspiration and uncertain absorption obtain when administered by NG tube, particularly in patients with gastric atony. Parenteral T4 preparations are available in vials containing 100 and 500 μg. A high single intravenous bolus dose (usually 300–600 μg) has been used for decades, based on a report suggesting that replacement of the entire extrathyroidal pool of T4 was desirable to restore near-normal hormonal status as rapidly as possible. An average estimate of total body T4 is 500 μg—hence, that initial dose. Thereafter, the body T4 pool is maintained by administration of 50 to 100 μg daily given intravenously or orally [32]. With the large initial dosage, serum T4 concentrations rapidly rise to supranormal values and then fall to within the normal reference range in 24 hours. In sequence, as T4 is converted to T3, the serum T3 concentrations begin to rise and serum TSH concentrations start falling [33].

In a relatively recent report, Rodriguez and colleagues [34] described their success using a large initial loading dose of T4 as recommended by Nicoloff and LoPresti [5] and Holvey and coworkers [32]. Patients randomly received a loading dose of 500 μg administered intravenously, followed by a daily maintenance dose of 100 μg administered intravenously, or just the maintenance dose. Four of the 11 patients had a fatal outcome, only 1 of whom had received high-dose T4. Mortality correlated with the severity of concomitant illness, with an Acute Physiology, Age, Chronic Health Evaluation (APACHE) score of greater than 20 indicating a potentially poor outcome. Surviving patients tended to be younger and to have better Glasgow Coma Scale scores. T3 is available for intravenous administration in vials containing 10 μg. When given alone, the usual dose is 10 to 20 μg, followed by 10 μg every 4 hours for the first 24 hours and then 10 μg every 6 hours for 1 or 2 days; by that time, the patient should be alert enough to continue therapy by the oral route. Measurable increases in body temperature and oxygen consumption occur within 2 to 3 hours after intravenous administration of T3 but may take 8 to 14 hours or longer after intravenous administration of T4. These changes after T3 therapy are likely to be accompanied by significant clinical improvement within 24 hours [35] but at a greater risk of adverse cardiovascular side effects. In fact, in one report, high serum T3 concentrations during treatment with T3 alone were associated with a fatal outcome in several patients [36]. This outcome is difficult to assess, because, as mentioned previously, myxedema coma may be associated with high mortality rates in spite of treatment. Thus, in another series of 8 patients, 2 of 3 patients treated with high-dose T3 died of pneumonia, whereas the other 5 who were treated with smaller doses of T4 or T3 survived [37]. When reported cases in the literature were analyzed for associations with mortality, it was seen that advanced age, high-dose T4 therapy, and cardiac complications had the highest association with mortality. The authors concluded that a 500-μg dose of T4 should be safe in younger patients but that lower doses should be considered in elderly patients. Consequently, I have personally adopted what I believe to be a prudent but effective approach to therapy, and that is to administer T4 and T3. T4 is given intravenously at a dose of 4 μg/kg of lean body weight (or approximately 200–250 μg), followed by 100 μg 24 hours later and then 50 μg daily intravenously or orally, as appropriate. Adjustment of the dose is based on subsequent clinical and laboratory results, as in any other hypothyroid patient. With respect to T3, the initial intravenous dose is 10 μg, and the same dose is given every 8 to 12 hours until the patient can take maintenance oral doses of T4.

This approach is not offered as the optimal or preferred manner of treatment with thyroid hormone but rather as one that makes physiologic sense in regard to safety and efficacy. No general guide to treatment can take into account all the factors that might affect sensitivity to thyroid hormone, such as age, intrinsic cardiovascular function, neuropsychiatric status, and comorbid conditions that may affect drug dosages because of alterations in drug distribution and metabolism. Hence, patients should be monitored closely before each dose of thyroid hormone is administered.

With aggressive comprehensive treatment, most patients with myxedema coma should recover. It is better, however, that it be prevented by the early recognition and treatment of hypothyroidism.

Summary

Myxedema coma is the term given to the most severe presentation of profound hypothyroidism and is often fatal in spite of therapy. Decompensation of the hypothyroid patient into a coma may be precipitated by a number of drugs, systemic illnesses (eg, pneumonia), and other causes.

It typically presents in older women in the winter months and is associated with signs of hypothyroidism, hypothermia, hyponatremia, hypercarbia, and hypoxemia. Treatment must be initiated promptly in an intensive care unit setting. Although thyroid hormone therapy is critical to survival, it remains uncertain whether it should be administered as T4, T3, or both. Adjunctive measures, such as ventilation, warming, fluids, antibiotics, pressors, and corticosteroids, may be essential for survival.

References

[1] Report of a Committee of the Clinical Society of London to investigate the subject of myxedema. Trans Clin Soc (Lond) 1888;(Suppl):21.
[2] Fliers E, Wiersinga WM. Myxedema coma. Rev Endocr Metabol Disord 2003;4:137–41.
[3] Wall CR. Myxedema coma: diagnosis and treatment. Am Fam Phys 2000;62:2485–90.
[4] Ringel MD. Management of hypothyroidism and hyperthyroidism in the intensive care unit. Crit Care Clin 2001;17:59–74.
[5] Nicoloff JT, LoPresti JS. Myxedema coma: a form of decompensated hypothyroidism. Endocrinol Metab Clin North Am 1993;22:279–90.
[6] Mazonson PD, Williams ML, Cantley LK, et al. Myxedema coma during long-term amiodarone therapy. Am J Med 1984;77:751–4.
[7] Cullen MJ, Mayne PD, Sliney I. Myxoedema coma. Ir J Med Sci 1979;148:201–6.
[8] Reinhardt W, Mann K. Incidence, clinical picture, and treatment of hypothyroid coma: results of a survey. Med Klin 1997;92:521–4.
[9] Sanders V. Neurologic manifestations of myxedema. N Engl J Med 1962;266:547–51.
[10] Schenck JB, Rizvi AA, Lin T. Severe primary hypothyroidism manifesting with torsades de pointes. Am J Med Sci 2006;331:154–6.
[11] Zwillich CW, Pierson DJ, Hofeldt FD, et al. Ventilatory control in myxedema and hypothyroidism. N Engl J Med 1975;292:662–5.
[12] Martinez FJ, Bermudez-Gomez M, Celli BR. Hypothyroidism: a reversible cause of diaphragmatic dysfunction. Chest 1989;96:1059–63.
[13] Wilson WR, Bedell GM. The pulmonary abnormalities in myxedema. J Clin Invest 1960; 39:42–55.
[14] Massumi RA, Winnacker JL. Severe depression of the respiratory center in myxedema. Am J Med 1964;36:876–82.
[15] Ladenson PW, Goldenheim PD, Ridgway EC. Prediction of reversal of blunted respiratory responsiveness in patients with hypothyroidism. Am J Med 1988;84:877–83.
[16] Domm BB, Vassallo CL. Myxedema coma with respiratory failure. Am Rev Respir Dis 1973; 107:842–5.
[17] Yamamoto T. Delayed respiratory failure during the treatment of myxedema coma. Endocrinol Jpn 1984;31:769–75.
[18] Urquhart AD, Rea IM, Lawson LT, et al. A new complication of hypothyroid coma: neurogenic dysphagia: Presentation, diagnosis, and treatment. Thyroid 2001;11:595–8.
[19] Lindberger K. Myxoedema coma. Acta Med Scand 1975;198:87–90.
[20] DeRubertis FR Jr, Michelis MF, Bloom MG, et al. Impaired water excretion in myxedema. Am J Med 1971;51:41–53.
[21] Skowsky RW, Kikuchi TA. The role of vasopressin in the impaired water excretion of myxedema. Am J Med 1978;64:613–21.
[22] Wartofsky L, Burman KD. Alterations in thyroid function in patients with systemic illness: the euthyroid sick syndrome. Endocr Rev 1982;3:164–217.
[23] Hooper MJ. Diminished TSH secretion during acute non-thyroidal illness in untreated primary hypothyroidism. Lancet 1976;1:48–9.

[24] Mathes DD. Treatment of myxedema coma for emergency surgery. Anesth Analg 1997;85: 30–6.

[25] Pereira VG, Haron ES, Lima-Neto N, et al. Management of myxedema coma: report on three successfully treated cases with nasogastric or intravenous administration of triiodothyronine. J Endocrinol Invest 1982;5:331–4.

[26] Turhan NO, Kockar MC, Inegol I. Myxedematous coma in a laboring woman suggested a pre-eclamptic coma: a case report. Acta Obstet Gynecol Scand 2004;83:1089–91.

[27] Stathatos N, Wartofsky L. Perioperative management of patients with hypothyroidism. Endocrinol Metab Clin North Am 2003;32:503–18.

[28] Bennett-Guerrero E, Kramer DC, Schwinn DA. Effect of chronic and acute thyroid hormone reduction on perioperative outcome. Anesth Analg 1997;85:30–6.

[29] Benfar G, de Vincentiis M. Postoperative airway obstruction: a complication of a previously undiagnosed hypothyroidism. Otolaryngol Head Neck Surg 2005;132:343–4.

[30] Batniji RK, Butehorn HF, Cevera JJ, et al. Supraglottic myxedema presenting as acute upper airway obstruction. Otolaryngol Head Neck Surg 2006;134:348–50.

[31] Chernow B, Burman KD, Johnson DL, et al. T3 may be a better agent than T4 in the critically ill hypothyroid patient: evaluation of transport across the blood–brain barrier in a primate model. Crit Care Med 1983;11:99–104.

[32] Holvey DN, Goodner CJ, Nicoloff JT, et al. Treatment of myxedema coma with intravenous thyroxine. Arch Intern Med 1964;113:139–46.

[33] Ridgway EC, McCammon JA, Benotti J, et al. Metabolic responses of patients with myxedema to large doses of intravenous L-thyroxine. Ann Intern Med 1972;77:549–55.

[34] Rodriguez I, Fluiters E, Perez-Mendez LF, et al. Factors associated with mortality of patients with myxoedema coma: prospective study in 11 cases treated in a single institution. J Endocrinol 2004;180:347–50.

[35] MacKerrow SD, Osborn LA, Levy H, et al. Myxedema-associated cardiogenic shock treated with intravenous triiodothyronine. Ann Intern Med 1992;117:1014–5.

[36] Hylander B, Rosenqvist U. Treatment of myxoedema coma: factors associated with fatal outcome. Acta Endocrinol (Copenh) 1985;108:65–71.

[37] Yamamoto T, Fukuyama J, Fujiyoshi A. Factors associated with mortality of myxedema coma: report of eight cases and literature survey. Thyroid 1999;9:1167–74.

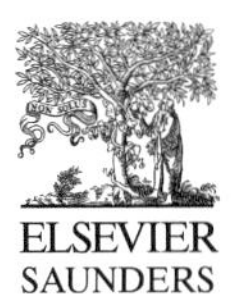

ELSEVIER
SAUNDERS

Endocrinol Metab Clin N Am
35 (2006) 699–724

ENDOCRINOLOGY AND METABOLISM CLINICS OF NORTH AMERICA

Emergencies Caused by Pheochromocytoma, Neuroblastoma, or Ganglioneuroma

Frederieke M. Brouwers, MD[a], Graeme Eisenhofer, PhD[b], Jacques W.M. Lenders, MD, PhD[c], Karel Pacak, MD, PhD, DSc[a,*]

[a]*Section on Medical Neuroendocrinology, Reproductive Biology and Medicine Branch, National Institute of Child Health and Human Development, 10 Center Drive MSC 1109, Building 10, CRC, Room 1E-1-3140, Bethesda, MD 20892-1109, USA*

[b]*Clinical Neurocardiology Section, National Institute of Neurological Disorders and Stroke, National Institutes of Health, 10 Center Drive MSC 1620, Building 10, Room 6N252, Bethesda, MD 20892-1620, USA*

[c]*Department of Internal Medicine, Division of General Internal Medicine, Radboud University Nijmegen Medical Centre, Geert Grooteplein Zuid 10, 6525 GA, Nijmegen Postbus 9101, Nijmegen 6500 HB, The Netherlands*

This article reviews emergency situations caused by diseases of the sympathetic nervous system. Pheochromocytoma is discussed first and most extensively, because there are numerous reports in the literature on patients with (unsuspected) pheochromocytoma presenting as an emergency. Two other tumors of the sympathetic nervous system are then discussed that less commonly result in endocrine emergencies: neuroblastoma and ganglioneuroma.

Pheochromocytoma

Paragangliomas are rare catecholamine-producing tumors derived from chromaffin cells that can be fatal if left undiagnosed. They occur mainly

Work for this article was supported by the intramural program of the National Institute of Child Health and Human Development and the National Institute of Neurological Disorders and Stroke, National Institutes of Health.

* Corresponding author. Section on Medical Neuroendocrinology, Reproductive Biology and Medicine Branch, National Institute of Child Health and Human Development, 10 Center Drive MSC 1109, Building 10, CRC, Room 1E-1-3140, Bethesda, MD 20892-1109.

E-mail address: karel@mail.nih (K. Pacak).

0889-8529/06/$ - see front matter
doi:10.1016/j.ecl.2006.09.014

within the adrenal gland, where they are referred to as pheochromocytomas, and less commonly at extra-adrenal sites [1,2]. Because the intra-adrenal and extra-adrenal tumors are histopathologically indistinguishable, the term *pheochromocytoma* is used herein for both extra-adrenal and intra-adrenal tumors. Although most pheochromocytomas occur sporadically without an obvious association with a familial syndrome, as many as 24% have a hereditary basis involving mutations of five different genes associated with different syndromes: the rearranged during transfection proto-oncogene (multiple endocrine neoplasia), the von Hippel-Lindau gene (von Hippel-Lindau disease), the neurofibromatosis type 1 gene (neurofibromatosis), and the genes encoding succinate dehydrogenase enzyme subunits B and D (familial paragangliomas) [3].

Characteristically, patients present with sustained or paroxysmal hypertension, and the triad of headaches, palpitations, and sweating is often seen. There are numerous reports in the literature of unusual presentations of benign or metastatic pheochromocytomas; for this reason, pheochromocytoma is sometimes labeled "the great mimic." Some of these unusual presentations require emergency intervention. In such situations, it is important to establish the correct diagnosis because any surgery in a patient with unsuspected pheochromocytoma carries a high risk for morbidity and mortality.

Emergency situations can occur owing to high levels of catecholamines secreted by the tumor (an overview of the organ-specific responses mediated by adrenergic receptors is shown in Table 1), or they can be the consequence of complications related to a local tumor mass effect. Symptoms related to tumor localization are not discussed herein because they are often nonspecific and similar in management to that of any other tumor at such a location.

The different ways in which a pheochromocytoma can occur as an emergency are discussed according to the following clinical settings: pheochromocytoma multisystem failure, cardiovascular emergencies, pulmonary emergencies, abdominal emergencies, neurologic emergencies, renal emergencies, and metabolic emergencies (Table 2). Treatment for these emergencies in patients with pheochromocytoma is only discussed if it is different from standard practice. In addition, a separate section describes the general perioperative management of patients with pheochromocytoma. Lastly, pheochromocytoma in pregnancy is discussed. This presentation is associated with a high morbidity and mortality if pheochromocytoma is unsuspected.

Multisystem failure

Even though multisystem failure is a rare presentation of pheochromocytoma, with few cases discussed in the literature to date [4–11], this entity is discussed first herein because early detection is crucial to improve the patient's chances of survival. Pheochromocytoma multisystem crisis is defined

Table 1
Organ-specific responses mediated by adrenergic receptors

Adrenergic impulses			Cholinergic impulses
Effector organs	Receptor type	Responses	Responses
Eye			
Radial muscle, iris	α_1	Contraction (mydriasis) + +	–
Sphincter muscle, iris		–	Contraction (miosis) +++
Ciliary muscle	β_2	Relaxation for far vision +	Contraction for near vision +++
Heart			
SA node	β_1, β_2	Increase in heart rate ++	Decrease in heart rate; vagal arrest +++
Atria	β_1, β_2	Increase in contractility and conduction velocity ++	Decrease in contractility, shortened AP duration +++
AV node	β_1, β_2	Increase in automaticity and conduction velocity +++	Decrease in conduction velocity, AV block +++
His-Purkinje system	β_1, β_2	Increase in automaticity and conduction velocity +++	Little effect
Ventricles	β_1, β_2	Increase in contractility, conduction velocity, automaticity, and rate of idioventricular pacemakers +++	Slight decrease in contractility
Arterioles			
Coronary	α_1, α_2; β_2	Constriction +, dilations ++	Constriction +
Skin and mucosa	α_1, α_2	Constriction +++	Dilation
Skeletal muscle	α; β_2	Constriction ++, dilations ++	Dilation +
Cerebral	α_1	Constriction (slight)	Dilation
Pulmonary	α_1, β_2	Constriction +, dilations	Dilation
Abdominal viscera	α_1, β_2	Constriction +++, dilations +	–
Salivary glands	α_1, α_2	Constriction +++	Dilation ++
Renal	α_1, α_2; β_1, β_2	Constriction +++, dilations +	–
Veins (systemic)	α_1, α_2; β_2	Constriction ++, dilations ++	–
Lung			
Tracheal and bronchial muscle	β_2	Relaxation +	Contraction ++
Bronchial glands	α_1; β_2	Decreased secretion; increased secretion	Stimulation +++

(*continued on next page*)

Table 1 (*continued*)

Adrenergic impulses			Cholinergic impulses
Effector organs	Receptor type	Responses	Responses
Stomach			
Motility and tone	α_1 α_2; β_2	Decrease (usually) +	Increase ++
Sphincters	α_1	Contraction (usually) +	Relaxation (usually) +
Secretion	Inhibition (?)	Stimulation +++	
Intestine			
Motility and tone	α_1, α_2; β_1, β_2	Decrease +	Increase +++
Sphincters	α_1	Contraction (usually) +	Relaxation (usually) +
Secretion	α_2	Inhibition	Stimulation ++
Gallbladder and ducts	β_2	Relaxation +	Contraction +
Kidney			
Renin secretion	α_1; β_1	Decrease +, increase ++	–
Urinary bladder			
Detrusor	β_2	Relaxation (usually) +	Contraction +++
Trigone and sphincter	α_1	Contraction ++	Relaxation ++
Ureter			
Motility and tone	α_1	Increase	Increase (?)
Uterus	α_1; β_2	Pregnant: contraction (α_1), relaxation (β_2) Nonpregnant: relaxation (β_2)	Variable
Sex organs, male	α_1	Ejaculation ++	Erection +++
Skin			
Pilomotor muscles	α_1	Contraction ++	–
Sweat glands	α_1	Localized secretion +	Generalized secretion +++
Spleen capsule	α_1; β_2	Contraction +++, relaxation +	–
Adrenal medulla		–	Secretion of epinephrine and norepinephrine (primarily nicotinic and secondarily muscarinic)
Skeletal muscle	β_2	Increased contractility, glycogenolysis, K^+ uptake	–
Liver	α_1; β_2	Glycogenolysis and gluconeogenesis +++	–
Pancreas			
Acini	α	Decreased secretion +	Secretion ++
Islets (β cells)	α_2	Decreased secretion +++	–
	β_2	Increased secretion +	–

(*continued on next page*)

Table 1 (*continued*)

Adrenergic impulses			Cholinergic impulses
Effector organs	Receptor type	Responses	Responses
Fat cells	α_2; β_1, (β_3)	Lipolysis +++ (thermogenesis)	–
Salivary glands	α_1	K^+ and water secretion +	K^+ and water secretion +++
	β	Amylase secretion +	
Lacrimal glands	α	Secretion +	Secretion +++
Nasopharyngeal glands		–	Secretion ++
Pineal gland	β	Melatonin synthesis	–
Posterior pituitary	β_1	Antidiuretic hormone secretion	–

+/– indicates response and its intensity.

Abbreviations: AV, atrioventricular; SA, sinoatrial.

Adapted from Pacak K, Keiser HR, Eisenhofer G. Pheochromocytoma. In: DeGroot LJ, Jameson JL, editors. Endocrinology. 5th edition. Philadelphia: Elsevier Saunders; 2006. p. 2501–34.

as multiple organ failure, a temperature often greater than 40°C, encephalopathy, and hypertension or hypotension [4]. Similar to hypertensive crises due to pheochromocytoma, the multisystem crisis may be provoked in a patient with unsuspected and untreated pheochromocytoma by manipulation of the tumor, by anesthetic agents at the induction of anesthesia, or by certain other drugs (corticosteroids, antiemetics [metoclopramide], imipramine). Patients often have pulmonary edema, sometimes necessitating ventilation [6,7,9–11], and acute (anuric) renal failure requiring hemodialysis [5,9,11]. Some patients also have intravascular disseminated coagulation [7,9]. The clinical presentation can be mistaken for septicemia, in which case appropriate treatment is delayed [5,7,10,12–14]. Fever and acute inflammatory symptoms may be due to interleukin-6 production by the tumor [15]; therefore, a pheochromocytoma should be included in the differential diagnosis if a patient with suspected septicemic shock is refractory to fluid and inotropic agents.

If the patient deteriorates despite vigorous medical treatment appropriate for pheochromocytoma, emergency tumor removal is indicated, even if the patient's condition is critical, because this may increase the chances for survival. If the patient can be stabilized, surgery should be delayed to allow adequate medical preparation because this improves survival [16,17]. The prognosis for these patients is grave if diagnosis is delayed.

Cardiovascular emergencies

Pheochromocytomas can present with a variety of life-threatening cardiovascular symptoms, such as hypertensive crisis, shock or profound

Table 2
Emergencies due to pheochromocytoma

Clinical setting	Most prominent symptoms/signs
Pheochromocytoma multisystem crisis	Multiple organ failure, temperature ≥40°C, hypertension and/or hypotension [4–12,14]
Cardiovascular	Collapse [180,181]
	Hypertensive crisis
	Upon induction of anesthesia [182–184]
	Medication induced or through other mechanisms [22,25,182,185–190]
	Shock or severe hypotension [8,13,22,24,26–30,87,102,111,191–194]
	Acute heart failure [44]
	Myocardial infarction [69,70,190,195–198]
	Arrhythmia [35–38,40,47]
	Cardiomyopathy [33,50,52,60,65,79,199–203]
	Myocarditis [204,205]
	Dissecting aortic aneurysm [80]
	Limb ischemia, digital necrosis or gangrene [74,77,78]
	Deep vein thrombosis [206]
Pulmonary	Acute pulmonary edema [31,64,83–85,190,207–212]
	Adult respiratory distress syndrome [14,213]
Abdominal	Abdominal bleeding [89,90,97,108,214,215]
	Paralytic ileus [74,95,96,216]
	Acute intestinal obstruction [94,217]
	Severe enterocolitis and peritonitis [99]
	Colon perforation [74,100,218–220]
	Bowel ischemia [50,218,221,222]
	Mesenteric vascular occlusion [223]
	Acute pancreatitis [104,224]
	Cholecystitis [102,103]
	Megacolon [225]
	Watery diarrhea syndrome with hypokalemia [91,226]
Neurologic	Hemiplegia [79,114–117,121]
	General muscle weakness [226,227]
	Generalized seizures [124,125]
Renal	Acute renal failure [33,49,106,109,111]
	Acute pyelonephritis [107]
	Severe hematuria [228]
	Renal artery stenosis by compression of tumor [112,113]
Metabolic	Diabetic ketoacidosis [229]
	Lactic acidosis [230]

Adapted from Brouwers FM, Lenders JW, Eisenhofer G, et al. Pheochromocytoma as an endocrine emergency. Rev Endocr Metab Disord 2003;4:126–8.

hypotension, acute heart failure, myocardial infarction, arrhythmia, cardiomyopathy, myocarditis, dissection of an aortic aneurysm, and acute peripheral ischemia.

Hypertensive crisis

Most patients with pheochromocytoma have hypertension, which can be sustained or paroxysmal. The latter is a result of episodic secretion of catecholamines by the tumor. In 75% of patients, paroxysms with severe hypertension occur at least weekly [18]. Often, these paroxysms may be precipitated by postural changes, exertion, intake of certain foods or beverages, emotion, and urination. Furthermore, they may be provoked by direct tumor stimulation and the use of certain drugs (eg, histamine, adrenocorticotropic hormone [ACTH], metoclopramide, phenothiazine, tricyclic antidepressants, or anesthetic agents). Intravenous urographic contrast media have also been implicated in such provocation; however, in a small study, the nonionic contrast medium iohexol did not appear to increase catecholamine levels significantly [19]. Blood pressure can reach high values. Such a situation is termed a *hypertensive crisis* when it is life threatening or compromises vital organ function. In all of the previously mentioned situations, the hypertensive crises are the result of a rapid and marked release of catecholamines from the tumor. Hypertensive crises may also develop as a consequence of administration of a beta-adrenoceptor blocker in patients who have a pheochromocytoma who are not on alpha-adrenoceptor blocking agents. In such a situation, unopposed stimulation of alpha-adrenoceptors could lead to a rise in blood pressure.

Patients may experience hypertensive crises in different ways. Some report severe headaches or diaphoresis, whereas others have visual disturbances, palpitations, encephalopathy, acute myocardial infarction, congestive heart failure, or cerebrovascular accidents. It is crucial to start proper antihypertensive therapy immediately.

Treatment of a hypertensive crisis due to pheochromocytoma should be based on administration of phentolamine. This drug is usually given as an intravenous bolus of 2.5 to 5 mg at 1 mg/min. The short half-life of phentolamine allows this dose to be repeated every 3 to 5 minutes until hypertension is adequately controlled. Phentolamine can also be given as a continuous infusion (100 mg of phentolamine in 500 mL of 5% dextrose in water) with an infusion rate adjusted to the patient's blood pressure during continuous blood pressure monitoring. Alternatively, control of blood pressure may be achieved by a continuous infusion of sodium nitroprusside (preparation similar to phentolamine) at 0.5 to 10.0 μg/kg per minute (with the infusion stopped if no results are seen after 10 minutes) [20,21].

Shock and hypotension

Severe hypotension is seen infrequently in patients who have pheochromocytoma and may be preceded by a paroxysm of hypertension. A few patients have been described in whom severe hypotension or shock occurred after treatment with imipramine [22,23], metoclopramide [24,25], or dexamethasone [26]. Hypotension may be accompanied by syncope and may be episodic [27]. In less than 2% of patients, profound shock is the presenting manifestation [28]. In these patients, shock is accompanied by significant abdominal pain, signs consistent with pulmonary edema, intense mydriasis unresponsive to stimulus, profound weakness, diaphoresis, cyanosis, hyperglycemia, and leukocytosis [28].

Although hypotension was thought to occur only in patients with predominantly epinephrine-secreting tumors [29,30], it has also been described in norepinephrine-secreting tumors [31]. The mechanisms that lead to hypotension and shock in patients with pheochromocytoma are not understood. Hypovolemia, impairment of the peripheral response to catecholamines, the ratio of epinephrine and norepinephrine secreted by the tumor (epinephrine-induced vasodilatation), myocardial contractile dysfunction, and baroreflex failure may all contribute to hypotension [27,32].

In some patients, severe hypotension occurs in the postoperative period following resection of a pheochromocytoma. This hypotension is thought to be the result of the sudden depletion of circulating catecholamines in the continuing presence of alpha-adrenoceptor blockade and can be treated by fluid replacement and rarely by intravenous ephedrine or vasopressin [33].

Arrhythmia

Stimulation of beta-adrenoceptors by high levels of catecholamines released from the tumor may result in severe arrhythmia. Although sinus tachycardia occurs most frequently, pheochromocytomas have been associated with a wide variety of arrhythmias, including supraventricular [34], nodal [35], broad complex [36], ventricular tachycardia [37–39], torsade de pointes [40], and Wolff-Parkinson-White syndrome [41]. Furthermore, atrial fibrillation [42] and ventricular fibrillation [5,43,44] have been reported. Because arrhythmias are associated with many other diseases, patients who harbor a pheochromocytoma may undergo multiple tests and examinations by multiple specialists to identify the cause of the arrhythmia. Clinicians should consider a pheochromocytoma if the arrhythmia is paroxysmal, or if it is accompanied with sweating, hypertension, anxiety, nervousness, or pallor.

For rapid control of tachycardia due to atrial fibrillation or flutter, intravenous esmolol, a cardioselective short-acting beta 1 blocker, can be used (0.5 mg/kg intravenously over 1 minute, followed by an intravenous infusion of 0.1–0.3 mg/kg/min [45]). Caution is warranted if alpha blockade has not been achieved before the use of beta blockers, because unopposed alpha-receptor stimulation can result in a hypertensive crisis. Ventricular arrhythmias can be treated with lidocaine [46].

Some patients who have pheochromocytoma present with bradyarrhythmia or asystolic arrest [10,47,48]. These situations are the result of a reflex mechanism in which sinus slowing occurs at the onset of a sudden rise in blood pressure during a paroxysm [48]. Rarely, atrioventricular dissociation and bigeminy [34,40], right bundle branch block [49], and sick sinus syndrome [50] occur in patients with pheochromocytoma. Their treatment is similar to that in patients who do not have pheochromocytoma.

Catecholamine-induced myocarditis and cardiomyopathy

In addition to the previously discussed changes in heart rate and rhythm, hypercatecholemia can also cause sterile myocarditis and cardiomyopathy.

Catecholamine-induced dilating cardiomyopathy is most frequently reported [51–55]; however, some patients may present with a catecholamine-induced obstructive hypertrophic cardiomyopathy [50,56,57]. Acute heart failure or pulmonary edema requires immediate treatment, because the prognosis for patients with pheochromocytoma presenting with acute heart failure is poor, and death due to pulmonary edema may occur within 24 hours of the onset of such complaints [58]. Cardiac changes were found to be reversible in most cases after the institution of appropriate medication or excision of the pheochromocytoma [33,59–63]. Improvement can occur shortly after treatment [53,64,65], but recovery can also be more slow and take over 2 years [57,62]. The mechanisms for catecholamine-induced myocarditis and cardiomyopathy have been studied extensively; the importance of the different factors contributing to myocardial injury is still debated. Myocardial ischemia is thought to be most important, together with direct toxic effects of catecholamine oxidation products [66]. Furthermore, cardiac contractility may be decreased by compensatory downregulation of beta receptors on the heart owing to chronic elevation of epinephrine levels. Cardiac contractility may be further compromised by pheochromocytoma-induced hypocalcemia (through calcium sequestration), resulting in cardiogenic shock [67].

Myocardial ischemia and myocardial infarction

Some patients who have pheochromocytoma present with symptoms associated with myocardial ischemia or myocardial infarction [43,68–70]. They may experience chest discomfort, tachycardia, sweating, and anxiousness. These symptoms are caused by catecholamines, which induce vasoconstriction of the coronary arteries while simultaneously increasing myocardial oxygen demand through stimulation of heart rate and cardiac contractility. The presentation and electrocardiographic changes, such as ST-segment elevation or depression [69,71,72], negative T-waves, and a prolonged QT-interval (present in 7%–35% of patients [40,73]), may resemble those of patients with myocardial ischemia or infarction due to heart disease; however, patients with pheochromocytoma may also have other symptoms due to catecholamine excess, such as severe hypertension or headache, profuse sweating, or intense pallor. A history of episodic attacks is even more helpful. Most importantly, if the coronary arteries appear normal at angiography and no changes over time can be observed in cardiac enzymes despite a severe initial presentation, pheochromocytoma should be suspected [39].

Acute peripheral ischemia

In rare instances, pheochromocytoma causes sudden peripheral ischemia, resulting in necrosis or gangrene [74–77]. In most cases, this ischemia is due to extreme vasoconstriction or diffuse arterial vasospasms induced by catecholamine overload. Some patients may already have a history of intermittent claudication [76,78]. Catecholamine-induced vasospasms are easily overlooked if patients report no other symptoms characteristic for pheochromocytoma. Such patients may undergo extensive operations including amputation [58]. This treatment is very dangerous because any surgery in a patient with unsuspected pheochromocytoma carries a high risk for morbidity and mortality.

Ischemia may also be due to arterial occlusion as a result of embolisms of cardiac thrombi in patients with catecholamine-induced arrhythmia [79]; however, this is a rare event. Occasionally, pheochromocytoma is found during the evaluation or emergency surgery for suspected ruptured aneurysms of the abdominal aorta [76]. Both dissecting and obstructive aneurysms of the abdominal aorta have been found in patients who have pheochromocytoma [80–82].

Pulmonary emergencies

Infrequently, pulmonary edema is the presenting feature of pheochromocytoma [31,83–85]. This event has even been documented following surgery for an unrelated illness [86]. More often, pulmonary edema occurs during the course of the disease and in some patients becomes manifest after tumor resection [43]. Although pulmonary edema is cardiogenic in origin in most patients, some patients have noncardiogenic pulmonary edema [31,84]. This edema is thought to be the result of a catecholamine-induced transient increase in pulmonary capillary pressure owing to pulmonary venoconstriction and increased pulmonary capillary permeability [31,43,87]. Recently, it has been suggested that increased pulmonary neutrophil accumulation caused by catecholamine excess may have a pathophysiologic role in the development of pulmonary edema. Neutrophil-mediated injury would, in turn, lead to increased vascular protein permeability and promote lung edema [85].

Gastrointestinal emergencies

Patients who have pheochromocytomas who present with an acute onset of abdominal symptoms can pose a real challenge. Generally, they experience severe abdominal pain and vomiting. Close monitoring is important, because the abdominal symptoms may indicate hemorrhage of the tumor, which could be accompanied by the excretion of vast amounts of catecholamines. This excretion, in turn, could result in hypertensive crisis [88,89], shock, and rapid deterioration of the patient. Moreover, emergency surgery may be required to stop associated arterial bleeding. Alternatively, angiographic embolization may be employed to stop bleeding [88,90].

Other abdominal catastrophes are the result of prolonged catecholamine excess. Emergency surgery could be indicated if vasoconstriction or spasms of the mesenterial arteries cause bowel ischemia. In other patients, high catecholamine levels seem to affect predominantly gastrointestinal motility. Peristalsis is inhibited through relaxation of the gastrointestinal muscles and contraction of the pyloric and ileocecal sphincters, resulting in constipation.

Conversely, patients with a composite pheochromocytoma that is also secreting vasoactive intestinal polypeptide can present with acute and severe secretory diarrheas, resulting in dehydration, acidosis, and hypokalemia [91].

Patients may also present with intestinal pseudo-obstruction [92,93], abdominal distension [94], severe paralytic ileus [74,89,95,96], dilated small bowel loops [97], or megacolon [94,98]. The latter may be complicated by enterocolitis [98,99], volvulus or colonic rupture [100], and fecal peritonitis [101]. Other abdominal emergencies in patients who have pheochromocytoma include acute cholecystitis [102,103], acute pancreatitis [104], and ruptured aneurysm of the abdominal aorta [82].

Nephrologic emergencies

Rarely, a pheochromocytoma manifests with the clinical presentation of acute renal failure [105,106] or acute pyelonephritis [107]. Acute renal failure is associated with rhabdomyolysis, which may occur after ischemia owing to extreme catecholamine-induced vasoconstriction. The rhabdomyolysis leads to acute myoglobinuric renal failure [105]. More frequently, renal failure occurs as a complication during the course of the disease [5,49,108–111]. Other complications include renal infarction as a consequence of renal ischemia due to (deep) systemic shock, vasoconstriction, or tumor compression of the renal artery [112,113]. In some patients, hemodialysis is required [111].

Neurologic emergencies

Cerebrovascular accidents are most frequently responsible for the neurologic symptoms seen in patients who have pheochromocytoma [79,114–121]. In some patients, cerebral hemorrhage has been reported during paroxysmal attacks of hypertension. In rare cases, subarachnoidal bleeding is found [118]. Hemiparesis, sometimes together with homonymous hemianopsy, is reported most frequently [117]. Cerebral bleeding may be accompanied by seizures [18,116,122,123]. Generalized seizures can also occur as a result of cerebral ischemia caused by vasospasm of the cerebral circulation owing to high levels of circulating catecholamines and may be the presenting symptom [124,125]. In young patients with cerebral hemorrhage without an apparent cause, pheochromocytoma should be suspected. Rarely, neurologic symptoms such as paresis occur due to spinal cord compression by metastases.

Management

Management of pheochromocytoma-related emergencies depends on the symptoms; however, it should always include pharmacologic treatment to block the effects of high levels of circulating catecholamines and prevent life-threatening catecholamine-induced complications.

The most effective drug regimen to prepare patients for surgery has not been established, and, currently, several approaches are used to stabilize patients and prepare them for (elective) surgery [2]. Patients must be prepared using pharmacologic blockade of adrenoceptors. Phenoxybenzamine is the drug of choice for alpha-adrenoceptor blockade. It is usually given in a starting dose of 10 mg two times a day and is gradually increased up to 1 mg/kg/d given in three to four separate doses [2,126]. Doses higher than 100 mg per day are necessary in a few patients. Adequate alpha-receptor blockade will be achieved within 10 to 14 days. Beta-adrenoceptor blockade (usually, atenolol, 25 mg once daily, or propranolol, 40 mg three times daily) is added after appropriate alpha blockade to prevent reflex tachycardia associated with alpha blockade [2,126]. It can also be indicated if arrhythmia or angina is present after alpha blockade has been achieved. In rare cases, successful selective alpha-adrenoceptor blockade can lead to unopposed beta-adrenergic overactivity that affects multiple organ systems. Patients may experience tachycardia, diastolic dysfunction, diffuse edema (heart), peripheral vasodilatation and hypotension (vascular system), somnolence owing to cerebral hypoperfusion, and oliguria owing to renal hypoperfusion [127]. Treatment consists of beta blockade tapered to alleviate clinical symptoms.

Other approaches to prepare patients for surgery include the use of other alpha 1-adrenoceptor blockers, calcium channel blockers alone or in combination with alpha-receptor blockade [51,128], or labetalol (a combined alpha- and beta-adrenoceptor blocker).

To assess whether a patient is adequately prepared for surgery, the following criteria have been proposed: blood pressure below 160/90 mm Hg for at least 24 hours; the presence of orthostatic hypotension, but with blood pressure in the upright position remaining above 80/45 mm Hg; no more than one ventricular extrasystole every 5 minutes; and no S-T segment changes and T-wave inversions on echocardiography for 1 week [129].

Postoperatively, patients should be monitored closely for 24 hours in an intensive or immediate care unit. Hypotension and hypoglycemia are the two most common major complications seen at this time [2]. Rarely, patients experience pulmonary edema or cardiomyopathy following surgery [43,63].

Pheochromocytoma in pregnancy

Pheochromocytoma in pregnancy warrants special consideration, because it is associated with high morbidity and mortality if pheochromocytoma is unsuspected (40.3% maternal mortality and 56% fetal mortality). Pregnancy-related life-threatening situations can occur owing to tumor stimulation by pressure from the enlarging uterus, by fetal movements, or during labor in a patient with unsuspected pheochromocytoma. If the diagnosis is made antenatal, maternal and fetal mortality can be greatly reduced [130,131]. Nevertheless, in two series, pheochromocytoma remained unrecognized antepartum in 47% to 65% of patients [130,131]. Diagnosis of pheochromocytoma during pregnancy can be difficult because the clinical presentation may resemble pre-eclampsia. Whereas pre-eclampsia occurs after the twentieth week of gestation and is associated with hypertension in combination with proteinuria, hypertension caused by pheochromocytoma can occur throughout the entire pregnancy, and proteinuria and edema are often absent. Furthermore, pheochromocytoma-associated hypertension can be paroxysmal and may be accompanied by postural hypotension [132].

Hypertensive crisis owing to pheochromocytoma in pregnancy is highly unpredictable. Direct tumor stimulation leading to marked catecholamine release can occur as the result of examination, postural changes, pressure from the uterus, labor contractions, fetal movements, and tumor hemorrhage. It is most frequently seen in the period surrounding delivery. Acute hypertensive crisis may manifest as severely elevated blood pressure, arrhythmia, or pulmonary edema.

The diagnosis can be confirmed biochemically. Biochemical diagnosis can be hindered if the patient is on methyldopa to control blood pressure during pregnancy, because this drug can result in a false-positive test. If pheochromocytoma is suspected, treatment with methyldopa should be suspended or delayed for the measurement of metanephrines.

Once the diagnosis of pheochromocytoma is confirmed, appropriate adrenergic blockade should be initiated in all patients regardless of gestational age, because maternal hypertensive crisis is always dangerous for the fetus. Commonly, it results in uteroplacental insufficiency, early separation of the placenta, or fetal death [133]. In situations of hypertensive crisis, intravenous phentolamine as a bolus of 1 to 5 mg or as a continuous infusion of 1 mg/min can be used to control blood pressure. As a final resort, sodium nitroprusside may be used, but this has to be infused at a rate of less than 1 μg/kg/min to avoid fetal cyanide toxicity [134].

To prevent hypertensive crisis or to treat catecholamine-induced high blood pressure in pregnancy, phenoxybenzamine is most commonly used. With the exception of mild perinatal depression and transient hypotension in the newborn, there have been no reports of adverse fetal effects during treatment [135]. If beta blockade is indicated, a selective beta-blocking agent is preferred to lessen the chances of fetal growth retardation.

The timing of tumor excision depends on the duration of pregnancy at the time of diagnosis. Early in pregnancy, the tumor can be resected after suction and curettage or with preservation of the fetus. After the twenty-fourth week of pregnancy, long-term blockade with phenoxybenzamine, combined with a beta blocker if clinically indicated, should be attempted to bring the fetus to term [134,135]. This treatment is not without risks, because blockade does not always prevent acute crisis. Labor and vaginal delivery should be avoided, because this may cause tumor stimulation and further catecholamine secretion with severe hypertensive crisis despite adrenergic blockade. Cesarean section and simultaneous removal of the tumor is the recommended approach [135]. Anesthetic management for this situation is discussed in detail in the article by Dugas and colleagues [136].

Neuroblastoma

Neuroblastomas and ganglioneuroblastomas (a more mature form of neuroblastoma) are tumors that derive from primitive cells (neuroblasts) from the sympathetic nervous system. These tumors comprise the most common malignant disease of childhood and account for 7% to 10% of all childhood cancers [137,138]. The prevalence is uniform throughout the (industrialized) world, occurring in 1 in 7000 live births [137,139]. Neuroblastoma is predominantly a tumor of young children, with a median age at diagnosis of 18 months (40% are diagnosed by 1 year of age, 75% by 4 years of age, and 98% by 10 years of age) [139,140].

Approximately 65% of neuroblastomas are located in the abdomen, most commonly in the adrenal medulla. Other tumor locations are the chest (20%), pelvis (2% to 3%), neck (1% to 5%), and other locations (6% to 12%) [141–143]. The tumor typically spreads to regional lymph nodes, bone, and bone marrow, but can also metastasize to skin, liver, and soft tissues. Approximately 50% of patients have disseminated disease (lymph node involvement outside the cavity of origin) at presentation [143].

Symptoms and signs at presentation depend on the size and location of the primary tumor and on whether the tumor has metastasized. They are often related to a local mass effect of the tumor or metastasis and include paraplegia (paraspinal tumors, sometimes extending through intervertebral foramina ["dumbbell tumors"]), Horner's syndrome (ie, ptosis, miosis, and anhydrosis owing to cervical masses), ecchymotic proptosis ("raccoon eyes" owing to orbital involvement), and limping (involvement of long bones). Furthermore, in some cases, the tumor is accompanied by remote effects called paraneoplastic phenomena, such as opsoclonus-myoclonus ataxia syndrome caused by an autoimmune process (2% to 3% of patients) [144], or secretory diarrhea if the tumor is producing vasoactive intestinal peptide. Rarely, catecholamines secreted by the tumor (approximately 92% of neuroblastomas have elevated levels of catecholamines) contribute to symptoms and signs at presentation (hypertension or paroxysmal phenomena like flushing or tachycardia). Neuroblastomas are clinically heterogeneous, and disease progression varies widely according to age and disease burden at diagnosis [138].

To stage neuroblastomas, a set of international criteria has been developed—the International Neuroblastoma Staging System (INSS) [145,146]. There are four stages in the INSS classification. The disease is localized in stages 1 to 3, with the stage depending on the extent of lymph node involvement and the presence of midline extension of the disease. In stage 4, the disease is disseminated [146]. Stage 4S is a special subcategory that applies to children under 1 year of age with a distinct pattern of disseminated disease (dissemination limited to skin, liver, or bone marrow) that is associated with spontaneous regression and a high cure rate with or without nonsurgical treatment [147,148].

Prognosis and treatment options are determined predominantly by patient age at diagnosis, INSS stage, tumor histopathology (Shimada system), and biologic features of the tumor, such as the MYCN status (whether or not MYCN amplification is present), the DNA index (near diploid or hyperdiploid karyotype), and the presence or absence of deletions at 1p36 or 11q23 [138,149]. Treatment options include surgery (performed in almost all patients to establish the diagnosis and procure tissue for staging and biologic studies), chemotherapy (the principal treatment modality) with or without supplemental radiotherapy and autologous bone marrow transplantation, radionuclide therapy with ^{131}I-labeled meta-iodo-benzyl-guanidine (^{131}I-MIBG), retinoid therapy, and immunotherapy [140,150].

Emergency conditions related to neuroblastoma

Emergency situations that occur owing to neuroblastomas are not common. When they occur, they are often the result of catecholamine excess, paraneoplastic phenomena, or related to local mass effects of the tumor.

In rare cases, patients who have neuroblastoma experience symptoms and signs owing to catecholamine excess requiring emergency intervention similar to patients with pheochromocytoma. Because the mechanisms behind these conditions are the same as discussed for pheochromocytoma, they are not discussed separately herein. Cardiovascular events are described most frequently as emergency situations owing to catecholamine excess in neuroblastoma. Hypertensive encephalopathy accompanied by seizures [151], cardiogenic shock requiring respiratory ventilation [152], or cardiac failure [153,154] accompanied by coagulopathy and acute renal and hepatic failure [155] have all been described. Furthermore, one patient presented with a condition mimicking sepsis, with hypertension, vasoconstriction, multiorgan failure, and metabolic acidosis [156].

Sometimes paraneoplastic phenomena can lead to emergency conditions. These paraneoplastic manifestations have an immunologic basis and are associated with IgG and IgM antibodies that bind to the cytoplasm of cerebellar Purkinje's cells and to some axons of the peripheral nerves [157]. In one patient with occult neuroblastoma, encephalitis-like features of ataxia, generalized seizures, decreased consciousness, and involuntary movements were seen; however, this patient did not have any signs of opsoclonus-myoclonus at any time during his illness [158]. Less urgent paraneoplastic manifestations of neuroblastoma include paraneoplastic papilloedema with blurring of vision [159] and bilateral ptosis and muscle weakness [160].

A local mass effect of the tumor can also lead to emergency presentations. One patient with a rapidly increasing massive hepatomegaly owing to metastatic infiltration of the liver required mechanical ventilation and urgent surgical decompression for severe respiratory embarrassment [161]. Other treatment options successfully applied to patients with life-threatening abdominal distension owing to liver involvement include chemotherapy and radiotherapy [150]. Patients may present with leg palsy or weakness of the lower extremities if the tumor involves the spinal cord or results in spinal cord compression [162,163]. Other tumor mass–related presentations include blindness owing to metastatic neuroblastoma [164] and protein-losing enteropathy as the result of lymphatic obstruction [165] or elevated catecholamines [166], resulting in periorbital edema and severe hypoproteinemia.

Early diagnosis of these cases may improve the outcome [162]. For example, the blindness due to metastatic neuroblastoma was reversed by surgery 7 days after onset [164].

Ganglioneuroma

Ganglioneuroma is a rare benign tumor that derives from the sympathetic chain. Controversy exists as to whether it may occur de novo (primary ganglioneuroma) or whether it is a result of maturation and differentiation of neuroblastomas, as suggested by the International Neuroblastoma Pathology Committee [167,168]. Ganglioneuromas occur most frequent in the posterior mediastinum (38%), followed by a retroperitoneal site. As many as half of patients are asymptomatic [169–171], and if patients do experience symptoms, these are often caused by a mass effect of the tumor. Infrequently, patients may have hypertension owing to excessive catecholamine secretion by the tumor (only 20% to 39% of ganglioneuromas are reported to secrete catecholamines or catecholamine metabolites [172–174]), or they can have watery diarrhea owing to the secretion of vasoactive intestinal protein by the tumor [175–177]. Patients can be cured by the complete excision of the tumor; however, even if resection of the ganglioneuroma is incomplete, the prognosis usually remains good.

Endocrine emergencies related to ganglioneuroma are rare. In one patient, a membranous glomerulonephritis resulting in nephrotic syndrome was associated with a ganglioneuroma. A circulating tumor antigen–specific antibody was detected in the patient's serum that cross-reacted with an antigen present on the podocyte membrane of the renal glomeruli [178].

Summary

Pheochromocytoma may lead to important emergency situations. It is vital to think about this disease in any emergency situation when conventional therapy fails to achieve control or symptoms occur that do not fit the initial diagnosis, especially if signs and symptoms occur paroxysmal. The crucial role of keeping this diagnosis in mind is made clear by the fact that, in 50% of patients who have pheochromocytoma, the diagnosis is initially overlooked. When pheochromocytoma is considered, appropriate approaches must be used for its diagnosis and localization. These approaches include measurement of urinary and plasma catecholamines and metanephrines and imaging techniques such as CT, MRI, and ^{123}I- or ^{131}I-labeled MIBG scintigraphy. Measurement of plasma metanephrines is the biochemical test of choice [179]. MRI is the recommended imaging modality in emergency situations, because it has a high sensitivity for localizing adrenal and extra-adrenal pheochromocytoma.

Occasionally, neuroblastoma and ganglioneuroma may cause emergency situations. These situations are related to catecholamine excess, paraneoplastic phenomena, or local tumor mass effects. Diagnosis of neuroblastoma can be confirmed by biopsy and measurement of urinary catecholamines [146]. Many imaging modalities are used for localization and assessment of the extent of the disease, including MRI or CT and ^{123}I- or ^{131}I-labeled MIBG scintigraphy [140,146,150].

References

[1] Manger WM, Gifford RW Jr, Hoffman BB. Pheochromocytoma: a clinical and experimental overview. Curr Probl Cancer 1985;9:1–89.

[2] Lenders JW, Eisenhofer G, Mannelli M, et al. Phaeochromocytoma. Lancet 2005;366: 665–75.

[3] Bryant J, Farmer J, Kessler LJ, et al. Pheochromocytoma: the expanding genetic differential diagnosis. J Natl Cancer Inst 2003;95:1196–204.

[4] Newell KA, Prinz RA, Pickleman J, et al. Pheochromocytoma multisystem crisis: a surgical emergency. Arch Surg 1988;123:956–9.

[5] Gordon DL, Atamian SD, Brooks MH, et al. Fever in pheochromocytoma. Arch Intern Med 1992;152:1269–72.

[6] Moran ME, Rosenberg DJ, Zornow DH. Pheochromocytoma multisystem crisis. Urology 2006;67(4) 846e19–20.

[7] Herbland A, Bui N, Rullier A, et al. Multiple organ failure as initial presentation of pheochromytoma. Am J Emerg Med 2005;23:565–6.

[8] De Wilde D, Velkeniers B, Huyghens L, et al. The paradox of hypotension and pheochromocytoma: a case report. Eur J Emerg Med 2004;11:237–9.

[9] Caputo C, Fishbane S, Shapiro L, et al. Pheochromocytoma multisystem crisis in a patient with multiple endocrine neoplasia type IIB and pyelonephritis. Am J Kidney Dis 2002;39: E23.

[10] Kizer JR, Koniaris LS, Edelman JD, et al. Pheochromocytoma crisis, cardiomyopathy, and hemodynamic collapse. Chest 2000;118:1221–3.

[11] Kolhe N, Stoves J, Richardson D, et al. Hypertension due to phaeochromocytoma—an unusual cause of multiorgan failure. Nephrol Dial Transplant 2001;16:2100–4.

[12] Fred HL, Allred DP, Garber HE, et al. Pheochromocytoma masquerading as overwhelming infection. Am Heart J 1967;73:149–54.

[13] Ford J, Rosenberg F, Chan N. Pheochromocytoma manifesting with shock presents a clinical paradox: a case report. CMAJ 1997;157:923–5.

[14] Mok CC, Ip TP, So CC. Phaeochromocytoma with adult respiratory distress syndrome mimicking septicaemic shock. Med J Aust 1997;166:634–5.

[15] Kang JM, Lee WJ, Kim WB, et al. Systemic inflammatory syndrome and hepatic inflammatory cell infiltration caused by an interleukin-6 producing pheochromocytoma. Endocr J 2005;52:193–8.

[16] Ulchaker JC, Goldfarb DA, Bravo EL, et al. Successful outcomes in pheochromocytoma surgery in the modern era. J Urol 1999;161:764–7.

[17] Kobayashi T, Iwai A, Takahashi R, et al. Spontaneous rupture of adrenal pheochromocytoma: review and analysis of prognostic factors. J Surg Oncol 2005;90:31–5.

[18] Manger WM, Gifford RW Jr. Pheochromocytoma: current diagnosis and management. Cleve Clin J Med 1993;60:365–78.
[19] Mukherjee JJ, Peppercorn PD, Reznek RH, et al. Pheochromocytoma: effect of non-ionic contrast medium in CT on circulating catecholamine levels. Radiology 1997;202: 227–31.
[20] Bravo EL, Gifford RW Jr. Pheochromocytoma. Endocrinol Metab Clin North Am 1993; 22:329–41.
[21] Pacak K, Chrousos GP, Koch CA, et al. Pheochromocytoma: progress in diagnosis, therapy and genetics. In: Margioris AN, Chrousos GP, editors. Adrenal disorders. Totowa (NJ): Humana Press; 2001. p. 379–413.
[22] Ferguson KL. Imipramine-provoked paradoxical pheochromocytoma crisis: a case of cardiogenic shock. Am J Emerg Med 1994;12:190–2.
[23] Brown K, Ratner M, Stoll M. Pheochromocytoma unmasked by imipramine in an 8-year-old girl. Pediatr Emerg Care 2003;19:174–7.
[24] Maxwell PH, Buckley C, Gleadle JM, et al. Nasty shock after an anti-emetic. Nephrol Dial Transplant 2001;16:1069–72.
[25] Leow MK, Loh KC. Accidental provocation of phaeochromocytoma: the forgotten hazard of metoclopramide? Singapore Med J 2005;46:557–60.
[26] Takagi S, Miyazaki S, Fujii T, et al. Dexamethasone-induced cardiogenic shock rescued by percutaneous cardiopulmonary support (PCPS) in a patient with pheochromocytoma. Jpn Circ J 2000;64:785–8.
[27] Ueda T, Oka N, Matsumoto A, et al. Pheochromocytoma presenting as recurrent hypotension and syncope. Intern Med 2005;44:222–7.
[28] Bergland BE. Pheochromocytoma presenting as shock. Am J Emerg Med 1989;7:44–8.
[29] Richmond J, Frazer SC, Millar DR. Paroxysmal hypotension due to an adrenaline-secreting phaeochromocytoma. Lancet 1961;2:904–6.
[30] Hamrin B. Sustained hypotension and shock due to an adrenaline-secreting phaeochromocytoma. Lancet 1962;2:123–5.
[31] de Leeuw PW, Waltman FL, Birkenhager WH. Noncardiogenic pulmonary edema as the sole manifestation of pheochromocytoma. Hypertension 1986;8:810–2.
[32] Ramsay ID, Langlands JHM. Phaeochromocytoma. Lancet 1962;2:126–8.
[33] Augoustides JG, Abrams M, Berkowitz D, et al. Vasopressin for hemodynamic rescue in catecholamine-resistant vasoplegic shock after resection of massive pheochromocytoma. Anesthesiology 2004;101:1022–4.
[34] Sode J, Getzen LC, Osborne DP. Cardiac arrhythmias and cardiomyopathy associated with pheochromocytomas: report of three cases. Am J Surg 1967;114:927–31.
[35] Lydakis C, Hollinrake K, Lip GYH. An unusual cause of palpitations requiring atrioventricular node ablation and pacemaker therapy. Blood Press 1997;6:368–71.
[36] Tzemos N, McNeill GP, Jung RT, et al. Post exertional broad complex tachycardia in a normotensive patient: a rare presentation of phaeochromocytoma. Scott Med J 2001; 46:14–5.
[37] Petit T, de Lagausie P, Maintenant J, et al. Thoracic pheochromocytoma revealed by ventricular tachycardia: clinical case and review of the literature. Eur J Pediatr Surg 2000; 10:142–4.
[38] Michaels RD, Hays JH, O'Brian JT, et al. Pheochromocytoma associated ventricular tachycardia blocked with atenolol. J Endocrinol Invest 1990;13:943–7.
[39] Brilakis ES, Young WF Jr, Wilson JW, et al. Reversible catecholamine-induced cardiomyopathy in a heart transplant candidate without persistent or paroxysmal hypertension. J Heart Lung Transplant 1999;18:376–80.
[40] Shimizu K, Miura Y, Meguro Y, et al. QT prolongation with torsade de pointes in pheochromocytoma. Am Heart J 1992;124:235–9.
[41] Gurlek A, Erol C. Pheochromocytoma with asymmetric septal hypertrophy and Wolff-Parkinson-White syndrome. Int J Cardiol 1991;32:403–5.

[42] Hicks RJ, Wood B, Kalff V, et al. Normalization of left ventricular ejection fraction following resection of pheochromocytoma in a patient with dilated cardiomyopathy. Clin Nucl Med 1991;16:413–6.
[43] Cohen CD, Dent DM. Phaeochromocytoma and acute cardiovascular death (with special reference to myocardial infarction). Postgrad Med J 1984;60:111–5.
[44] Gill PS. Acute heart failure in the parturient—do not forget phaeochromocytoma. Anaesth Intensive Care 2000;28:322–4.
[45] Nicholas E, Deutschman CS, Allo M, et al. Use of esmolol in the intraoperative management of pheochromocytoma. Anesth Analg 1988;67:1114–7.
[46] Manger WM, Gifford RW. Pheochromocytoma. J Clin Hypertens (Greenwich) 2002;4: 62–72.
[47] Zweiker R, Tiemann M, Eber B, et al. Bradydysrhythmia-related presyncope secondary to pheochromocytoma. J Intern Med 1997;242:249–53.
[48] Forde TP, Yormak SS, Killip T 3rd. Reflex bradycardia and nodal escape rhythm in pheochromocytoma. Am Heart J 1968;76:388–92.
[49] Hamada N, Akamatsu A, Joh T. A case of pheochromocytoma complicated with acute renal failure and cardiomyopathy. Jpn Circ J 1993;57:84–90.
[50] Grossman E, Knecht A, Holtzman E, et al. Uncommon presentation of pheochromocytoma: case studies. Angiology 1985;36:759–65.
[51] Serfas D, Shoback DM, Lorell BH. Phaeochromocytoma and hypertrophic cardiomyopathy: apparent suppression of symptoms and noradrenaline secretion by calcium-channel blockade. Lancet 1983;2:711–3.
[52] Schaffer MS, Zuberbuhler P, Wilson G, et al. Catecholamine cardiomyopathy: an unusual presentation of pheochromocytoma in children. J Pediatr 1981;99:276–9.
[53] Lam JB, Shub C, Sheps SG. Reversible dilatation of hypertrophied left ventricle in pheochromocytoma: serial two-dimensional echocardiographic observations. Am Heart J 1985;109:613–5.
[54] Shapiro LM, Trethowan N, Singh SP. Normotensive cardiomyopathy and malignant hypertension in phaeochromocytoma. Postgrad Med J 1982;58:110–1.
[55] Velasquez G, D'Souza VJ, Hackshaw BT, et al. Phaeochromocytoma and cardiomyopathy. Br J Radiol 1984;57:89–92.
[56] Jacob JL, da Silveira LC, de Freitas CG, et al. Pheochromocytoma with echocardiographic features of obstructive hypertrophic cardiomyopathy: a case report. Angiology 1994;45: 985–9.
[57] Huddle KR, Kalliatakis B, Skoularigis J. Pheochromocytoma associated with clinical and echocardiographic features simulating hypertrophic obstructive cardiomyopathy. Chest 1996;109:1394–7.
[58] Sardesai SH, Mourant AJ, Sivathandon Y, et al. Phaeochromocytoma and catecholamine induced cardiomyopathy presenting as heart failure. Br Heart J 1990;63:234–7.
[59] Quigg RJ, Om A. Reversal of severe cardiac systolic dysfunction caused by pheochromocytoma in a heart transplant candidate. J Heart Lung Transplant 1994;13:525–32.
[60] Wood R, Commerford PJ, Rose AG, et al. Reversible catecholamine-induced cardiomyopathy. Am Heart J 1991;121:610–3.
[61] Imperato-McGinley J, Gautier T, Ehlers K, et al. Reversibility of catecholamine-induced dilated cardiomyopathy in a child with a pheochromocytoma. N Engl J Med 1987;316: 793–7.
[62] Mishra AK, Agarwal G, Kapoor A, et al. Catecholamine cardiomyopathy in bilateral malignant pheochromocytoma: successful reversal after surgery. Int J Cardiol 2000;76: 89–90.
[63] Gordon RY, Fallon JT, Baran DA. Case report: a 32-year-old woman with familial paragangliomas and acute cardiomyopathy. Transplant Proc 2004;36:2819–22.
[64] Kaye J, Edlin S, Thompson I, et al. Pheochromocytoma presenting as life-threatening pulmonary edema. Endocrine 2001;15:203–4.

[65] Salathe M, Weiss P, Ritz R. Rapid reversal of heart failure in a patient with phaeochromocytoma and catecholamine-induced cardiomyopathy who was treated with captopril. Br Heart J 1992;68:527–8.
[66] Ganguly PK, Beamish RE, Dhalla NS. Catecholamine cardiotoxicity in pheochromocytoma. Am Heart J 1989;117:1399–400.
[67] Olson SW, Deal LE, Piesman M. Epinephrine-secreting pheochromocytoma presenting with cardiogenic shock and profound hypocalcemia. Ann Intern Med 2004;140:849–51.
[68] Murai K, Hirota K, Niskikimi T, et al. Pheochromocytoma with electrocardiographic change mimicking angina pectoris, and cyclic change in direct arterial pressure—a case report. Angiology 1991;42:157–61.
[69] Mirza A. Myocardial infarction resulting from nonatherosclerotic coronary artery diseases. Am J Emerg Med 2003;21:578–84.
[70] Darze ES, Von Sohsten RL. Pheochromocytoma-induced segmental myocardial dysfunction mimicking an acute myocardial infarction in a patient with normal coronary arteries. Arq Bras Cardiol 2004;82:178–80, 175–7.
[71] Yoshinaga K, Torii H, Tahara M. A serial echocardiographic observation of acute heart injury associated with pheochromocytoma crisis. Int J Cardiol 1998;66:199–202.
[72] Liao WB, Liu CF, Chiang CW, et al. Cardiovascular manifestations of pheochromocytoma. Am J Emerg Med 2000;18:622–5.
[73] Stenstrom G, Swedberg K. QRS amplitudes, QTc intervals and ECG abnormalities in pheochromocytoma patients before, during and after treatment. Acta Med Scand 1988; 224:231–5.
[74] Januszewicz W, Wocial B. Clinical and biochemical aspects of pheochromocytoma: report of 110 cases. Cardiology 1985;72:131–6.
[75] Radtke WE, Kazmier FJ, Rutherford BD, et al. Cardiovascular complications of pheochromocytoma crisis. Am J Cardiol 1975;35:701–5.
[76] Krane NK. Clinically unsuspected pheochromocytomas: experience at Henry Ford Hospital and a review of the literature. Arch Intern Med 1986;146:54–7.
[77] Tack CJ, Lenders JW. Pheochromocytoma as a cause of blue toes. Arch Intern Med 1993; 153:2061.
[78] Scharf Y, Nahir M, Plavnic Y, et al. Intermittent claudication with pheochromocytoma. JAMA 1971;215:1323–4.
[79] Dagartzikas MI, Sprague K, Carter G, et al. Cerebrovascular event, dilated cardiomyopathy, and pheochromocytoma. Pediatr Emerg Care 2002;18:33–5.
[80] Triplett JC, Atuk NO. Dissecting aortic aneurysm associated with pheochromocytoma. South Med J 1975;68:748–53.
[81] Cabot. Case 27022. N Engl J Med 1941;224:77–9.
[82] Ehata T, Karasawa F, Watanabe K, et al. Unsuspected pheochromocytoma with abdominal aortic aneurysm—a case report. Acta Anaesthesiol Sin 1999;37:27–8.
[83] Naeije R, Yernault JC, Goldstein M, et al. Acute pulmonary oedema in a patient with phaeochromocytoma. Intensive Care Med 1978;4:165–7.
[84] Takeshita T, Shima H, Oishi S, et al. Noncardiogenic pulmonary edema as the first manifestation of pheochromocytoma: a case report. Radiat Med 2005;23:133–8.
[85] Sukoh N, Hizawa N, Yamamoto H, et al. Increased neutrophils in bronchoalveolar lavage fluids from a patient with pulmonary edema associated with pheochromocytoma. Intern Med 2004;43:1194–7.
[86] Fahmy N, Assaad M, Bathija P, et al. Postoperative acute pulmonary edema: a rare presentation of pheochromocytoma. Clin Nephrol 1997;48:122–4.
[87] Baxter MA, Hunter P, Thompson GR, et al. Phaeochromocytomas as a cause of hypotension. Clin Endocrinol (Oxf) 1992;37:304–6.
[88] Hendrickson RJ, Katzman PJ, Queiroz R, et al. Management of massive retroperitoneal hemorrhage from an adrenal tumor. Endocr J 2001;48:691–6.

[89] Hatada T, Nakai T, Aoki I, et al. Acute abdominal symptoms caused by hemorrhagic necrosis of a pheochromocytoma: report of a case. Surg Today 1994;24:363–7.
[90] Park JH, Kang KP, Lee SJ, et al. A case of a ruptured pheochromocytoma with an intratumoral aneurysm managed by coil embolization. Endocr J 2003;50:653–6.
[91] Van Eeckhout P, Shungu H, Descamps FX, et al. Acute watery diarrhea as the initial presenting feature of a pheochromocytoma in an 84-year-old female patient. Horm Res 1999;52:101–6.
[92] Khafagi FA, Lloyd HM, Gough IR. Intestinal pseudo-obstruction in pheochromocytoma. Aust N Z J Med 1987;17:246–8.
[93] Turner CE. Gastrointestinal pseudo-obstruction due to pheochromocytoma. Am J Gastroenterol 1983;78:214–7.
[94] Bernstein A, Wright AC, Spencer D. Phaeochromocytoma as a cause of gastrointestinal distension. Postgrad Med J 1967;43:180–3.
[95] Noguchi M, Taniya T, Ueno K, et al. A case of pheochromocytoma with severe paralytic ileus. Jpn J Surg 1990;20:448–52.
[96] Sawaki D, Otani Y, Sekita G, et al. Pheochromocytoma complicated with refractory paralytic ileus dramatically improved with intravenous administration of alpha-adrenergic receptor antagonist, phentolamine. J Clin Gastroenterol 2003;37:194.
[97] Lee PH, Blute R Jr, Malhotra R. A clinically "silent" pheochromocytoma with spontaneous hemorrhage. J Urol 1987;138:1429–32.
[98] Rosati LA, Augur NA Jr. Ischemic enterocolitis in pheochromocytoma. Gastroenterology 1971;60:581–5.
[99] Fee HJ, Fonkalsrud EW, Ament ME, et al. Enterocolitis with peritonitis in a child with pheochromocytoma. Ann Surg 1977;185:448–50.
[100] Mazaki T, Hara J, Watanabe Y, et al. Pheochromocytoma presenting as an abdominal emergency: association with perforation of the colon. Digestion 2002;65:61–6.
[101] Mullen JP, Cartwright RC, Tisherman SE, et al. Pathogenesis and pharmacologic management of pseudo-obstruction of the bowel in pheochromocytoma. Am J Med Sci 1985;290:155–8.
[102] Mishra AK, Agarwal G, Agarwal A, et al. Cystic phaeochromocytoma presenting as an acute abdomen with shock. Eur J Surg 2001;167:863–5.
[103] Cho YU, Kim JY, Choi SK, et al. A case of hemorrhagic gallbladder paraganglioma causing acute cholecystitis. Yonsei Med J 2001;42:352–6.
[104] Dugal Perrier NA, van Heerden JA, Wilson DJ, et al. Malignant pheochromocytoma masquerading as acute pancreatitis—a rare but potentially lethal occurrence. Mayo Clin Proc 1994;69:366–70.
[105] Shemin D, Cohn PS, Zipin SB. Pheochromocytoma presenting as rhabdomyolysis and acute myoglobinuric renal failure. Arch Intern Med 1990;150:2384–5.
[106] Gillett MJ, Arenson RV, Yew MK, et al. Diagnostic challenges associated with a complex case of cystic phaeochromocytoma presenting with malignant hypertension, microangiopathic haemolysis and acute renal failure. Nephrol Dial Transplant 2005;20:1014.
[107] Winter C, Schmidt-Mutter C, Cuny R, et al. Fatal form of phaeochromocytoma presenting as acute pyelonephritis. Eur J Anaesthesiol 2001;18:548–53.
[108] Evans JP, Bambach CP, Andrew S, et al. MEN type 2a presenting as an intra-abdominal emergency. Aust N Z J Surg 1997;67:824–6.
[109] Takabatake T, Kawabata M, Ohta H, et al. Acute renal failure and transient, massive proteinuria in a case of pheochromocytoma. Clin Nephrol 1985;24:47–9.
[110] Scully RE, Mark EJ, McNeely BU. Case records of the Massachusetts General Hospital. Weekly clinicopathological exercises. Case 6–1986. A 34-year-old man with hypertension and episodes of flushing, nausea, and vomiting. N Engl J Med 1986;314:431–9.
[111] Raman GV. Phaeochromocytoma presenting with cardiogenic shock and acute renal failure. J Hum Hypertens 1987;1:237–8.

[112] Crowe AV, Jones NF, Carr P. Five ways to be fooled by phaeochromocytoma—renal and urological complications. Nephrol Dial Transplant 1997;12:337–40.
[113] Kuzmanovska D, Sahpazova E, Kocova M, et al. Phaeochromocytoma associated with reversible renal artery stenosis. Nephrol Dial Transplant 2001;16:2092–4.
[114] Hill JB, Schwartzman RJ. Cerebral infarction and disseminated intravascular coagulation with pheochromocytoma. Arch Neurol 1981;38:395.
[115] Moritani H, Sakamoto M, Yoshida Y, et al. Pheochromocytoma of the urinary bladder revealed with cerebral hemorrhage. Intern Med 2001;40:638–42.
[116] Chuang HL, Hsu WH, Hsueh C, et al. Spontaneous intracranial hemorrhage caused by pheochromocytoma in a child. Pediatr Neurosurg 2002;36:48–51.
[117] Goswami R, Tandon N, Singh B, et al. Adrenal tumour, congestive heart failure and hemiparesis in an 18-year-old male: a clinical-pathological conference. Int J Cardiol 1995;49: 233–8.
[118] Beatty OL, Russell CF, Kennedy L, et al. Phaeochromocytoma in Northern Ireland: a 21 year review. Eur J Surg 1996;162:695–702.
[119] Favia G, Lumachi F, Polistina F, et al. Pheochromocytoma, a rare cause of hypertension: long-term follow-up of 55 surgically treated patients. World J Surg 1998;22:689–93.
[120] Plouin PF, Duclos JM, Soppelsa F, et al. Factors associated with perioperative morbidity and mortality in patients with pheochromocytoma: analysis of 165 operations at a single center. J Clin Endocrinol Metab 2001;86:1480–6.
[121] Fox JM, Manninen PH. The anaesthetic management of a patient with a phaeochromocytoma and acute stroke. Can J Anaesth 1991;38:775–9.
[122] Wilkenfeld C, Cohen M, Lansman SL, et al. Heart transplantation for end-stage cardiomyopathy caused by an occult pheochromocytoma. J Heart Lung Transplant 1992;11:363–6.
[123] Thomas JE, Rooke ED, Kvale WF. The neurologist's experience with pheochromocytoma: a review of 100 cases. JAMA 1966;197:754–8.
[124] Leiba A, Bar-Dayan Y, Leker RR, et al. Seizures as a presenting symptom of phaeochromocytoma in a young soldier. J Hum Hypertens 2003;17:73–5.
[125] Reichardt P, Apel TW, Domula M, et al. Recurrent polytopic chromaffin paragangliomas in a 9-year-old boy resulting from a novel germline mutation in the von Hippel-Lindau gene. J Pediatr Hematol Oncol 2002;24:145–8.
[126] Pacak K, Linehan WM, Eisenhofer G, et al. Recent advances in genetics, diagnosis, localization, and treatment of pheochromocytoma. Ann Intern Med 2001;134:315–29.
[127] Kantorovich V, Pacak K. A new concept of unopposed beta-adrenergic overstimulation in a patient with pheochromocytoma. Ann Intern Med 2005;142:1026–8.
[128] Proye C, Thevenin D, Cecat P, et al. Exclusive use of calcium channel blockers in preoperative and intraoperative control of pheochromocytomas: hemodynamics and free catecholamine assays in ten consecutive patients. Surgery 1989;106:1149–54.
[129] Roizen MF, Schreider BD, Hassan SZ. Anesthesia for patients with pheochromocytoma. Anesthesiol Clin North America 1987;5:269–75.
[130] Harper MA, Murnaghan GA, Kennedy L, et al. Phaeochromocytoma in pregnancy: five cases and a review of the literature. Br J Obstet Gynaecol 1989;96:594–606.
[131] Oishi S, Sato T. Pheochromocytoma in pregnancy: a review of the Japanese literature. Endocr J 1994;41:219–25.
[132] Schenker JG, Chowers I. Pheochromocytoma and pregnancy: review of 89 cases. Obstet Gynecol Surv 1971;26:739–47.
[133] Brunt LM. Phaeochromocytoma in pregnancy. Br J Surg 2001;88:481–3.
[134] Molitch ME. Endocrine emergencies in pregnancy. Baillieres Clin Endocrinol Metab 1992; 6:167–91.
[135] Ahlawat SK, Jain S, Kumari S, et al. Pheochromocytoma associated with pregnancy: case report and review of the literature. Obstet Gynecol Surv 1999;54:728–37.
[136] Dugas G, Fuller J, Singh S, et al. Pheochromocytoma and pregnancy: a case report and review of anesthetic management. Can J Anaesth 2004;51:134–8.

[137] Gurney JG, Ross JA, Wall DA, et al. Infant cancer in the US: histology-specific incidence and trends, 1973 to 1992. J Pediatr Hematol Oncol 1997;19:428–32.
[138] Maris JM. The biologic basis for neuroblastoma heterogeneity and risk stratification. Curr Opin Pediatr 2005;17:7–13.
[139] Brodeur GM. Neuroblastoma: biological insights into a clinical enigma. Nat Rev Cancer 2003;3:203–16.
[140] Brodeur GM, Maris JM. Neuroblastoma. In: Pizzo PA, Poplack DG, editors. Principles and practice of pediatric oncology. 5th edition. Philadelphia: Lippincott Williams & Wilkins; 2006. p. 895–939.
[141] Brossard J, Bernstein ML, Lemieux B. Neuroblastoma: an enigmatic disease. Br Med Bull 1996;52:787–801.
[142] Castleberry RP. Biology and treatment of neuroblastoma. Pediatr Clin North Am 1997;44: 919–37.
[143] Haase GM, Perez C, Atkinson JB. Current aspects of biology, risk assessment, and treatment of neuroblastoma. Semin Surg Oncol 1999;16:91–104.
[144] Rudnick E, Khakoo Y, Antunes NL, et al. Opsoclonus-myoclonus-ataxia syndrome in neuroblastoma: clinical outcome and antineuronal antibodies—a report from the Children's Cancer Group Study. Med Pediatr Oncol 2001;36:612–22.
[145] Brodeur GM, Seeger RC, Barrett A, et al. International criteria for diagnosis, staging, and response to treatment in patients with neuroblastoma. J Clin Oncol 1988;6:1874–81.
[146] Brodeur GM, Pritchard J, Berthold F, et al. Revisions of the international criteria for neuroblastoma diagnosis, staging, and response to treatment. J Clin Oncol 1993;11:1466–77.
[147] Evans AE, Baum E, Chard R. Do infants with stage IV-S neuroblastoma need treatment? Arch Dis Child 1981;56:271–4.
[148] Evans AE, Chatten J, D'Angio GJ, et al. A review of 17 IV-S neuroblastoma patients at the Children's Hospital of Philadelphia. Cancer 1980;45:833–9.
[149] Attiyeh EF, London WB, Mosse YP, et al. Chromosome 1p and 11q deletions and outcome in neuroblastoma. N Engl J Med 2005;353:2243–53.
[150] Kushner BH. Neuroblastoma: a disease requiring a multitude of imaging studies. J Nucl Med 2004;45:1172–88.
[151] El-Hayek M, Trad O, Hardy D, et al. The triad of seizures, hypertension, and neuroblastoma: the first described case. J Pediatr Hematol Oncol 2004;26:523–5.
[152] Chauty A, Raimondo G, Vergeron H, et al. Discovery of a neuroblastoma producing cardiogenic shock in a 2-month-old child. Arch Pediatr 2002;9:602–5.
[153] Sendo D, Katsuura M, Akiba K, et al. Severe hypertension and cardiac failure associated with neuroblastoma: a case report. J Pediatr Surg 1996;31:1688–90.
[154] Kedar A, Glassman M, Voorhess ML, et al. Severe hypertension in a child with ganglioneuroblastoma. Cancer 1981;47:2077–80.
[155] Steinmetz JC. Neonatal hypertension and cardiomegaly associated with a congenital neuroblastoma. Pediatr Pathol 1989;9:577–82.
[156] Lindner W, Behnisch W, Kunz U, et al. Congenital neuroblastoma mimicking early onset sepsis. Eur J Pediatr 2001;160:436–8.
[157] Russo C, Cohn SL, Petruzzi MJ, et al. Long-term neurologic outcome in children with opsoclonus-myoclonus associated with neuroblastoma: a report from the Pediatric Oncology Group. Med Pediatr Oncol 1997;28:284–8.
[158] Yeung WL, Li CK, Nelson EA, et al. Unusual neurological presentation of neuroblastoma. Hong Kong Med J 2003;9:142–4.
[159] Scott JX, Moses PD, Somashekar HR, et al. Paraneoplastic papilloedema in a child with neuroblastoma. Indian J Cancer 2005;42:102–3.
[160] Tatli B, Saribeyoglu ET, Aydinli N, et al. Neuroblastoma: an unusual presentation with bilateral ptosis. Pediatr Neurol 2004;30:284–6.
[161] Lee EW, Applebaum H. Abdominal expansion as a bridging technique in stage IV-S neuroblastoma with massive hepatomegaly. J Pediatr Surg 1994;29:1470–1.

[162] Christiansen GM, Pulley SA. Two cases of neuroblastoma presenting to the emergency department. J Emerg Med 1999;17:265–8.
[163] Nejat F, Zabihyan Sigarchi S, IzadYar M. Congenital dumbbell neuroblastoma mimicking birth trauma. J Neurol Neurosurg Psychiatry 2005;76:143–4.
[164] McGirt MJ, Cowan JA Jr, Gala V, et al. Surgical reversal of prolonged blindness from a metastatic neuroblastoma. Childs Nerv Syst 2005;21:583–6.
[165] D'Amico MA, Weiner M, Ruzal-Shapiro C, et al. Protein-losing enteropathy: an unusual presentation of neuroblastoma. Clin Pediatr (Phila) 2003;42:371–3.
[166] Gerdes JS, Katz AJ. Neuroblastoma appearing as protein-losing enteropathy. Am J Dis Child 1982;136:1024–5.
[167] Shimada H, Ambros IM, Dehner LP, et al. The International Neuroblastoma Pathology Classification (the Shimada system). Cancer 1999;86:364–72.
[168] Shimada H, Ambros IM, Dehner LP, et al. Terminology and morphologic criteria of neuroblastic tumors: recommendations by the International Neuroblastoma Pathology Committee. Cancer 1999;86:349–63.
[169] Stowens D. Neuroblastoma and related tumors. Arch Pathol 1957;63:451–3.
[170] Radin R, David CL, Goldfarb H, et al. Adrenal and extra-adrenal retroperitoneal ganglioneuroma: imaging findings in 13 adults. Radiology 1997;202:703–7.
[171] Carpenter WB, Kernohan JW. Retroperitoneal ganglioneuromas and neurofibromas: a clinicopathological study. Cancer 1963;16:788–97.
[172] Geoerger B, Hero B, Harms D, et al. Metabolic activity and clinical features of primary ganglioneuromas. Cancer 2001;91:1905–13.
[173] Hamilton JP, Koop CE. Ganglioneuromas in children. Surg Gynecol Obstet 1965;121:803–12.
[174] Lucas K, Gula MJ, Knisely AS, et al. Catecholamine metabolites in ganglioneuroma. Med Pediatr Oncol 1994;22:240–3.
[175] Hansen LP, Lund HT, Fahrenkrug J, et al. Vasoactive intestinal polypeptide (VIP)-producing ganglioneuroma in a child with chronic diarrhea. Acta Paediatr Scand 1980;69:419–24.
[176] Scheibel E, Rechnitzer C, Fahrenkrug J, et al. Vasoactive intestinal polypeptide (VIP) in children with neural crest tumours. Acta Paediatr Scand 1982;71:721–5.
[177] Koch CA, Brouwers FM, Rosenblatt K, et al. Adrenal ganglioneuroma in a patient presenting with severe hypertension and diarrhea. Endocr Relat Cancer 2003;10:99–107.
[178] Wadhwa NK, Gupta M, Afolabi A, et al. Membranous glomerulonephritis in a patient with an adrenal ganglioneuroma. Am J Kidney Dis 2004;44:363–8.
[179] Lenders JW, Pacak K, Walther MM, et al. Biochemical diagnosis of pheochromocytoma: which test is best? JAMA 2002;287:1427–34.
[180] Spencer E, Pycock C, Lytle J. Phaeochromocytoma presenting as acute circulatory collapse and abdominal pain. Intensive Care Med 1993;19:356–7.
[181] Preuss J, Woenckhaus C, Schwesinger G, et al. Non-diagnosed pheochromocytoma as a cause of sudden death in a 49-year-old man: a case report with medico-legal implications. Forensic Sci Int 2006;156:223–8.
[182] Jones SE, Redfern N, Shaw IH, et al. Exaggerated cardiovascular response to anaesthesia—a case for investigation. Anaesthesia 1999;54:882–4.
[183] Diamond JA. Pheochromocytoma in a symptomatic patient with severe hypertension upon anesthesia induction. Am J Hypertens 2001;14:729–30.
[184] Myklejord DJ. Undiagnosed pheochromocytoma: the anesthesiologist nightmare. Clin Med Res 2004;2:59–62.
[185] Achong MR, Keane PM. Pheochromocytoma unmasked by desipramine therapy. Ann Intern Med 1981;94:358–9.
[186] Montminy M, Teres D. Shock after phenothiazine administration in a pregnant patient with a pheochromocytoma: a case report and literature review. J Reprod Med 1983;28:159–62.

[187] Raisanen J, Shapiro B, Glazer GM, et al. Plasma catecholamines in pheochromocytoma: effect of urographic contrast media. AJR Am J Roentgenol 1984;143:43–6.
[188] Korzets A, Floro S, Ori Y, et al. Clomipramine-induced pheochromocytoma crisis: a near fatal complication of a tricyclic antidepressant. J Clin Psychopharmacol 1997; 17:428–30.
[189] Pineda Pompa LR, Barrera-Ramirez CF, Martinez-Valdez J, et al. Pheochromocytoma-induced acute pulmonary edema and reversible catecholamine cardiomyopathy mimicking acute myocardial infarction. Rev Port Cardiol 2004;23:561–8.
[190] Brown H, Goldberg PA, Selter JG, et al. Hemorrhagic pheochromocytoma associated with systemic corticosteroid therapy and presenting as myocardial infarction with severe hypertension. J Clin Endocrinol Metab 2005;90:563–9.
[191] Delaney JP, Paritzky AZ. Necrosis of a pheochromocytoma with shock. N Engl J Med 1969;280:1394–5.
[192] Mohamed HA, Aldakar MO, Habib N. Cardiogenic shock due to acute hemorrhagic necrosis of a pheochromocytoma: a case report and review of the literature. Can J Cardiol 2003;19:573–6.
[193] Guzik P, Wykretowicz A, Wesseling IK, et al. Adrenal pheochromocytoma associated with dramatic cyclic hemodynamic fluctuations. Int J Cardiol 2005;103:351–3.
[194] Schifferdecker B, Kodali D, Hausner E, et al. Adrenergic shock—an overlooked clinical entity? Cardiol Rev 2005;13:69–72.
[195] Zangrillo A, Valentini G, Casati A, et al. Myocardial infarction and death after caesarean section in a woman with protein S deficiency and undiagnosed phaeochromocytoma. Eur J Anaesthesiol 1999;16:268–70.
[196] Biccard BM, Gopalan PD. Phaeochromocytoma and acute myocardial infarction. Anaesth Intensive Care 2002;30:74–6.
[197] Dinckal MH, Davutoglu V, Soydinc S, et al. Phaeochromocytoma-induced myocarditis mimicking acute myocardial infarction. Int J Clin Pract 2003;57:842–3.
[198] Katechis D, Makaryus AN, Spatz A, et al. Acute myocardial infarction in a patient with pheochromocytoma and neurofibromatosis. J Invasive Cardiol 2005;17:331–3.
[199] Gatzoulis KA, Tolis G, Theopistou A, et al. Cardiomyopathy due to a pheochromocytoma: a reversible entity. Acta Cardiol 1998;53:227–9.
[200] Mootha VK, Feldman J, Mannting F, et al. Pheochromocytoma-induced cardiomyopathy. Circulation 2000;102:E11–3.
[201] Dalby MC, Burke M, Radley-Smith R, et al. Pheochromocytoma presenting after cardiac transplantation for dilated cardiomyopathy. J Heart Lung Transplant 2001;20: 773–5.
[202] Attar MN, Moulik PK, Salem GD, et al. Phaeochromocytoma presenting as dilated cardiomyopathy. Int J Clin Pract 2003;57:547–8.
[203] Vahdat A, Vahdat O, Chandraratna PA. Pheochromocytoma presenting as reversible acute cardiomyopathy. Int J Cardiol 2006;108:395–6.
[204] Baratella MC, Menti L, Angelini A, et al. An unusual case of myocarditis. Int J Cardiol 1998;65:305–10.
[205] Magalhaes LC, Darze ES, Ximenes A, et al. Acute myocarditis secondary to pheochromocytoma. Arq Bras Cardiol 2004;83:346–8, 343–5.
[206] Stevenson S, Ramani V, Nasim A. Extra-adrenal pheochromocytoma: an unusual cause of deep vein thrombosis. J Vasc Surg 2005;42:570–2.
[207] Munk Z, Tolis G, Jones W, et al. Pheochromocytoma presenting with pulmonary edema and hyperamylasemia. Can Med Assoc J 1977;116:357–9.
[208] Joshi R, Manni A. Pheochromocytoma manifested as noncardiogenic pulmonary edema. South Med J 1993;86:826–8.
[209] Okada Y, Suchi M, Takeyama H, et al. Noncardiogenic pulmonary edema as the chief manifestation of a pheochromocytoma: a case report of MEN 2A with pedigree analysis of the RET proto-oncogene. Tohoku J Exp Med 1999;188:177–87.

[210] Bos JC, Toorians AW, van Mourik JC, et al. Emergency resection of an extra-adrenal phaeochromocytoma: wrong or right? A case report and a review of literature. Neth J Med 2003;61:258–65.
[211] Baguet JP, Hammer L, Mazzuco TL, et al. Circumstances of discovery of phaeochromocytoma: a retrospective study of 41 consecutive patients. Eur J Endocrinol 2004;150:681–6.
[212] Grinda JM, Bricourt MO, Salvi S, et al. Unusual cardiogenic shock due to pheochromocytoma: recovery after bridge-to-bridge (extracorporeal life support and DeBakey ventricular assist device) and right surrenalectomy. J Thorac Cardiovasc Surg 2006;131:913–4.
[213] O'Hickey S, Hilton AM, Whittaker JS. Phaeochromocytoma associated with adult respiratory distress syndrome. Thorax 1987;42:157–8.
[214] Chan MK, Tse HW, Mok FP. Ruptured phaeochromocytoma—a lesson in acute abdomen. Hong Kong Med J 2003;9:221–3.
[215] Orikasa K, Namima T, Ohnuma T, et al. Spontaneous rupture of adrenal pheochromocytoma with capsular invasion. Int J Urol 2004;11:1013–5.
[216] Cruz SR, Colwell JA. Pheochromocytoma and ileus. JAMA 1972;219:1050–1.
[217] Blecha M, Galanopolous C, Dharkar D, et al. Massive organ of Zuckerkandl inducing small bowel obstruction. J Am Coll Surg 2005;201:480–1.
[218] Carr ND, Hulme A, Sheron N, et al. Intestinal ischaemia associated with phaeochromocytoma. Postgrad Med J 1989;65:594–6.
[219] Hashimoto Y, Motoyoshi S, Maruyama H, et al. The treatment of pheochromocytoma associated with pseudo-obstruction and perforation of the colon, hepatic failure, and DIC. Jpn J Med 1990;29:341–6.
[220] Karri V, Khan SL, Wilson Y. Bowel perforation as a presenting feature of pheochromocytoma: case report and literature review. Endocr Pract 2005;11:385–8.
[221] Salehi A, Legome EL, Eichhorn K, et al. Pheochromocytoma and bowel ischemia. J Emerg Med 1997;15:35–8.
[222] Sohn CI, Kim JJ, Lim YH, et al. A case of ischemic colitis associated with pheochromocytoma. Am J Gastroenterol 1998;93:124–6.
[223] Morris K, McDevitt B. Phaeochromocytoma presenting as a case of mesenteric vascular occlusion. Ir Med J 1985;78:356–7.
[224] Greaves DJ, Barrow PM. Emergency resection of phaeochromocytoma presenting with hyperamylasaemia and pulmonary oedema after abdominal trauma. Anaesthesia 1989;44:841–2.
[225] Sweeney AT, Malabanan AO, Blake MA, et al. Megacolon as the presenting feature in pheochromocytoma. J Clin Endocrinol Metab 2000;85:3968–72.
[226] Onozawa M, Fukuhara T, Minoguchi M, et al. Hypokalemic rhabdomyolysis due to WDHA syndrome caused by VIP-producing composite pheochromocytoma: a case in neurofibromatosis type 1. Jpn J Clin Oncol 2005;35:559–63.
[227] Smith JC, Meehan C, Lyons P, et al. A man presenting with limb weakness and electrolyte imbalance. Postgrad Med J 1999;75:691–3.
[228] Dewan M, Rasshid M, Elmalik EM, et al. Lessons to be learned: a case study approach. Paraganglioma of the urinary bladder. J R Soc Health 2001;121:193–8.
[229] Ishii C, lnoue K, Negishi K, et al. Diabetic ketoacidosis in a case of pheochromocytoma. Diabetes Res Clin Pract 2001;54:137–42.
[230] Bornemann M, Hill SC, Kidd GS 2nd. Lactic acidosis in pheochromocytoma. Ann Intern Med 1986;105:880–2.

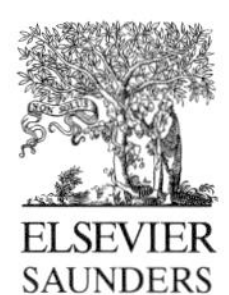
ELSEVIER
SAUNDERS

Endocrinol Metab Clin N Am
35 (2006) 725–751

ENDOCRINOLOGY
AND METABOLISM
CLINICS
OF NORTH AMERICA

Hyperglycemic Crises in Diabetes Mellitus: Diabetic Ketoacidosis and Hyperglycemic Hyperosmolar State

Abbas E. Kitabchi, PhD, MD*,
Ebenezer A. Nyenwe, MD

Division of Endocrinology, Diabetes and Metabolism,
University of Tennessee Health Science Center, 956 Court Avenue,
Suite D334, Memphis, TN 38163, USA

Diabetic ketoacidosis (DKA) and hyperglycemic hyperosmolar state (HHS) potentially are fatal acute metabolic complications of diabetes [1–6]. DKA accounts for 8% to 29% of all hospital admissions with a primary diagnosis of diabetes. The annual incidence of DKA from population-based studies is estimated to range from 4 to 8 episodes per 1000 patient admissions with diabetes [7]. The incidence of DKA continues to increase, with DKA accounting for approximately 115,000 hospitalizations in the United States in 2003 (Fig. 1A) [8]. The rate of hospital admissions for HHS is lower than for DKA and is less than 1% of all diabetic-related admissions [6,7]. DKA also is economically burdensome, with an average cost of $13,000 per patient per hospitalization [9]. Thus, the annual expenditure for the care of patients who have DKA may exceed $1 billion. The mortality rate for DKA has been falling over the years. Age-adjusted mortality rates in the United States dropped by 22% between 1980 and 2001 (from 32 to 20 per 100,000 diabetic population, respectively) (Fig. 1B) [10]. Contrary to the trend in DKA mortality, the mortality rate of HHS has remained alarmingly high and may exceed 40%, compared with less than 5% in patients who have DKA [11,12].

DKA consists of the biochemical triad of hyperglycemia, ketonemia, and metabolic acidosis (Fig. 2) [13]. The terms, hyperglycemic hyperosmolar nonketotic coma and hyperglycemic hyperosmolar nonketotic state, have

The works of Dr. Kitabchi cited in this article were supported in part by grant number RR 00211 from the National Institutes of Health, Division of Research Resources, Bethesda, Maryland.

* Corresponding author.
E-mail address: akitabchi@utmem.edu (A.E. Kitabchi).

doi:10.1016/j.ecl.2006.09.006

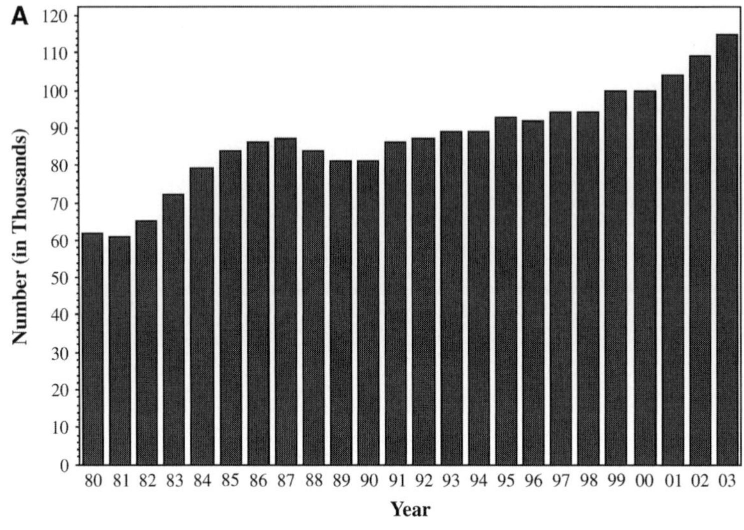

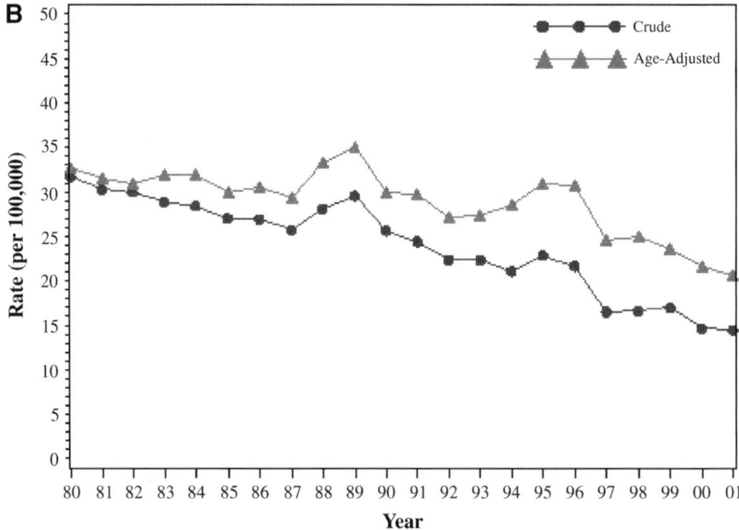

Fig. 1. (*A*) Incidence of DKA. (Centers for Disease Control and Prevention. Diabetes surveillance system. Atlanta: US Department of Health and Human Services; 2003. Available at: www.cdc.gov/diabetes/statistics/index.htm. Accessed June 10, 2006.) (*B*) Mortality rate of DKA. (*Adapted from* Centers for Disease Control and Prevention. Diabetes Surveillance System. Atlanta GA: US Department of Health and Human Services; 2003. Available at; www.cdc.gov/diabetes/statistics/mortalitydka. Accessed June 23, 2006.)

been replaced with HHS [11,14] to reflect that (1) alterations of sensoria often may be present without coma and (2) HHS may consist of moderate to variable degrees of clinical ketosis. Although DKA and HHS often are discussed as separate entities, they represent points along a spectrum of

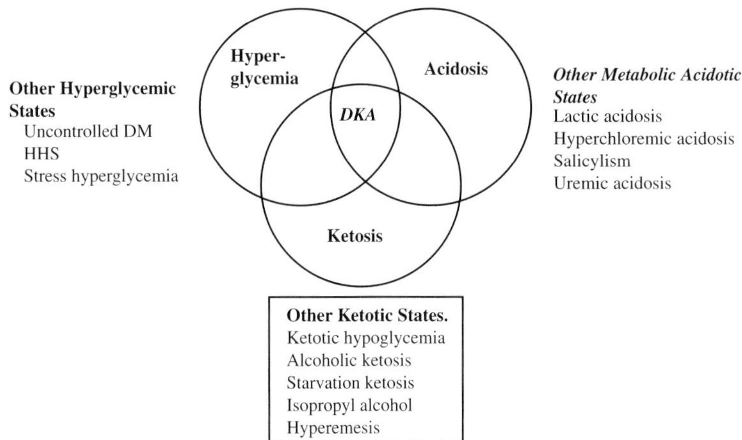

Fig. 2. Differential diagnosis of DKA. (*Adapted from* Kitabchi AE, Fisher JN. Diabetes mellitus. In: Glew RA, Peters SP, editors. Clinical studies in medical biochemistry. New York: Oxford University Press; 1987. p. 105.)

emergencies caused by poorly controlled diabetes. DKA and HHS are characterized by absolute or relative insulinopenia. Clinically, they differ only by the severity of dehydration, ketosis, and metabolic acidosis [2,4,6]. DKA occurs most often in patients who have type 1 diabetes mellitus (T1DM), although it also can occur in type 2 diabetes mellitus (T2DM), especially in patients from ethnic minority groups [15–18]. Similarly, although HHS occurs most commonly in T2DM, it can be seen in T1DM in conjunction with DKA [19]. Table 1 summarizes the biochemical criteria for DKA and HHS and water and electrolyte deficits in these two conditions. It also provides a simple method for calculating anion gap and serum osmolality from serum electrolytes and glucose [20].

Precipitating factors

A diligent search for the precipitating causes of all episodes of DKA and HHS should be made, as the correction of these factors contributes to better outcome. Omission or inadequate dosing of insulin and infection are the most common precipitants of DKA and HHS [11,14,21–24]. Other causes include pancreatitis, silent myocardial infarction, cerebrovascular accident, and drugs. Restricted water intake resulting from ill health or immobilization, compounded by altered thirst response of the elderly, contributes to severe dehydration and HHS. Approximately 30% of patients ages 65 and above presenting with HHS do not have prior history of diabetes [22]; delayed recognition of hyperglycemic symptoms in such patients may lead to severe dehydration. Drugs that affect carbohydrate metabolism, such as

Table 1
Diagnostic criteria and typical total body deficits of water and electrolytes in diabetic ketoacidosis and hyperglycemic hyperosmolar syndrome

	Diabetic ketoacidosis			Hyperglycemic hyperosmolar syndrome
	Mild	Moderate	Severe	
Diagnostic criteria and classification				
Plasma glucose (mg/dL)	>250	>250	>250	>600
Arterial pH	7.25–7.30	7.00–<7.24	<7.00	>7.30
Serum bicarbonate (mEq/L)	15–18	10–<15	<10	>15
Urine ketone[a]	Positive	Positive	Positive	Small
Serum ketone[a]	Positive	Positive	Positive	Small
Effective serum osmolality[b]	Variable	Variable	Variable	>320
Anion gap[c]	>10	>12	>12	Variable
Mental status	Alert	Alert/drowsy	Stupor/coma	Variable
Typical deficits				
Total water (L)	6			9
Water (mL/kg)[d]	100			100–200
Na+ (mEq/kg)	7–10			5–13
Cl− (mEq/kg)	3–5			5–15
K+ (mEq/kg)	3–5			4–6
PO4 (mmol/kg)	5–7			3–7
Mg++ (mEq/kg)	1–2			1–2
Ca++ (mEq/kg)	1–2			1–2

[a] Nitroprusside reaction method.
[b] Calculation: effective serum osmolality: 2[measured Na^+ (mEq/L)+glucose (mg/dL)/18 [mOsm/Kg].
[c] Calculation: anion gap: (Na^+)–(Cl^-+$HCO3^-$ (mEq/L) [normal = 12 ± 2].
[d] per kg of body weight.

Data from Kitabchi AE, Fisher JN, Murphy MB, et al. Diabetic ketoacidosis and the hyperglycemic hyperosmolar nonketotic state. In: Kahn CR, Weir GC, editors. Joslin's diabetes mellitus. 13th ed. Philadelphia: Lea & Febiger; 1994. p. 738–70; and Kitabchi AE, Murphy MB. Hyperglycemic crises in adult patients with diabetes mellitus. In: Wass JA, Shalet SM, Amiel SA, editors. Oxford textbook of endocrinology. New York: Oxford University Press; 2002. p. 1734–47.

corticosteroids, thiazides, sympathomimetic agents (such as dobutamine and terbutaline) [21], and second-generation antipsychotics agents [25], may precipitate HHS or DKA. Cocaine also is associated with recurrent DKA [23,26]. A retrospective study of more than 200 cases of DKA in an inner-city community hospital showed active use of cocaine to be an independent risk factor for recurrent DKA [23]. In patients who have T1DM, psychologic problems and eating disorders may contribute to 20% of recurrent DKA [27]. Factors associated with omission of insulin include fear of weight gain, hypoglycemia, rebellion from authority, and the stress of chronic disease. Mechanical problems with continuous subcutaneous insulin infusion devices also can precipitate DKA [28]. A recent report suggests a relationship between low-carbohydrate dietary intake and metabolic acidosis [29]. Also, there are case reports of patients presenting with DKA as the primary manifestation of acromegaly [30–33]. Important precipitants of DKA and HHS are shown in Table 2. As indicated by the studies listed in Table 2, omission of insulin therapy is becoming a more frequent precipitant of DKA than infection [34–39].

Increasing numbers of DKA cases are reported in patients who have T2DM. Available evidence shows that up to 50% of African American and Hispanic patients presenting with DKA as the initial manifestation of diabetes have T2DM [18,40–43]. These patients who have ketosis-prone T2DM develop sudden-onset impairment in insulin secretion and action, resulting in profound insulinopenia, but recover β-cell function with resolution of DKA [16,40,41,44,45], with 40% of them remaining noninsulin dependent 10 years after the initial episode of DKA [40–42]. The reason

Table 2
Precipitating factors for diabetic ketoacidosis

Study location/dates	Number of cases	Infection	Cardiovascular disease	Noncompliance	New onset	Other conditions	Unknown
Frankfurt, Germany Petzold et al, 1971 [34]	472	19	6	38	+[a]	+	+
Birmingham, UK Soler et al, 1968–72 [35]	258	28	3	23	+	+	+
Erfurt, Germany Panzram, 1970–71 [36]	133	35	4	21	+	+	+
Basel, Switzerland Berger et al, 1968–78 [37]	163	56	5	31	+	+	+
Rhode Island Faich et al, 1975–79 [38]	152	43	—	26	+	+	+
Memphis, TN Kitabchi et al, 1974–85 [1]	202	38	—	28	22	10	4
Atlanta, GA Umpierez et al, 1993–94 [15]	144	28	—	41	17	10	4
Bronx, NY Nyenwe et al, 2001–04 [39]	219	25	3	44	25	12	15

Data are percentages of all cases except in Nyenwe et al, where new-onset disease was not included in the percentage.

[a] + indicates complete data on these items were not given; therefore, the total is less than 100%.

Data from Kitabchi AE, Umpierrez GE, Murphy MB, et al. Management of hyperglycemic crises in patients with diabetes. Diabetes Care 2001;24:131–53.

for acute transient β-cell failure is not known with certainty. Postulated mechanisms include glucotoxicity, lipotoxicity, and genetic predisposition. A genetic mechanism involving glucose-6-phosphate dehydrogenase deficiency is associated with ketosis-prone diabetes [46].

Pathogenesis of diabetic ketoacidosis and hyperglycemic hyperosmolar state

The underlying defects in DKA and HHS are (1) reduced net effective action of circulating insulin as a result of decreased insulin secretion (DKA) or ineffective action of insulin, (2) elevated levels of counterregulatory hormones—glucagon, catecholamines, cortisol, and growth hormone, resulting in (3) inability of glucose to enter insulin-sensitive tissues (liver, muscle, and adipocytes) [14,15,20,21].

Diabetic ketoacidosis

In DKA, there is severe alteration of carbohydrate, protein, and lipid metabolism. Hyperglycemia and lipolysis play central roles in the genesis of this metabolic decompensation [47–49].

Carbohydrate metabolism

The hyperglycemia in DKA is the result of three events: (1) increased gluconeogenesis; (2) increased glycogenolysis; and (3) decreased glucose use by liver, muscle, and fat. Decreased insulin and elevated cortisol levels also result in decreased protein synthesis and increased proteolysis with increased production of amino acids (alanine and glutamine), which serve as substrates for gluconeogenesis [47]. Furthermore, muscle glycogen is catabolized to lactic acid via glycogenolysis. The lactic acid so produced is transported to the liver in the Cori cycle, where it serves as carbon skeleton for gluconeogenesis [47]. Increased levels of glucagon, cathecholamines, and cortisol with concurrent insulinopenia stimulate gluconeogenic enzymes, especially phosphoenolpyruvate carboxykinase (PEPCK) [1,6,20,47,48]. Decreased glucose use is exaggerated further by increased levels of circulating catecholamines and free fatty acids (FFA) [50].

Lipid metabolism

Excess catecholamines coupled with effective insulinopenia promote triglyceride breakdown (lipolysis) to FFA and glycerol, the latter providing carbon skeleton for gluconeogenesis and the former providing the substrate for the formation of ketone bodies [20,47,48]. Elevated FFA level leads to increased production of ketone bodies via beta oxidation and very low-density lipoprotein by the liver. Severe hypertriglyceridemia may be evident clinically as lipemia retinalis [6]. Ketogenesis is enhanced further by decreased concentrations of malonyl coenzyme A (CoA), which occurs as a result of the increased ratio of glucagon to insulin in DKA [48,50].

Malonyl CoA inhibits carnitine palmitoyl acyltransferase (CPT1), the rate-limiting enzyme of ketogenesis. Therefore, reduction in malonyl CoA leads to stimulation of CPT1 and effective increase in ketogenesis [48]. Increased production of ketone bodies (acetoacetate and β-hydroxybutyrate [BOHB]) leads to ketonemia [46,50,51]. There also is decreased clearance of ketone bodies in DKA, which contributes to ketonemia [50]. These ketoacids are neutralized by extracellular and cellular buffers, resulting in their loss and subsequent anion gap metabolic acidosis [49]. Studies in diabetic and pancreatectomized patients demonstrate the cardinal role of hyperglucagonemia in an insulinopenic internal milieu in the genesis of DKA [52,53]. In the absence of stressful situations, such as dehydration, vomiting, or intercurrent illness, ketosis usually is mild, whereas glucose levels increase with simultaneous rise in serum potassium level [54].

Elevated levels of proinflammatory cytokines, lipid peroxidation markers, and procoagulant factors, such as plasminogen activator inhibitor-1 and C-reactive protein, are demonstrated in DKA. The levels of these factors return to normal with insulin therapy and correction of hyperglycemia [55]. This inflammatory and procoagulant state may explain the well-known association between hyperglycemic crisis and thrombotic state.

Hyperglycemic hyperosmolar state

The pathogenesis of DKA and HHS are similar; however, they differ in that in HHS there is (1) enough insulin to prevent lipolysis (as it takes one tenth as much insulin to suppress lipolysis as it does to stimulate glucose use), (2) greater dehydration, and (3) possible smaller increases in counterregulatory hormones [3,4,6,22,56]. Table 3 demonstrates biochemical differences between DKA and HHS [22,56]. Fig. 3 shows the pathogenetic pathways in the evolution of DKA and HHS, whereas Fig. 4 depicts the biochemical changes in the pathogenesis of DKA.

Fluid and electrolyte abnormalities

Severe derangement of water and electrolyte balance occurs in DKA and HHS, resulting from insulin deficiency, hyperglycemia, and hyperketonemia. Osmotic diuresis resulting from hyperglycemia promotes net loss of multiple minerals and electrolytes, including sodium, potassium, calcium, magnesium, chloride, and phosphate. Although some of these electrolytes (sodium, potassium, and chloride) can be replaced rapidly during treatment, others require days or weeks to restore losses and achieve balance [57–59]. Ketoanion excretion, which obligates urinary cation excretion, also contributes to electrolyte derangement, albeit less than hyperglycemia. Insulin deficiency per se also may contribute to renal losses of water and electrolytes because of deficient water and salt resorptive effect of insulin in the renal tubule [58,59]. Intracellular dehydration occurs as hyperglycemia, and water loss leads to increased plasma tonicity, causing a shift of

Table 3
Admission biochemical data in patients who have hyperglycemic hyperosmolar syndrome and diabetic ketoacidosis

Parameters measured	Hyperglycemic hyperosmolar syndrome	Diabetic ketoacidosis
Glucose (mg/dL)	930 ± 83	616 ± 36
Na+ (mEq/L)	149 ± 3.2	134 ± 1.0
K+ (mEq/L)	3.9 ± 0.2	4.5 ± 0.13
SUN (mg/dL)	61 ± 11	32 ± 3
Creatinine (mg/dL)	1.4 ± 0.1	1.1 ± 0.1
pH	7.3 ± 0.03	7.12 ± 0.04
Bicarbonate (mEq/L)	18 ± 1.1	9.4 ± 1.4
BOHB (mmol/L)	1.0 ± 0.2	9.1 ± 0.85
Total osmolality (mosm/kg)	380 ± 5.7	323 ± 2.5
IRI (nmol/L)	0.08 ± 0.01	0.07 ± 0.01
C peptide (nmol/L)	1.14 ± 0.1	0.21 ± 0.03
FFA (nmol/L)	1.5 ± 0.19	1.6 ± 0.16
Human growth hormone (ng/L)	1.9 ± 0.2	6.1 ± 1.2
Cortisol (ng/L)	570 ± 49	500 ± 61
IRI (nmol/l)*	0.27 ± 0.05	0.09 ± 0.01
C peptide (nmol/L)	1.75 ± 0.23	0.25 ± 0.05
Glucagon (pg/L)	689 ± 215	580 ± 147
Catecholamines (ng/L)	0.28 ± 0.09	1.78 ± 0.4
Anion gap	11	17

Data are presented as mean ± SEM.

Abbreviation: IRI, immuno reactive insulin.

* Values after intravenous tolbutamide.

Data from Kitabchi AE, Umpierrez GE, Murphy MB, et al. Management of hyperglycemic crises in patients with diabetes. Diabetes Care 2001;24:131–53.

water out of cells. This is associated with movement of potassium from the cell to the extracellular compartment, a phenomenon that is aggravated by acidosis and breakdown of intracellular protein [60]. Furthermore, the entry of potassium into the cell is impaired by lack of effective insulin action. Other factors that may contribute to excessive volume losses include diuretic use, fever, diarrhea, nausea, and vomiting. Severe dehydration, older age, and the presence of comorbid conditions in patients who have HHS account for the higher mortality in these patients.

Diagnosis

History and physical examination

Obtaining a concise but relevant history is an important aspect of diagnosis and management. The symptoms of DKA begin rapidly within a few hours of precipitating events. In many cases, patients are not aware of the disease. Development of HHS, alternatively, is insidious in onset and may occur over days or weeks. Final symptoms may include clouding of sensorium, which progresses to mental obtundation and coma. Only 30% of

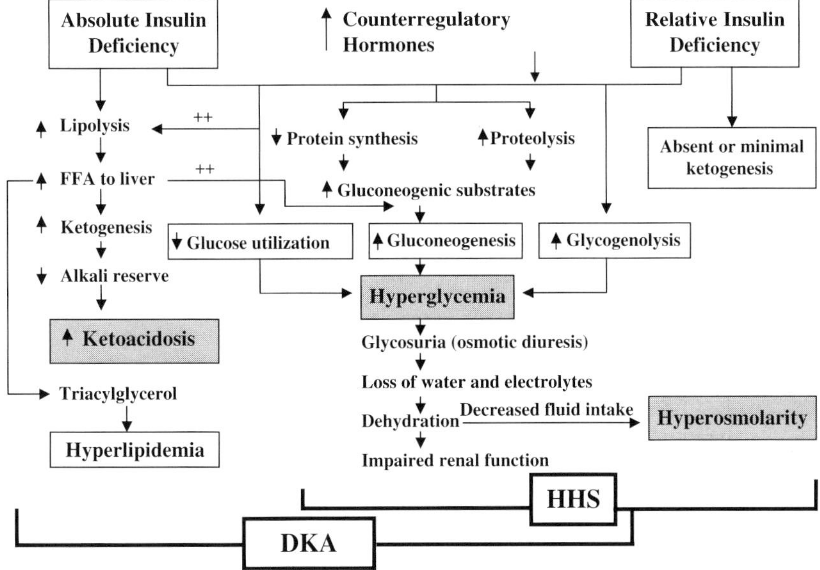

Fig. 3. Pathogenesis of DKA and HHS. (*Adapted from* Kitabchi AE, Murphy MB. Hyperglycemic crises in adult patients with diabetes mellitus. In: Wass JA, Shalet SM, Amiel SA, editors. Oxford textbook of endocrinology. New York: Oxford University Press; 2002. p. 1734–47.)

HHS patients are comatose [3,6,11,22], however. Occasionally, patients who have HHS may present with focal neurologic deficit and seizure disorder. The common clinical picture in DKA and HHS are symptoms of hyperglycemia, such as polyuria, polyphagia, polydipsia, weight loss, weakness, and physical signs of dehydration, such as dry buccal mucosa, sunken eyeballs, poor skin turgor, tachycardia, hypotension, and shock in severe cases. Kussmaul respiration, acetone breath, nausea, vomiting, and abdominal pain also may occur in DKA. Abdominal pain, which correlates with the severity of acidosis [11], may be severe enough to be confused with acute abdomen in 50% to 75% of cases [11,61,62]. Therefore, in the absence of acidosis, a cause of abdominal pain other than DKA should be pursued. Gastrointestinal hemorrhage of DKA may result in hematemesis. Approximately 30% of DKA patients also may present in a hyperosmolar state [19]. Patients often present as normothermic or with mild hypothermia, even when harboring an infection [6]. The majority of patients who have an effective osmolarity of greater than 330 mOsm/kg are severely obtundated or comatose, but altered mental status rarely exists in patients who have osmolarity of less than 320 mOsm/kg (see Fig. 5). Therefore, severe alteration in the level of consciousness in the latter situation requires evaluation for other causes, including cerebrovascular accident and other catastrophic events, such as myocardial and bowel infarctions. Signs and symptoms of the precipitating cause of DKA or HHS may be present and should be sought in each case.

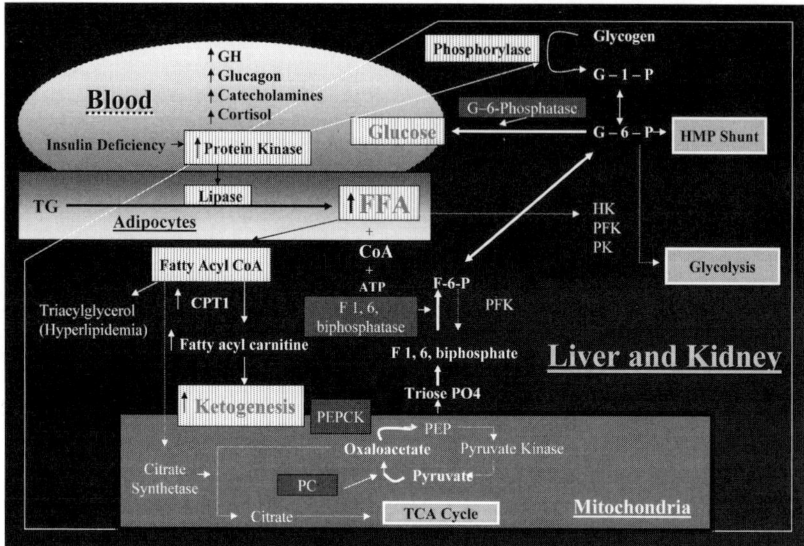

Fig. 4. Biochemical changes that occur during DKA. ATP, adenosine triphosphate; CoA, acetyl CoA; F 1,6, frutose 1,6; G-1-P, glucose-1-phosphatase; G-6-P, glucose-6-phosphatase; GH, growth hormone; HK, hexokinase; HMP, hexose monophosphate shunt; PC, pyruvate carboxylase; PFK, phosphofrutokinase; PK, pyruvate kinase; PEP, phosphoenolpyruvate; TCA, tricarboxylic acid cycle; TG, triglyceride. (*From* Kitabchi AE, Murphy MB. Consequences of insulin deficiency. Skyler JS, editor. In: Atlas of diabetes. 3rd edition. Philadelphia: Williams and Wilkins; 2005; with permission.)

Laboratory evaluation

A prompt physical examination and high blood glucose (by finger stick) in association with ketonuria can suggest strongly the presence of DKA. A definitive diagnosis, however, must be established by laboratory tests. The initial laboratory evaluation for DKA or HHS should include a stat metabolic profile (including plasma glucose, serum urea nitrogen [SUN]/creatinine, serum ketones, electrolytes [with calculated anion gap], osmolality, urinalysis, urine ketones by dipstick, and initial arterial blood gases and complete blood count with differential). Other ancillary investigations include electrocardiogram, chest radiograph, and culture of body fluids as indicated clinically. Glycosylated hemoglobin (HbA1c) may be useful in differentiating chronic hyperglycemia of uncontrolled diabetes from acute metabolic decompensation in a previously well-controlled patient who has diabetes. The diagnostic criteria for DKA and HHS are shown in Table 1. DKA is classified as mild, moderate, or severe based on the severity of metabolic acidosis and the presence of altered mental status [11]. More than 30% of patients have features of DKA and HHS [11,15,19]. Patients who have HHS typically have pH greater than 7.30, bicarbonate level

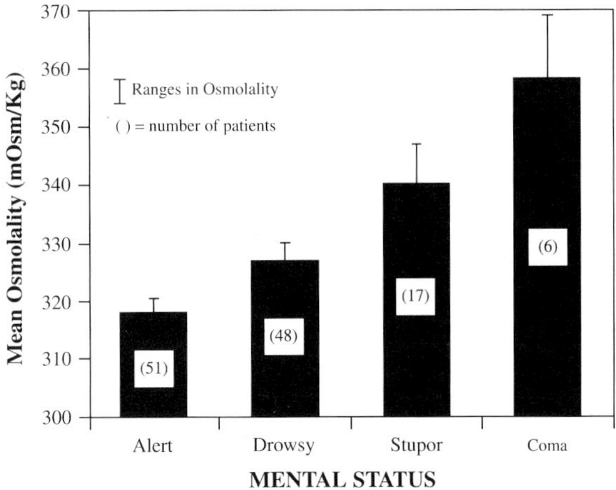

Fig. 5. Relationship between serum osmolality and level of consciousness. (*Adapted from* Kitabchi AE, Wall B. Diabetic ketoacidosis. Med Clin North Am 1995;79(1):10–37.)

greater than 20 mEq/L, and negative ketone bodies in plasma and urine. Some of them, however, may have ketonemia.

Leukocytosis is a common finding in patients who have DKA or HHS [6,21]. Leukocytosis greater than 25,000/μL suggests ongoing infection requiring further work-up [63]. The admission serum sodium usually is low because of the osmotic flux of water from the intracellular to the extracellular space in the presence of hyperglycemia. An increase in serum sodium concentration in the presence of hyperglycemia indicates a profound degree of water loss. Furthermore, if the plasma is not cleared of chylomicrons, pseudonormoglycemia and pseudohyponatremia may occur in DKA [64,65]. Serum potassium concentration may be elevated because of an extracellular shift of potassium. Low normal or frankly low serum potassium level on initial evaluation suggests severe total-body potassium deficit, requiring cardiac monitoring and more diligent potassium repletion to prevent cardiac arrhythmia. The total body loss of sodium and potassium could be as high as 500 to 700 mEq [57,66].

Hyperamylasemia, which correlates with pH and serum osmolality [67] and elevated level of lipase, may occur in 16% to 25% of patients who have DKA [67,68]. The origin of amylase in DKA may be nonpancreatic tissue, such as the parotid gland [68]. Therefore, pancreatic enzymes may not be reliable tools for the diagnosis of pancreatitis in the setting of DKA [67]. Other pitfalls include artificial elevation of serum creatinine, either as a result of dehydration or interference from ketone bodies if a colorimetric method is used [69]. Most of the laboratory tests for ketone bodies use the nitroprusside method, which detects acetoacetate, but not BOHB, the more abundant ketone body. Newer glucose meters have the capability to measure BOHB, which overcomes this problem. In most clinical laboratories, however, the initial measurement of ketone bodies is done by the nitroprusside method. The follow-up measurement of ketones by nitroprusside method, therefore, is not recommended, because BOHB is converted to acetoacetate during treatment and the ketones test may show high values, suggesting erroneously that ketonemia is deteriorating [1]. Drugs that have sulfhydryl groups can interact with the reagent in the nitroprusside reaction, giving a false-positive result [70]. Particularly important in this regard is captopril, an angiotensin-converting enzyme inhibitor used for the treatment of hypertension and diabetic nephropathy. Clinical judgment and consideration of other biochemical data are required to interpret the value of positive nitroprusside reaction in patients taking captopril and suspected of having DKA.

Differential diagnosis

DKA consists of the biochemical triad of hyperglycemia, ketonemia, and anion gap metabolic acidosis (see Fig. 2). Each of these components can be caused by other metabolic conditions [5]. Therefore, patients may present with metabolic conditions resembling DKA or HHS. For example, in alcoholic ketoacidosis, total ketone bodies are much greater than in DKA, with a higher BOHB-to-acetoacetate ratio of 7:1 versus a ratio of 3:1 in DKA [2]. Patients who have alcoholic ketoacidosis seldom present with hyperglycemia. It also is possible that patients who have a low intake of food present with mild ketoacidosis (starvation ketosis). This may not occur in individuals on prolonged fasting, however, unless they have a problem with ketone metabolism. Patients who have starvation ketosis rarely present with serum bicarbonate concentration less than 18 and do not exhibit hyperglycemia. Additionally, DKA has to be distinguished from other causes of high anion gap acidosis, including lactic acidosis, advanced chronic renal failure, and ingestion of drugs, such as salicylate, methanol, and ethylene glycol. Isopropyl alcohol, which is available commonly as rubbing alcohol, can cause considerable ketosis and high osmolar gap without metabolic acidosis; however, it has a tendency to cause hypoglycemia rather than hyperglycemia. These conditions with their laboratory findings are enumerated in Table 4 [71,72]. Finally, patients who have diabetes insipidus presenting with severe polyuria and dehydration and who are treated with dextrose water can have hyperglycemia, presenting a clinical picture that can be confused with HHS [73].

Treatment

The goals of therapy in patients who have DKA and HHS [6,12,21] include (1) improvement of circulatory volume and tissue perfusion, (2) gradual reduction of serum glucose and plasma osmolarity, (3) correction of

Table 4
Laboratory evaluation of metabolic causes of acidosis and coma

	Starvation or high fat intake	Diabetic ketoacidosis	Lactic acidosis	Uremic acidosis	Alcoholic ketosis (starvation)	Salicylate intoxication	Methanol or ethylene glycol intoxication	Hyperosmolar coma	Hypoglycemic coma	Rhabdomyolysis	Isoproproply alcohol
pH	Normal	↓	↓	Mild ↓	↓↑	↓↑[a]	↓	Normal	Normal	Mild ↓ may be ↓↓	Normal
Plasma glucose	Normal	↑	Normal	Normal	↓ or normal	Normal or ↓	Normal	↑↑ > 500 mg/dL	↓↓ < 30 mg/dL	Normal	↓
Glycosuria	Negative	++	Negative	Negative	Negative	Negative[c]	Negative	++	Negative	Negative	Negative
Total plasma ketones[b]	Slight ↑	↑↑	Normal	Normal	Slight to moderate ↑	Normal	Normal	Normal or slight ↑	Normal or slight ↑	Normal	↑↑
Anion gap	Slight ↑	↑	↑	Slight ↑	↑	↑	↑	Normal	Normal or slight	↑↑	Normal
Osmolality	Normal	↑	Normal	↑	Normal	Normal	↑↑	↑↑ > 330 mOsm/kg	Normal	Normal or slight ↑	↑
Uric acid	Mild (starvation)	↑	Normal	Normal	↑	Normal	Normal	Normal	Normal	↑	Normal
Miscellaneous	False positive	May give lactate for ethylene glycol	Serum > 200 > 7 mmol/L	SUN mg/dL	Salicylate	Serum levels positive	Serum positive		Hemoglobinuria	Myoglobinuria	

[a] Positive.
[b] Acetest and Ketostix measure acetoacetic acid only; thus, misleading low values may be obtained because the majority of "ketone bodies" are BOHB.
[c] Respiratory alkalosis/metabolic acidosis; may get false-positive or false-negative urinary glucose caused by the presence of salicylate or its metabolites.

Adapted from Kitabchi AE, Fisher JN, Murphy MB, et al. Diabetic ketoacidosis and the hyperglycemic hyperosmolar nonketotic state. In: Kahn CR, Weir GC, editors. Joslin's diabetes mellitus. 13th ed. Philadelphia: Lea & Febiger; 1994. p. 738–70.

electrolyte imbalance and, in DKA, steady resolution of ketosis, and (4) identification and prompt treatment of comorbid precipitating causes. The recommended protocols for the treatment of patients who have DKA and HHS are summarized in Box 1 [12,74]. It must be emphasized that successful treatment of DKA and HHS requires frequent monitoring, within clinical and laboratory parameters, of patients regarding these goals. A flow sheet, such as the one illustrated in Fig. 6, should be maintained [1].

Fluids

DKA and HHS are volume-depleted states [4,21,49,75,76] with water deficits of approximately 6 L in DKA and 9 L in HHS (see Table 1). Therefore, the initial fluid therapy is directed toward expansion of interstitial and intravascular volume and restoration of renal perfusion. The initial fluid of choice is isotonic saline, which the authors recommend to be infused at the rate of 15 to 20 mL/kg body weight per hour or 1 to 1.5 L during the first hour. This expands the extracellular volumes. The choice of fluid for continued repletion depends on hydration status, serum electrolyte levels, and urinary output. In patients who are hypernatremic or eunatremic, 0.45% sodium chloride (infused at 4 to 14 mL/kg/h) is appropriate; 0.9% sodium chloride at a similar rate is preferred in patients who have hyponatremia. The goal is to replace half of the estimated water deficit over a period of 12 to 24 hours. In patients who have hypotension, aggressive fluid repletion with isotonic saline should continue until blood pressure is stabilized.

The administration of insulin without fluid replacement in such patients with hypotension may aggrevate hypotension. Furthermore, the use of hydrating fluid in the first hour of therapy before insulin has multiple advantages in that it (1) provides a chance to obtain serum potassium value before insulin administration, (2) prevents possible deterioration of hypotensive patients with the use of insulin without adequate hydration, and (3) is well known that insulin effectiveness is lessened in hyperosmolar state [77]. Therefore, expanding intravascular and intracellular volumes by hydration renders the body less resistant to low-dose insulin. Hydration alone also may reduce the level of counterregulatory hormones and hyperglycemia [78]. Hydration reduces serum blood glucose, SUN, and potassium levels without significant changes in pH or HCO3 [19]. The mechanism for lowering glucose is believed due to osmotic diuresis [48,78]. Patients who have DKA and HHS require calories for proper metabolism of ketone bodies. Therefore, in DKA, as soon as blood glucose falls below 200 mg/dL, the sodium chloride solution should be replaced with 5% glucose-containing saline solution with a reduced rate of insulin administration until acidosis and ketosis are controlled while avoiding hypoglycemia. In HHS, the use of D5 ½ NSS should start when blood glucose reaches 300 mg/dL, bearing in mind that overzealous replacement with hypotonic fluids is implicated in

Box 1. Outline for treatment of diabetic ketoacidosis and hyperglycemic hyperosmolar state

Laboratory evaluation

After a brief history and physical examination, initial laboratory evaluation should include determination of complete blood count, blood glucose, serum electrolytes, SUN, creatinine, serum ketones, osmolality, arterial blood gases, and urinalysis. Admission electrocardiogram, chest radiograph, and cultures of blood, urine, and sputum may be ordered if indicated clinically. During therapy, capillary blood glucose should be determined every hour at the bedside using a glucose oxidase reagent strip, and blood should be drawn every 2 to 4 hours for determination of serum electrolytes, glucose, SUN, creatinine, phosphorus, and venous pH.

Fluids

Administer 1000 mL normal saline (0.9% sodium chloride) first hour, then normal or 0.45% saline at 250 to 500 mL/h, depending on serum sodium concentration. When plasma glucose is less than 200 mg/dL, change to 5% dextrose in .45% saline to allow continued insulin administration until ketonemia is controlled, while avoiding hypoglycemia.

Insulin

Administer 0.1 U/kg body weight as intravenous bolus followed by 0.1 U/kg/h as a continuous infusion. The goal is to achieve a rate of decline of glucose between 50 and 70 mg/h. When plasma glucose is equal to 200 mg/dL, change fluid to D5 ½ NSS and reduce insulin rate to 0.05 U/kg/h. Thereafter, adjust insulin rate to maintain glucose levels to between 150 and 200 mg/dL until serum is greater than or equal to 18 mEq/L and pH is greater than 7.30. In patients who have mild to moderate DKA, subcutaneous rapid-acting analogs may be an alternative to intravenous insulin (see caveats discussed later).

Potassium

If serum K+ greater than 5.0 mEq/L, no supplementation is required. If serum K+ is equal to 4 to 5 mEq/L, add 20 mEq/L to each liter of replacement fluid after adequate renal function is established (urine flow at least 50 mL/h). If serum K+ equal to 3 to 4 mEq/L, add 40 mEq/L to each liter of replacement fluid. If serum K+ is less than 3 mEq/L, hold insulin and give 10 to 20 mEq/h until K+ is greater than 3.3, then add 40 mEq/L to each liter of replacement fluid.

Bicarbonate
If arterial pH is less than 7.0 or bicarbonate is less than 5 mEq, give 50 mEq in 200 mL of H_2O over 1 hour until pH increases to greater than 7.0. Do not give bicarbonate if pH is greater than 7.0. For pH less than 6.9, give 100 mEq of bicarbonate and 20 mEq of KCl in 400 mL of H_2O to run for 2 hours.

Phosphate
If indicated (serum levels < 1 mg/dL), administer 20 to 30 mmol potassium phosphate over 24 hours. Monitor serum calcium level.

Transition to subcutaneous insulin
Insulin infusion should be continued until resolution of ketoacidosis (glucose < 200 mg/dL, bicarbonate > 18 mEq/L, and pH > 7.30). When this occurs, start subcutaneous insulin regimen. To prevent recurrence of DKA during the transition period to subcutaneous insulin, intravenous insulin should be continued for 1 to 2 hours after subcutaneous insulin is given.
Similar protocol should be used for HHS except that no bicarbonate is needed for HHS and switching to glucose-containing fluid is done when blood glucose reaches 300 mg/dL. HHS is resolved when glucose is greater than or equal to 300 mg/dL osmolality is less than 320, and patient is alert.

Data from Kitabchi AE. Medical guidelines for clinical practice. Hyperglycemic crises in diabetes mellitus. Diabetic ketoacidosis and hyperglycemic hyperosmolar state. Endocr Pract, in press; *From* Kitabchi AE, Murphy MB. Consequences of insulin deficiency. In: Skyler JS, editor. Atlas of diabetes. 3rd edition. Philadelphia: Current Medicine; 2005; with permission.

the development of cerebral edema. It should be emphasized that the replacement of urinary losses also is important, as failure to do this leads to delay in the restoration of sodium, potassium, and water deficits [1,11].

Insulin therapy

The cornerstone of DKA and HHS therapy is insulin in physiologic doses [76,79]. Insulin should not be given to patients unless the serum potassium value is greater than 3.3 mEq/L. The authors recommend the use of intravenous bolus of regular insulin (0.1 U/kg body weight) and continuous infusion of regular insulin (at a dose of 0.1U/kg/h) as the method of choice. The optimal rate of glucose decrement should be between 50 and 70 mg/h. If this is not achieved in the first hour, the insulin dose may be doubled to

Height:________________

SUGGESTED Weight:

Initially:________________

DKA / HHS FLOWSHEET After 24hr:________________

	DATE: HOUR:												
	MENTAL STATUS*												
	TEMPERATURE												
	PULSE												
	RESPIRATION/DEPTH**												
	BLOOD PRESSURE												
	SERUM GLUCOSE (MG/DL)												
	SERUM KETONES												
	URINE KETONES												
ELECTROLYTES	SERUM Na^+ (mEq/L)												
	SERUM K^+ (mEq/L)												
	SERUM CL^- (mEq/L)												
	SERUM HCO_3^- (mEq/L)												
	SERUM BUN (mg/dl)												
	EFFECTIVE OSMOLALITY 2 [measured Na (mEq/L)] + Glucose (mg/dl)/18												
	ANION GAP												
ARTERIAL/VENOUS BLOOD GASES	pH VENOUS(V) ARTERIAL (A)												
	pO_2												
	pCO_2												
	O_2 SAT												
INSULIN	UNITS in PAST HOUR												
	ROUTE												
INTAKE FLUID/METABOLITES	0.45% NaCl (ml) PAST HOUR												
	0.9% NaCl (ml) PAST HOUR												
	5% DEXTROSE (ml) PAST HOUR												
	KCL (mEq) PAST HOUR												
	PO_4 (mMOLES) PAST HOUR												
	OTHER												
OUTPUT	URINE (ml)												
	OTHER												

* A-ALERT D-DROWSY S-STUPOROUS C-COMATOSE

** D-DEEP S-SHALLOW N-NORMAL

Fig. 6. Sample flow sheet used for the monitoring of patients who have DKA and HHS. (*Adapted from* Kitabchi AE, Umpierrez GE, Murphy MB, et al. Management of hyperglycemic crises in patients with diabetes. Diabetes Care 2001;24:131–53; with permission.)

maintain steady decline in glucose level. When plasma glucose reaches 200 mg/dL for DKA or 300 for HHS, the hydration fluid should be changed to D5 ½ NSS, and insulin rate should be decreased to 0.05 U/kg/h. The rate of insulin should be adjusted to maintain blood glucose between 150 and 200 mg/dL in DKA and 250 to 300 mg/dL for HHS until DKA is resolved or mental obtundation and hyperosmolar state are corrected in HHS.

A study that investigated the optimum route of insulin therapy in DKA [80] demonstrated that the time for resolution of DKA was identical in patients who received regular insulin via intravenous, intramuscular, or subcutaneous routes. Patients who received intravenous insulin, however, showed a more rapid decline in blood glucose and ketone bodies in the first 2 hours of treatment [80]; they also attained immediate pharmacologic level of insulin concentration. Thus, it was established that intravenous loading dose of insulin was desirable regardless of the subsequent route of administration. A follow-up study [81] demonstrated that a priming dose given half by intravenous route and half by intramuscular route was as effective as one dose given intravenously in lowering the level of ketone bodies in the first hour and that the addition of albumin to the infusate, which was a routine practice in the past to prevent adsorption of insulin to the tubing and containers, was not necessary. Recent clinical studies show the potency and cost effectiveness of subcutaneous rapid-acting insulin analogs (lispro or aspart) in the management of patients who have uncomplicated mild to moderate DKA. The patients received subcutaneous rapid-acting insulin dose of 0.2 U/kg initially, followed by 0.1 U/kg every hour or an initial dose of 0.3 U/kg followed by 0.2 U/kg every 2 hours until blood glucose was less than 250 mg/dL, then the insulin dose was decreased by half to 0.05 or 0.1 U/kg, respectively, and administered every 1 or 2 hours until resolution of DKA [82,83]. There were no differences in length of hospital stay, total amount of insulin needed for resolution of hyperglycemia or ketoacidosis, or in the incidence of hypoglycemia among treatment groups. The use of insulin analogs allowed treatment of DKA in general wards or the emergency department, reducing cost of hospitalization by 30% [82–84]. The use of fast-acting insulin analogs is not recommended for patients who have severe DKA or HHS, as there are no studies to support their use. Again these agents may not be effective in patients who have severe fluid depletion, as they are given subcutaneously.

During the follow-up period, blood should be drawn every 2 to 4 horus for determination of serum electrolytes, glucose, SUN, creatinine, osmolality, and venous pH. After the initial arterial pH is drawn, venous pH can be used to assess the acid/base status. An equivalent arterial pH value is calculated by adding 0.03 to the venous pH value [85]. The resolution of DKA is reached when the blood glucos is less than or equal to 200 mg/dL, serum bicarbonate is greater than or equal to 18, pH is greater than 7.30, and anion gap is less than 12. HHS is resolved when osmolarity is less than 320 mOsm/kg with a gradual recovery to mental alertness. The latter, however, may take twice as long as blood glucose control to attain. Ketonemia typically takes longer to clear than hyperglycemia. Once DKA is resolved, patients who are able to eat can be started on a multiple-dose insulin regimen with a long-acting insulin to cover basal insulin requirements and short- or rapid-acting insulin given before meals as needed to control plasma glucose. Intravenous insulin infusion should be continued for 1 to 2 hours after the subcutaneous insulin is given to ensure adequate plasma insulin levels. Immediate discontinuation of intravenous insulin coupled with delayed initiation of a subcutaneous insulin regimen may lead to hyperglycemia or recurrence of ketoacidosis. If patients are unable to eat, it is preferable to continue the intravenous insulin infusion and fluid replacement. Patients who have known diabetes may be given insulin at the dose they were receiving before the onset of DKA or HHS. In patients who have new-onset diabetes, a multidose insulin regimen should be started at a dose of 0.5 to 0.8 U/kg per day, including regular or rapid-acting and basal insulin; the dose is adjusted until an optimal dose is established.

Potassium

Although total-body potassium is depleted [66,86], mild to moderate hyperkalemia frequently is seen in patients who have DKA because of acidosis, proteolysis, and insulinopenia. Insulin therapy, correction of acidosis, and volume expansion decrease serum potassium concentration. To prevent hypokalemia, potassium replacement is initiated after serum levels fall below 5.3 mEq/L in patients who have adequate urine output (50 mL/h). An addition of 20 to 30 mEq potassium to each liter of infused fluid is sufficient to maintain a serum potassium concentration within the normal range of 4 to 5 mEq/L. Occasionally, patients who have DKA may present with significant hypokalemia, especially if they have been vomiting or had been on diuretics. In such cases, potassium replacement should begin with fluid therapy, and insulin treatment should be delayed until potassium concentration is restored to greater than 3.3 mEq/L to avoid arrhythmias and respiratory muscle weakness [86,87].

Bicarbonate

There is no clear role for the routine use of bicarbonate in DKA [88], as the use of bicarbonate remains controversial [89]. In patients who have pH greater than 7.0, insulin therapy inhibits lipolysis and also corrects ketoacidosis without use of bicarbonate [48,49]. Bicarbonate therapy is associated with some adverse effects, such as hypokalemia [84], decreased tissue oxygen uptake and cerebral edema [90], and delay in the resolution of ketosis [90,91]. Patients who have stretched their compensatory mechanism to its limits (low bicarbonate < 10 or $P_{CO_2} < 12$), however, may experience deterioration of their pH if not treated with bicarbonate [90]. A prospective randomized study in patients who had pH between 6.9 and 7.1 showed that bicarbonate therapy conferred no risk or benefit in DKA [92]. Therefore, in patients who have pH between 6.9 and 7.0, it may be prudent to give 50 mmol of bicarbonate in 200 mL of sterile water with 10 mEq of potassium chloride over 2 hours to maintain the pH at greater than 7.0 [74]. Considering the deleterious effects of severe acidosis, including impaired myocardial contractility, adult patients who have pH less than 6.9 should be given 100 mmol sodium bicarbonate in 400 mL sterile water (an isotonic solution) with 20 mEq potassium chloride administered at a rate of 200 mL/h for 2 hours until the venous pH is greater than 7.0 [74]. Venous pH should be assessed every 2 hours until the pH rises to 7.0; treatment can be repeated every 2 hours if necessary.

Phosphate

In addition to sodium and potassium, there also is a deficit of phosphate in patients who have DKA and HHS, which is approximately 1 mmol/kg body weight on average. As with potassium, however, serum levels of phosphate at presentation usually are normal or increased and decrease rapidly after initiation of insulin therapy. Randomized studies in patients who have DKA [93–95] show that phosphate repletion confers no benefit on clinical outcome. In patients who have potential complications of hypophosphatemia, however, which includes cardiac and skeletal muscle weaknesses, the use of phosphate may be justified [96]. Phosphate administration may result in hypocalcemia when used in high doses [93,94]. Considering that potassium chloride overload may cause hyperchloremic acidosis [97], it would be prudent to recommend that potassium be given as one-third potassium phosphate and two-thirds potassium chloride for adequate provision of phosphate, although this has not been investigated officially.

Box 1 summarizes, in stepwise fashion, the procedures for management of DKA [98]. A similar protocol should be used for HHS except that no bicarbonate is needed for HHS and switching to glucose-containing fluid is done when blood glucose reaches 300 mg/dL.

Complications

Hypoglycemia and hypokalemia were the most common complications of DKA and HHS, resulting from overenthusiastic treatment with insulin and bicarbonate (hypokalemia), but these sequelae occur infrequently with current low-dose insulin regimen. During the recovery phase, patients who have DKA frequently develop a short-lived hyperchloremic nonanion gap acidosis, which usually is of little clinical consequence [74,97,99,100]. Hyperchloremic acidosis is caused by the loss of large amounts of ketoanions (which usually are metabolized to bicarbonate) during the evolution of DKA [101] and excess infusion of chloride-containing fluids during treatment [100].

Cerebral edema, a frequently fatal complication of DKA, occurs in 0.7% to 1.0% of children, in particular those who have newly diagnosed diabetes. It also may occur in patients who have known diabetes and in young adults, usually those under 20 years of age [74,90,102,103]. Cerebral edema also is reported in patients who have HHS. Headache is the earliest clinical manifestation of cerebral edema. This is followed by altered level of consciousness and lethargy. Neurologic deterioration may be rapid owing to brainstem herniation. If the clinical symptoms are well established, mortality rate may higher than 70%, with only 7% to 14% of patients recovering without permanent neurologic deficit. Manitol infusion and mechanical ventilation may be used to combat cerebral edema.

The cause of cerebral edema is not known with certainty; however, it is believed that rapid decline in plasma osmolality with the treatment of DKA or HHS results in an efflux of water into the brain cells [89,90–92,101,103]. Although this osmotically mediated mechanism sounds plausible, a recent study using MRI shows that cerebral edema was the result of increased cerebral perfusion [90]. Another postulated mechanism for cerebral edema in patients who have DKA involves the cell membrane Na^+/H^+ exchanger, which is activated in DKA. The high H^+ level allows more Na^+ into the cells, thus attracting more water into cells with consequent edema [88,104]. Acetoacetate and β-hydoxybutyrate also may play a role in the pathogenesis of cerebral edema [88,105,106]. These ketone bodies are shown to affect vascular integrity and permeability, thus contributing to edema formation. There may be interplay of these factors in the pathogenesis of cerebral edema in patients who have hyperglycemic crisis. Avoidance of overzealous hydration, reduction of plasma osmolality, and hemodynamic monitoring are reasonable precautionary measures to decrease the risk of cerebral edema in high-risk patients. Hypoxemia and noncardiogenic pulmonary edema may occur during the treatment of DKA. The pathogenesis of pulmonary edema may be similar to that of cerebral edema, suggesting that the sequestration of fluid in the tissues may be more widespread than is believed. Thrombotic conditions, including disseminated intravascular coagulation, contribute to the morbidity and mortality of hyperglycemic emergencies [88,107]. Prophylactic use of heparin, if there is no gastrointestinal hemorrhage, should be helpful.

Prevention

Recent studies [6,15,23,108,109] suggest that the omission of insulin is the most common precipitant of DKA. This partly is because patients with recurrent DKA are socioeconomically underprivileged and may not have the power to access and afford medical care. In addition, they have a propensity to using illicit drugs, which is associated with recurrent DKA [23,26]. Therefore, it is important that medical care be made available to these patients. Education of patients about sick day management is vital to preventing DKA and should include information on when to contact a health care provider, blood glucose goals, use of insulin, and initiation of appropriate nutrition during illness. Patients must be advised to continue insulin and to seek professional advice early in the course of the illness. Close follow-up is important, as it is shown that quarterly visits to the endocrine clinic in such circumstances reduce the number of emergency department admissions for DKA [110]. Close observation, early recognition of symptoms, and medical care are helpful in preventing HHS in the elderly. A recent study [111] of adolescents who had T1DM suggests that some of the risk factors for DKA may be related to higher HbA1c, uninsured children, and psychologic problems, all of which need to be dealt with. Considering that DKA and HHS potentially are fatal and are economically burdensome complications of diabetes, every effort toward their prevention would be worthwhile.

Summary

DKA and HHS potentially are fatal but largely are preventable acute metabolic complications of uncontrolled diabetes, the incidence of which continues to increase. Mortality from DKA has declined remarkably over the years because of better understanding of its pathophysiology and treatment. The mortality rate of HHS, however, remains alarmingly high owing to older age and mode of presentation of the patients and associated comorbid conditions. DKA and HHS also are burdensome economically; therefore, any resources invested in their prevention would be rewarding.

References

[1] Kitabchi AE, Fisher JN, Murphy MB, et al. Diabetic ketoacidosis and the hyperglycemic hyperosmolar nonketotic state. In: Kahn CR, Weir GC, editors. Joslin's diabetes mellitus. 13th ed. Philadelphia: Lea & Febiger; 1994. p. 738–70.

[2] Alberti KGMM. Diabetic acidosis, hyperosmolar coma, and lactic acidosis. In: Becker KL, editor. Principles and practice of endocrinology and metabolism. 3rd edition. Philadelphia: Lippincott Williams & Wilkins; 2001. p. 1438–50.

[3] Matz R. Management of hyperosmolar hyperglycemic syndrome. Am Fam Physician 1999; 60:1468–76.

[4] Kitabchi AE, Murphy MB. Hyperglycemic crises in adult patients with diabetes mellitus. In: Wass JA, Shalet SM, Amiel SA, editors. Oxford textbook of endocrinology. New York: Oxford University Press; 2002. p. 1734–47.

[5] Kitabchi AE, Wall B. Diabetic ketoacidosis. Med Clin North Am 1995;79(1):10–37.

[6] Kitabchi AE, Umpierrez GE, Murphy MB, et al. Management of hyperglycemic crises in patients with diabetes. Diabetes Care 2001;24:131–53.

[7] Johnson DD, Palumbo PJ, Chu CP. Diabetic ketoacidosis in a community-based population. Mayo Clin Proc 1980;55:83–8.

[8] Centers for Disease Control and Prevention. Diabetes surveillance system. Atlanta: US Department of Health and Human Services; 2003. Available at:www.cdc.gov/diabetes/statistics/index.htm. Accessed June 10, 2006.

[9] Javor KA, Kotsanos JG, McDonald RC, et al. Diabetic ketoacidosis charges relative to medical charges of adult patients with type I diabetes. Diabetes Care 1997;20:349–54.

[10] Centers for Disease Control and Prevention. Diabetes surveillance system. Atlanta: US Department of Health and Human Services; 2003. Available at:www.cdc.gov/diabetes/statistics/mortalitydka. Accessed June 23, 2006.

[11] Ennis ED, Stahl EJVB, Kreisberg RA. The hyperosmolar hyperglycemic syndrome. Diabetes Rev 1994;2:115–26.

[12] Kitabchi AE. Medical guidelines for clinical practice: hyperglycemic crises in diabetes mellitus—diabetic ketoacidosis and hyperglycemic hyperosmolar state. Endocr Pract, in press.

[13] Kitabchi AE, Fisher JN. Diabetes mellitus. In: Glew RA, Peters SP, editors. Clinical studies in medical biochemistry. New York: Oxford University Press; 1987. p. 102–17.
[14] Fishbein HA. Diabetic ketoacidosis, hyperosmolar nonketotic coma, lactic acidosis and hypoglycemia. In: Harris MI, Hamman RF, editors. Diabetes in America (National Diabetes Group). Washington, DC: US Department of Health and Human Sciences; 1985. p. XII-1–16.
[15] Umpierrez GE, Kelly JP, Navarrete JE, et al. Hyperglycemic crises in urban blacks. Arch Intern Med 1997;157:669–75.
[16] Umpierrez GE, Woo W, Hagopian WA, et al. Immunogenetic analysis suggests different pathogenesis for obese and lean African Americans with diabetic ketoacidosis. Diabetes Care 1999;22(9):1517–23.
[17] Kitabchi AE. Editorial: ketosis-prone diabetes—a new subgroup of patients with atypical type 1 and type 2 diabetes? J Clin End Metab 2003;88:5087–9.
[18] Nyenwe EA, Loganathan RS, Blum S, et al. Characteristics of patients admitted with diabetic ketoacidosis in an inner city hospital [abstract]. J Invest Med 2006;54(Suppl 1): S267.
[19] Kitabchi AE, Fisher JN. Insulin therapy of diabetic ketoacidosis: physiologic versus pharmacologic doses of insulin and their routes of administration. In: Brownlee M, editor. Handbook of diabetes mellitus, vol. 5. New York: Garland ATPM Press; 1981. p. 95–149.
[20] Kitabchi AE, Umpierrez GE, Murphy MB, et al. American Diabetes Association. Hyperglycemic crises in diabetes. Diabetes Care 2004;27(Suppl 1):S94–102.
[21] Kitabchi AE, Umpierrez GE, Murphy MB. Diabetic ketoacidosis and hyperglycemic hyperosmolar state. In: DeFronzo RA, Ferrannini E, Keen H, Zimmet P, editors. International textbook of diabetes mellitus. 3rd edition. Chichester (UK): John Wiley & Sons; 2004. p. 1101–19.
[22] Wachtel TJ, Silliman RA, Lamberton P. Predisposing factors for the diabetic hyperosmolar state. Arch Intern Med 1987;147:499–501.
[23] Nyenwe EA, Loganathan RS, Blum S, et al. Active use of cocaine: an independent risk factor for recurrent diabetic ketoacidosis in a city hospital. Endocrine Practice, in press.
[24] Westphal SA. The occurrence of diabetic ketoacidosis in non-insulin dependent diabetes and newly diagnosed diabetic adults. Am J Med 1996;101:19–24.
[25] Newcomer JW. Second generation (atypical) antipsycotics and metabolic effects: a comprehensive literature review. CNS Drugs 2005;19(Suppl 1):1–93.
[26] Warner GA, Greene GS, Buschsbaum MS, et al. Diabetic ketoacidosis associated with cocaine use. Arch Intern Med 1998;158:1799–802.
[27] Polonsky WH, Anderson BJ, Lohrer PA, et al. Insulin omission in women with IDDM. Diabetes Care 1994;17:1178–85.
[28] Peden NR, Broatan JT, McKenry JB. Diabetic ketoacidosis during long-term treatment with continuous subcutaneous insulin infusion. Diabetes Care 1984;7:1–5.
[29] Shah P, Isley WL. Ketoacidosis during a low carbohydrate diet. N Engl J Med 2006;354: 97–8.
[30] Soveid M, Ranjbar-Omrani G. Ketoacidosis as the primary manifestation of acromegaly. Arch Iranian Med 2005;8:326–8.
[31] Katz JR, Edwards R, Kahn M, et al. Acromegaly presenting with diabetic ketoacidosis. Postgrad Med J 1996;72:682–3.
[32] Vidal-Cortada J, Conget-Donlo JI, Navarro-Tellex MP, et al. Diabetic ketoacidosis as the first manifestation of acromegaly. Ann Med Intern 1995;12:76–8.
[33] Szeto CC, Li KY, Ko GT, et al. Acromegaly presenting in a woman with diabetic ketoacidosis and insulin resistance. Int J Clin Pract 1997;51:476–7.
[34] Petzoldt R, Trabert C, Walther A, et al. [Etiology and prognosis of diabetic coma: a retrospective study]. Verh Dtsch Ges Inn Med 1971;77:637–40 [in German].
[35] Soler NG, Bennett MA, Fitzgerald MG, et al. Intensive care management of diabetic ketoacidosis. Lancet 1973;5:951–4.

[36] Panzram G. [Epidemiology of diabetic coma]. Schweiz Med Wochenschr 1973;103:203–8 [in German].
[37] Berger W, Keller U, Voster D. [Mortality from diabetic coma at the Basle Cantonal Hospital during 2 consecutive observation periods 1968–1973 and 1973–1978, using conventional insulin therapy and treatment with low dose insulin]. Schweiz Med Wochenschr 1979;109:1820–4 [in German].
[38] Faich GA, Fishbein HA, Ellis SE. The epidemiology of diabetic acidosis: a population-based study. Am J Epidemiol 1983;117:551–8.
[39] Nyenwe EA, Loganathan R, Blum S, et al. Admissions for diabetic ketoacidosis in ethnic minority group in a city hospital. Metabolism, in press.
[40] Umpierrez GE, Smiley D, Kitabchi AE. Ketosis-prone type 2 diabetes mellitus. Ann Intern Med 2006;144:350–7.
[41] Maldonado M, Hampe CS, Gaur LK, et al. Ketosis-prone diabetes: dissection of a heterogeneous syndrome using an immunogenetic and beta-cell functional classification, prospective analysis, and clinical outcomes. J Clin Endocrinol Metab 2003;88:5090–8.
[42] Mauvais-Jarvis F, Sobngwi E, Porcher R, et al. Ketosis-prone type 2 diabetes in patients of sub-Saharan African origin: clinical pathophysiology and natural history of beta-cell dysfunction and insulin resistance. Diabetes 2004;53:645–53.
[43] Umpierrez GE, Casals MM, Gebhart SP, et al. Diabetic ketoacidosis in obese African-Americans. Diabetes 1995;44:790–5.
[44] Banerji MA, Chaiken RL, Huey H, et al. GAD antibody negative NIDDM in adult black subjects with diabetic ketoacidosis and increased frequency of human leukocyte antigen DR3 and DR4. Flatbush diabetes. Diabetes 1994;43:741–5.
[45] Kitabchi AE. Editorial: ketosis-prone diabetes—a new subgroup of patients with atypical type 1 an type 2 diabetes? JCEM 2003;88:5087–9.
[46] Sobngwi E, Gautier JF, Kevorkian JP, et al. High prevalence of glucose 6-phosphate dehydrogenase deficiency without gene mutation suggests a novel genetic mechanism predisposed to ketosis-prone diabetes. J Clin End Metab 2005;90:4446–51.
[47] Exton JH. Mechanisms of hormonal regulation of hepatic glucose metabolism. Diabetes Metab Rev 1987;3:163–83.
[48] McGarry JD, Woeltje KF, Kuwajima M, et al. Regulation of ketogenesis and the renaissance of carnitine palmitoyltransferase. Diabetes Metab Rev 1989;5:271–84.
[49] DeFronzo RA, Matzuda M, Barret E. Diabetic ketoacidosis: a combined metabolic-nephrologic approach to therapy. Diabetes Rev 1994;2:209–38.
[50] Reichard GA Jr, Skutches CL, Hoeldtke RD, et al. Acetone metabolism in humans during diabetic ketoacidosis. Diabetes 1986;35:668–74.
[51] Balasse EO, Fery F. Ketone body production and disposal: effects of fasting, diabetes and exercise. Diabetes Metab Rev 1989;5:247–70.
[52] Unger RH, Orci L. Glucagon and the A cell. Physiology and pathophysiology. N Engl J Med 1981;304:1518.
[53] Barnes AJ, Bloom SR, George K, et al. Ketoacidosis in pancreatectomized man. N Engl J Med 1977;296:1250.
[54] Kitabchi AE. Low dose insulin therapy in diabetic ketoacidosis: facts or fiction? Diabetes Metab Rev 1989;5:337–63.
[55] Stentz FB, Umpierrez GE, Cuervo R, et al. Proinflammatory cytokines, markers of cardiovascular risks, oxidative stress, and lipid peroxidation in patients with hyperglycemic crises. Diabetes 2004;53:2079–86.
[56] Chupin M, Charbonnel B, Chupin F. C-peptide blood levels in ketoacidosis and in hyperosmolar nonketotic diabetic coma. Acta Diabetol Lat 1981;18:123–8.
[57] Atchley DW, Loeb RF, Richards DW, et al. A detailed study of electrolyte balances following withdrawal and reestabilishment of insulin therapy. J Clin Invest 1933;12:681–95.
[58] Howard RL, Bichet DG, Shrier RW. Hypernatremic polyuric states. In: Seldin D, Giebisch G, editors. The kidney: physiology and pathophysiology. New York: Raven; 1991. p. 1578.

[59] DeFronzo RA, Cooke CR, Andres R, et al. The effect of insulin on renal handling of sodium, potassium, calcium and phosphate in man. J Clin Invest 1975;55:845–55.
[60] Castellino P, Luzi L, Haymond M, et al. Effect of insulin and plasma amino acid concentrations on leucine turnover in man. J Clin Invest 1987;80:1784–93.
[61] Umpierrez G, Freire AX. Abdominal pain in patients with hyperglycemic crises. J Crit Care 2002;17:63–7.
[62] Campbell IW, Duncan LJ, Innes JA, et al. Abdominal pain in diabetic metabolic decompensation. Clinical significance. JAMA 1975;233:166–8.
[63] Slovis CM, Mark VG, Slovis RJ, Bain RP. Diabetic ketoacidosis & infection leukocyte count and differential as early predictors of infection. Am J Emerg Med 1987;5:1–5.
[64] Kaminska ES, Pourmoabbed G. Spurious laboratory values in diabetic ketoacidosis and hyperlipidaemia. Am J Emerg Med 1993;11:77–80.
[65] Rumbak MJ, Hughes TA, Kitabchi AE. Pseudonormoglycaemia in diabetic ketoacidosis with elevated triglycerides. Am J Emerg Med 1991;9:61–3.
[66] Adrogue HJ, Lederer ED, Suki WN, et al. Determinants of plasma potassium levels in diabetic ketoacidosis. Medicine 1986;65:163–71.
[67] Vinicor F, Lehrner LM, Karn RC, et al. Hyperamylasemia in diabetic ketoacidosis: sources and significance. Ann Intern Med 1979;91:200–4.
[68] Yadav D, Nair S, Norkus EP. Nonspecific hyperamylasemia in diabetic ketoacidosis: incidence and correlation with biochemical abnormalities. Am Coll Gastroenterol 2000;95: 3123.
[69] Gerard SK, Rhayam-Bashi H. Characterization of creatinine error in ketotic patients: a prospective comparison of alkaline picrate methods with an enzymatic method. Am J Clin Pathol 1985;84:659–61.
[70] Csako G, Elin RJ. Unrecognized false-positive ketones from drugs containing free sulfhydryl groups. JAMA 1993;269:1634.
[71] Bjellerup P, Kaliner A, Kollind M. GLC determination of serum-ethylene glycol interferences in ketotic patients. J Toxicol Clin Toxicol 1994;32:85–7.
[72] Morris LE, Kitabchi AE. Coma in the diabetic. In: Schnatz JD, editor. Diabetes mellitus: problems in management. Menlo Park (CA): Addison-Wesley; 1982. p. 234–51.
[73] Freidenberg GR, Kosnik EJ, Sotos JF. Hyperglycemic coma after suprasellar surgery. N Engl J Med 1980;303:863.
[74] Kitabchi AE, Umpierrez GE, Murphy MB, et al. Hyperglycemic crisis in adult patients with diabetes mellitus. Diabetes Care, in press.
[75] Hillman K. Fluid resuscitation in diabetic emergencies–a reappraisal. Intensive Care Med 1987;13:4–8.
[76] Alberti KG, Hockaday TD, Turner RC. Small doses of intramuscular insulin in the treatment of diabetic "coma". Lancet 1973;II:515–22.
[77] Bratusch-Marrain PR, Komajati M, Waldhausal W. The effect of hyperosmolarity on glucose metabolism. Pract Cardiol 1985;11:153–63.
[78] Waldhausl W, Kleinberger G, Korn A, et al. severe hyperglycemia: effects of rehydration on endocrine derangements and blood glucose concentration. Diabetes 1979;28:577–84.
[79] Kitabchi AE, Ayyagari V, Guerra SMO. Medical house staff. The efficacy of low dose versus conventional therapy of Insulin for treatment of diabetic ketoacidosis. Ann Intern Med 1976;84:633–8.
[80] Fisher JN, Shahshahani MN, Kitabchi AE. Diabetic ketoacidosis: low dose insulin therapy by various routes. N Engl J Med 1977;297:238–47.
[81] Sacks HS, Shahshahani MN, Kitabchi AE, et al. Similar responsiveness of diabetic ketoacidosis to low-dose insulin by intramuscular injection and albumin-free infusion. Ann Intern Med 1979;90:36–42.
[82] Umpierrez GE, Latif K, Stoever J, et al. Efficacy of subcutaneous insulin lispro versus continuous intravenous regular insulin for the treatment of patients with diabetic ketoacidosis. Am J Med 2004;117:291–6.

[83] Umpierrez GE, Cuervo R, Karabell A, et al. Treatment of diabetic ketoacidosis with subcutaneous insulin aspart. Diabetes Care 2004;27:1873–8.
[84] Della Manna T, Steinmetz L, Campos PR, et al. Subcutaneous use of a fast-acting insulin analog: an alternative treatment for pediatric patients with diabetic ketoacidosis. Diabetes Care 2005;28:1856–61.
[85] Kelly AM. The case for venous rather than arterial blood gases in diabetic ketoacidosis. Emerg Med Australas 2006;18:64–7.
[86] Beigelman PM. Potassium in severe diabetic ketoacidosis [editorial]. Am J Med 1973;54: 419–20.
[87] Abramson E, Arky R. Diabetic acidosis with initial hypokalemia: therapeutic implications. JAMA 1966;196:401–3.
[88] Ennis ED, Kreisberg RA. Diabetic ketoacidosis and hyperosmolar syndrome. In: Leroith D, Taylor SI, Olefsky JM, editors. Diabetes mellitus. A fundamental and clinical text. 3rd edition. Philadelphia: Lippincott Williams & Wilkins; 2004. p. 627–42.
[89] Viallon A, Zeni F, Lafond P, et al. Does bicarbonate therapy improve the management of severe diabetic ketoacidosis? Crit Care Med 1999;27:2690–3.
[90] Glaser NS, Wooten-Gorges SL, Marcin JP, et al. Mechanism of cerebral edema in children with diabetic ketoacidosis. J Pediar 2004;145:149–50.
[91] Okuda Y, Adrogue HJ, Field JB, et al. Counterproductive effects of sodium bicarbonate in diabetic ketoacidosis in childhood. J Clin Endocrinol Metab 1996;81:314.
[92] Morris LR, Murphy MB, Kitabchi AE. Bicarbonate therapy in severe diabetic ketoacidosis. Ann Intern Med 1986;105:836–40.
[93] Winter RJ, Harris CJ, Phillips LS, et al. Diabetic ketoacidosis: induction of hypocalcemia and hypomagnesemia by phosphate therapy. Am J Med 1979;67:897–900.
[94] Fisher JN, Kitabchi AE. A randomized study of phosphate therapy in the treatment of diabetic ketoacidosis. J Clin Endocrinol Metab 1983;57:177–80.
[95] Keller V, Berger W. Prevention of hypophosphalemia by phosphate infusion during treatment of diabetic ketoacidosis and hyperosmolar coma. Diabetes 1980;29:87–95.
[96] Kreisberg RA. Phosphorus deficiency and hypophosphatemia. Hosp Pract 1977;12: 121–8.
[97] Adrogue HJ, Wilson H, Boyd AE, et al. Plasma acid-base patterns in diabetic ketoacidosis. N Engl J Med 1982;307:1603–10.
[98] Kitabchi AE, Murphy MB. Consequences of insulin deficiency. In: Skyler JS, editor. Atlas of diabetes. 3rd edition. Philadelphia: Current Medicine; 2005.
[99] Oh MS, Carroll HJ, Goldstein DA, et al. Hyperchloremic acidosis during the recovery phase of diabetic ketosis. Ann Intern Med 1978;89:925–7.
[100] Oh MS, Carroll HJ, Uribarri J. Mechanism of normochloremic and hyperchloremic acidosis in diabetic ketoacidosis. Nephron 1990;54:1–6.
[101] Fleckman AM. Diabetic ketoacidosis. Endocrinol Metabol Clin North Am 1993;22: 181–207.
[102] Duck SC, Wyatt DT. Factors associated with brain herniation in the treatment of diabetic ketoacidosis. J Pediatr 1988;113:10–4.
[103] Silver SM, Clark EC, Schroeder BM, et al. Pathogenesis of cerebral edema after treatment of diabetic ketoacidosis. Kidney Int 1997;51:1237–44.
[104] Smedman L, Escobar R, Hesser V, et al. Sub-clinical cerebral edema does not occur regularly during treatment for diabetic ketoacidosis. Acta Paediatr 1997;86:1172.
[105] Isales CM, Min L, Hoffman WH. Acetoacetate and betahydroxybutyrate differentially regulate endothelin-1 and vascular endothelial growth factor in mouse brain microvascular endothelial cells. J Diabet Complications 1993;13:91.
[106] Edge JA. Cerebral oedema during treatment of diabetic ketoacidosis. Are we any nearer finding a cause? Diabetes Metab Res Rev 2000;16:316.
[107] Buyukasik Y, Illeri NS, Haznedarogu IC, et al. Enhanced subclinical coagulation activation during diabetic ketoacidosis. Diabetes Care 1998;21:868.

[108] Musey VC, Lee JK, Crawford R, et al. Diabetes in urban African-Americans. Cessation of insulin therapy is the major precipitating cause of diabetic ketoacidosis. Diabetes Care 1995;18:483–9.
[109] Maldonado MR, Chong ER, Oehl MA, et al. Economic impact of diabetic ketoacidosis in a multiethnic indigent population: analysis of costs based on the precipitating cause. Diabetes Care 2003;26:1265–9.
[110] Laffel LM, Brackett J, Ho J, et al. Changing the process of diabetes care improves metabolic outcomes and reduces hospitalizations. Qual Manag Health Care 1998;6:53–62.
[111] Rewers A, Chase HP, Mackenzie T, et al. Predictors of acute complications in children with type 1 diabetes. JAMA 2002;287:2511–8.

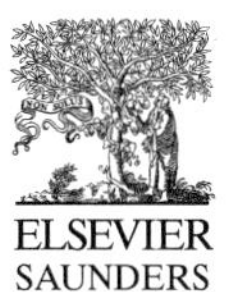

ELSEVIER
SAUNDERS

Endocrinol Metab Clin N Am
35 (2006) 753–766

ENDOCRINOLOGY
AND METABOLISM
CLINICS
OF NORTH AMERICA

Hypoglycemia

Jean-Marc Guettier, MD*, Phillip Gorden, MD

National Institute of Diabetes and Digestive and Kidney Disease, National Institutes of Health, 9600 Rockville Pike, Bethesda, MD 20892, USA

Hypoglycemia always constitutes an emergency because it signals an inability of the central nervous system (CNS) to meet its energy needs. Resultant mental status impairment places the patient and others at risk for accidents and traumatic injury. Left untreated, hypoglycemia can result in permanent neurologic damage and death. To make the diagnosis of hypoglycemia, documentation of plasma glucose below the normal range is necessary. Conditions that present with similar symptoms without low plasma glucose are thus excluded. This biochemical criterion is not sufficient, however, because plasma glucose values below the normal range do not always distinguish between normal and pathologic forms of hypoglycemia [1] and may reflect laboratory error or artifactual hypoglycemia from glycolysis within the collected sample (eg, erythrocytosis, leukocytosis). The definition proposed by Whipple [2] in 1938 is still the most useful and defines pathologic hypoglycemia as a triad of low plasma glucose, hypoglycemic symptoms, and resolution of symptoms with correction of the blood sugar. Symptoms caused by a sudden drop in blood glucose [3,4] are associated with increased autonomic nervous system outflow (adrenergic and cholinergic symptoms) and include anxiety, tremulousness, palpitation, sweating, nausea, and hunger. Hypoglycemia is also commonly associated with symptoms of compromised CNS function because of brain glucose deprivation (neuroglycopenic symptoms). Symptoms include weakness, fatigue, confusion, seizures, focal neurologic deficit, and coma.

Predisposing factors

Although there are many conditions that can predispose to hypoglycemia, it is most often observed in those treated for diabetes [5–8]. Because of the high prevalence of diabetes in the population, hypoglycemia is the

* Corresponding author.
E-mail address: guettierj@mail.nih.gov (J.-M. Guettier).

0889-8529/06/$ - see front matter Published by Elsevier Inc.
doi:10.1016/j.ecl.2006.09.005

most frequently encountered endocrine emergency in the ambulatory and inpatient care settings [5,8–11]. In the Diabetes Control and Complications Trial (DCCT), an estimated 10% to 30% of type1 diabetes patients experienced one hypoglycemic episode requiring third-party assistance for treatment per year [12]. Previous hypoglycemic episodes, lower glycosylated hemoglobin levels, and intensive therapy predicted hypoglycemic events in this population. In the first 10 years of the United Kingdom Prospective Diabetes Study (UKPDS), hypoglycemic episodes requiring third-party intervention occurred at an incidence of 1.2% for type 2 patients treated with insulin [13]. More recent studies suggest an incidence of severe hypoglycemia in type 2 diabetes approximating that of type 1 diabetes [6,14]. In a retrospective analysis of an elderly population with type 2 diabetes, recent hospitalization, advanced age, African-American ancestry, and use of five or more medications independently predicted hypoglycemia [15]. As levels of glycemia in the general population of patients with type 1 or 2 diabetes approximate target levels, an increased incidence of hypoglycemic events in this population can be expected [7,12,13]. Hypoglycemia is less common in the nondiabetic population (reviewed in the article by Service [16]), and its etiologic basis and risk factors differ. In the nondiabetic hospitalized patient, the risk of developing hypoglycemia is associated with malnutrition, malignancy, renal disease, congestive heart failure, and sepsis [9,17]. In the ambulatory patient, predisposing factors may not be readily apparent. In this population, the clinician should be aware of risk factors, such as poly pharmacy, advanced age, ingestion of specific foods (eg, unripened ackee fruit), an undiagnosed underlying psychiatric disorder, or previous gastrointestinal surgery.

General principles

Role of counterregulation in glucose homeostasis

In the nonfasting state, glucose is the preferred substrate for the brain. The brain relies on a continuous external supply of glucose to meet its energy requirements because it lacks the capacity to store a significant amount or produce this substrate de novo. Redundant counterregulatory mechanisms to insulin's glucose lowering action have evolved to maintain systemic glucose balance so as to ensure its continuous supply to the brain. The response involves both behavioral and physiologic mediators. The latter include hormones, the autonomic nervous system, and glucose itself. The CNS plays an important role in processing and coordinating the response to an acute drop in systemic blood glucose. Hormonal mechanisms that orchestrate the hypoglycemic response have been well characterized [18,19] and involve a decrease in the secretion of insulin (decreased glucose uptake from insulin-dependent tissue and increased glycogenolysis), followed by a concomitant rise in systemic glucagon (increased glycogenolysis), epinephrine (increased glycogenolysis, increased gluconeogenesis, decreased glucose uptake from insulin-dependent tissue, and decreased insulin secretion), growth hormone, and cortisol. In concert, these mechanisms limit glucose use by peripheral tissues and increase endogenous glucose production with resultant recovery from hypoglycemia. Drugs (eg, subcutaneously administered insulin, beta-blockers) or disease states (eg, diabetes, liver or renal failure) can overcome or modulate the behavioral or physiologic mediators of the counterregulatory response and impair recovery from hypoglycemia. The phenomenon of "hypoglycemia unawareness" that follows frequent recurrent hypoglycemic episodes in the setting of tightly controlled diabetes [20] or insulinoma [21] is an example of such modulation. The dysregulation of the counterregulatory response in diabetes has been extensively studied and recently reviewed [22].

Pathophysiologic mechanisms of hypoglycemia

Conceptually, hypoglycemia results from an absolute or relative imbalance between the rate of glucose appearance and disappearance from the circulation. Excess glucose utilization by peripheral tissues favors disappearance and usually results from a circulating insulin concentration inappropriate for the level of glycemia. In rare cases, however, it may be caused by antibodies or incompletely processed insulin-like growth factors (IGFs) that act on insulin receptors. Increased glucose metabolism by tissues as seen in intense exercise, weight loss, sepsis, or pregnancy also favors disappearance of circulating glucose and can lead to hypoglycemia if circulating glucose can not be replenished as quickly as it is used (eg, compromised endogenous glucose production). The rate of glucose appearance is determined by oral intake of substrate and, in the fasting state, by the rate of endogenous glucose production (eg, glycogenolysis, gluconeogenesis). In the fasting adult, diseases associated predominantly with compromised endogenous glucose production include malnutrition, liver failure, renal failure, endocrine deficiencies, and enzymatic defects in glycometabolic pathways (eg, congenital [glucose-6-phosphatase deficiency] or acquired [ethanol, unripened ackee fruit]).

Classification of hypoglycemia and clinical implications

The hypoglycemic syndromes can be divided into two classes: fasting (also termed *postabsorptive*) hypoglycemia and reactive (also termed *postprandial*) hypoglycemia. Fasting hypoglycemia occurs in the postabsorptive period (ie, hours after a meal), and reactive hypoglycemia occurs in relation to ingestion of a mixed meal or a glucose load. Fasting hypoglycemia is a manifestation of a major health problem that necessitates diagnostic and therapeutic intervention.

The subject of reactive hypoglycemia is more controversial. In practice, many patients are told that they have reactive hypoglycemia, but not many have a low plasma glucose at the time of symptoms [23,24]. In addition, low postprandial plasma glucose levels alone are not sufficient to define pathologic reactive hypoglycemia. Indeed, an estimated 10% to 30% of normal individuals undergoing oral glucose tolerance testing have plasma glucose levels less than 50 mg/dL at the end of the test without ever developing symptoms [25–27]. As a general rule, any patient who has had a severe adverse event (eg, loss of consciousness, traumatic injury or accident) attributed to postprandial hypoglycemia requires further workup. One of the least disputed causes of reactive hypoglycemia is termed *alimentary hypoglycemia* and was most commonly observed in patients after a gastrectomy for peptic ulcer disease [28]. The pathophysiology of this disorder is presumed to involve disruption of controlled gastric emptying, which results in decreased transit time of aliments from the stomach to the small intestine, causing a rapid elevation in plasma glucose that triggers a quick and exaggerated insulin response. The abnormal insulin response can cause a precipitous drop in blood glucose with consequent adrenergic and neuroglycopenic symptoms. Alimentary hypoglycemia is most frequently observed 2 hours after a meal and has been described as a component of the dumping syndrome. An ongoing debate over the causative basis for reactive hypoglycemia after roux-en-Y surgery for morbid obesity exists. Nesidioblastosis or islet hyperplasia has been proposed by some as causative [29,30], whereas others consider it to be a consequence of the well-established dumping syndrome [31].

Specific causes of fasting hypoglycemia in adults

Drug-induced hypoglycemia

Drugs account for the most frequent cause of hypoglycemia in adults. The most commonly implicated drugs are insulin, sulfonylurea, and ethanol [5,8–11].

Insulin

Insulin-induced hypoglycemia usually occurs in patients with diabetes treated with insulin. Factors to consider in assessing hypoglycemia in a patient with diabetes include errors in the type, dose, or timing of insulin injection; failure to account for changes in nutrition affecting the peripheral action (eg, weight loss, exercise) or clearance of insulin (eg, renal failure); and altered counterregulation as a result of underlying disease or drugs (eg, beta-blockers). Some patients with psychiatric illness inject insulin surreptitiously, thereby inducing hypoglycemia. These patients have usually acquired their familiarity with insulin through a relative with insulin-treated diabetes or through employment as a health care worker [32].

Sulfonylurea

As with insulin, sulfonylurea-associated hypoglycemia can occur as a result of volitional or inadvertent overdose [33], surreptitious use [34,35], or criminally intended administration [36,37]. Risk factors associated with an inadvertent overdose in a patient taking sulfonylurea to treat diabetes include advanced age, drug-drug interaction, and decreased renal (eg, chlorpropamide) or hepatic clearance (eg, tolbutamide, glipizide, glyburide) [15,33]. Accidental overdoses can also occur in patients unknowingly taking sulfonylurea as a result of dispensing error [38,39].

Ethanol

Ethanol inhibits gluconeogenesis [40]. This phenomenon has been attributed to consumption of a rate-limiting cofactor required for gluconeogenesis as a result of ethanol metabolism [41–43]. Ethanol-induced hypoglycemia occurs after glycogen stores have been depleted (12–72 hours), when levels of circulating glucose reflect de novo synthesis from an alternate substrate. Ethanol levels in plasma may be normal or no longer detectable at the time of hypoglycemia. Hypoglycemia should be excluded before attributing impaired cognition to inebriation in the setting of ethanol ingestion.

Other drugs

Many other drugs have been reported to cause hypoglycemia. High-dose salicylates [43–45], beta-blockers [46], and sulfa-based drugs [47] are commonly implicated. Pentamidine at doses used to treat P*neumocystis carinii* pneumonia can also cause hypoglycemia [48]. Quinine [49,50] and antiarrhythmics (eg, quinidine [51], disopyramide [52]) have been associated with hypoglycemia. Quinolone antibiotics [53,54] (eg, gatifloxacin, levofloxacin) have received recent attention for their propensity to cause dysglycemia. Increased insulin secretion is postulated as the underlying mechanism behind pentamidine, quinine derivatives (including quinolones), and antiarrhythmic-induced hypoglycemia.

Organ failure

Liver disease

The liver, through glycogenolysis and gluconeogenesis, supplies most of the glucose to the circulation in the fasting state. The normal liver has a large functional reserve [55], and it is estimated that as little as 20% residual function would suffice to prevent hypoglycemia. This large reserve likely accounts for the fact that most patients with liver disease never develop hypoglycemia. Liver diseases most commonly associated with hypoglycemia include hepatocellular carcinoma [56] and fulminant hepatitis caused by hepatotoxic agents or viruses [57]. Genetic defects in glycometabolic pathways can also lead to hypoglycemia as a consequence of deficient hepatic glycogenolysis and gluconeogenesis, and most are diagnosed in childhood. Finally, liver dysfunction can contribute to hypoglycemia through compromised drug metabolism (eg, tolbutamide, glyburide, glipizide).

Renal disease

The kidney is second only to the liver as a gluconeogenic organ [58]. Factors associated with renal disease that predispose to hypoglycemia include caloric deprivation from anorexia, vomiting, or protein restriction; depletion of gluconeogenic substrate from the latter or hemodialysis treatment; use of glucose-free dialysate; and decreased clearance of renally excreted drugs or their metabolites (eg, insulin, chlorpropamide, metabolite of glyburide).

Endocrinopathies

Deficiencies in cortisol and growth hormone have been causally linked to hypoglycemia [59–64]. Although these hormones do not play a major role in the recovery from acute hypoglycemia, they play an important role in long-term support of counterregulation by contributing to gluconeogenesis [65–68]. Pituitary disease that results in combined corticotropin and growth hormone deficiency particularly predisposes to the development of hypoglycemia.

Neoplasm

Non–islet-cell tumors

Mesenchymal tumors, hepatocellular carcinoma, adrenocortical tumors, carcinoid tumors, leukemia, and lymphomas are the tumors most commonly associated with hypoglycemia. These tumors cause hypoglycemia by secreting a factor with insulin-like action that is chemically distinct from insulin [69,70]. An incompletely processed IGF-II molecule, termed *Big IGF-II* [71–73], with decreased affinity to IGF-binding proteins has been established as the cause of hypoglycemia in some tumors [74,75]. A case of reactive hypoglycemia caused by a tumor secreting glucagon-like peptide-1 (GLP-1) and somatostatin has also been reported [76]. Finally, ectopic insulin secretion from tumors is a rare phenomenon. Although sporadic case reports exist in the literature, few reports [77–79] have conclusively excluded the possibility of a concomitant insulinoma.

Insulinoma

Pancreatic β-cell tumors are rare and can cause hypoglycemia by secreting insulin autonomously. Most of these tumors are small, solitary, and benign (<10% are malignant) [80,81]. The central defect is an inability of insulinoma cells to suppress insulin secretion appropriately in response to a decreasing circulating glucose concentration. This relative excess of insulin in relation to glucose leads to fasting hypoglycemia. Although development of hypoglycemia in the postprandial period does not rule out the presence of an insulinoma, a negative supervised fast does, because virtually all patients with insulinomas develop hypoglycemia after a 48-hour supervised fast [82]. Thus, demonstrating fasting hypoglycemia is essential for the diagnosis of insulinoma.

Islet hyperplasia

In adults, a variety of histologic patterns in islets have been linked to hypoglycemia. This condition has been called nesidioblastosis or diffuse islet hyperplasia or the syndrome of noninsulinoma pancreatogenous hyperinsulinism [29,30,83,84]. There is no doubt that these histologic patterns exist, but their relation to hypoglycemia is controversial. Adding to the confusion is the fact that similar histologic patterns are observed in cases of persistent hyperinsulinemic hypoglycemia of infancy (PHHI). In contrast to adults, however, many of these infants have an identifiable genetic basis for their hyperinsulinemia in the form of sulfonylurea receptor 1 (SUR1) [85,86] potassium channel Kir6.2 [87,88], glucokinase [89], or glutamate dehydrogenase [90] mutations. Finally, nesidioblastosis as a cause of hypoglycemia after bariatric surgery is confounded by the fact that gastric surgery can result in alimentary hypoglycemia.

Autoimmune causes

Anti-insulin receptor antibody

Rarely, hypoglycemia is caused by autoantibodies that bind the insulin receptor and mimic the biologic action of insulin [91–93] (reviewed in article by Taylor and colleagues [94]). Most patients with this syndrome have an antecedent diagnosis of autoimmune disease. In some patients, an elevated erythrocyte sedimentation rate or positive anti-nuclear antibody titer may be the only finding suggestive of an autoimmune cause.

Anti-insulin antibody

Development of hypoglycemia has also been associated with autoantibodies directed against insulin itself [94–97]. These antibodies bind free circulating plasma insulin when its concentration is high and release insulin when the concentration of free plasma insulin drops. Release of insulin at inappropriate times can cause hypoglycemia. Hypoglycemia in this setting is typically observed in the postprandial period, but fasting hypoglycemia has been reported.

Diagnostic approach to fasting hypoglycemia

Establishing fasting hypoglycemia

The first step in the diagnosis is to establish the presence of fasting hypoglycemia. The supervised fast is used for this purpose. This test is performed in the hospital setting to mitigate the risk to the patient if hypoglycemia develops. The patient is fasted and monitored from 48 to 72 hours for biochemical and symptomatic evidence of hypoglycemia. A retrospective review of surgically proven insulinomas showed that hypoglycemia develops within the first 48 hours of the fast in 95% of cases [82].

Establishing the cause

History

Once fasting hypoglycemia has been established, the next step is to identify the cause. The history frames the clinical context (eg, liver failure, sepsis, autoimmune disease, neoplasm, no past health problems) and should be reviewed for a potential drug etiology (including ethanol). The history also may provide important clues to suggest dispensing error as a cause of the hypoglycemia (eg, onset of hypoglycemia after a recent refill).

Biochemistry

Biochemical tests to assess for potential liver, renal, adrenal, and anterior pituitary dysfunction should be obtained. Growth hormone and cortisol levels in the normal range at the time of hypoglycemia are not uncommon, especially if the problem has been long-standing. Hormonal deficiency as a cause should be established in the usual manner (eg, cosyntropin or insulin tolerance test). Blood and urine should be screened for the presence of hypoglycemic agents to rule out surreptitious use. If positive, the screen should be repeated to rule out the presence of interfering substances. The presence of insulin antibodies usually suggests that the patient has received insulin by injection but may represent autoantibodies against insulin in rare cases. The current highly purified insulin preparations used for the treatment of diabetes are less immunogenic than in the past. Thus, the absence of insulin antibodies does not reliably exclude surreptitious injection of insulin.

Specific to insulinoma

If the initial evaluation fails to reveal a cause for the hypoglycemia, the possibility of insulinoma should next be considered. Several different approaches to demonstrate the presence of an insulinoma exist, but the most useful is the 48-hour supervised fast with measurement of plasma insulin and proinsulin. Demonstrating abnormal insulin suppression at the time the patient develops fasting hypoglycemia establishes the diagnosis of insulinoma. This test is based on the premise that insulin secretion in normal β cells is suppressed, before the onset of symptoms, when the plasma glucose level reaches 40 to 50 mg/dL. In contrast, the threshold for insulin suppression in insulinoma may be absent or shifted to a lower plasma glucose level and symptoms may arise before insulin suppression. Thus, a plasma insulin level that fails to suppress to less than 6 microIU/mL at the time of hypoglycemia strongly suggests the presence of an insulin-secreting tumor [80], whereas a plasma insulin level that suppresses to less than 6 microIU/mL favors another etiology. The sensitivity of this test is not 100%; in rare cases, suppression of plasma insulin levels to less than 5 microIU/mL is seen in patients with an insulin-secreting tumor. Presumably, the tumors in these patients have retained some glucose sensing ability. In addition, newer more specific insulin assays no longer measure insulin precursors. When compared with the old assay used to establish the 6 microIU/mL cutoff, these new assays would be expected to yield lower values. In these rare patients, measurement of proinsulin at the termination of the fast is extremely useful. An elevated fasting proinsulin level in this setting strongly suggests a diagnosis of insulinoma. A study using a gel filtration radioimmunoassay to measure proinsulin plasma levels in insulinoma found that proinsulin made up 25% or more of the total immunoreactive insulin in 87% of cases [98]. Only two other conditions that are easily distinguished from insulinoma present with a similarly high ratio of proinsulin to total measured insulin (eg, familial hyperproinsulinemia [99] and hyperglycemia). For the newer commercially available direct proinsulin sandwich assay, a fasting proinsulin plasma level above the assay's normal range is seen in 85% of insulinoma cases (22 pmol/L or 0.2 ng/mL) [98] and is specific for the presence of an insulinoma in the fasting state. This test should be reserved for patients with equivocal plasma insulin levels.

C-peptide levels

Measurement of the plasma C-peptide level at the time of hypoglycemia is useful to diagnose patients injecting insulin surreptitiously. The distinguishing biochemical features in these patients are low C-peptide levels accompanied by high insulin levels. A similar pattern may be seen in patients with autoantibodies directed against the insulin receptor. In these patients, antibodies interfere with insulin binding to its receptor, thereby affecting its clearance from the circulation. Because C-peptide clearance is unaffected, these patients can present with elevated insulin levels and low C-peptide levels.

Insulin-like growth factor-II levels

It has been suggested that at least 50% of non–islet-cell tumors that cause hypoglycemia produce incompletely processed IGF-II (Big IGF-II) and that IGF-II is directly responsible for causing hypoglycemia. The correlation between circulating IGF-II levels and IGF-II hypoglycemic activity is complex. The interaction between circulating IGF-II and specific binding proteins is believed to determine IGF-II hypoglycemic activity. Protein profiles that permit egress of IGF-II from the circulation and allow tissue entry are postulated to result in hypoglycemia. Measurement of circulating IGF-II levels in isolation is thus not a useful routine diagnostic test.

Principles of therapy

The first priority in treating hypoglycemia is to administer a quantity of glucose sufficient to maintain a plasma glucose level greater than 50 mg/dL. This can be accomplished by oral carbohydrate replacement through frequent meals and snacks. In some patients, however, intravenous glucose replacement is necessary. The second priority is to address the underlying cause. Examples of interventions include removal or adjustment of the offending drug, appropriate hormone replacement for patients with deficiency, or confrontation and psychiatry referral for patients with a factitious disorder. In the case of insulinoma, resection of the tumor is usually curative. For nonresectable malignant insulinoma, diazoxide may provide some benefit [100]. Hypoglycemia resulting from non–islet-cell tumors is usually treated by interventions aimed at reducing tumor burden. If this cannot be achieved, glucose administration is the only therapy. The syndrome of autoantibodies against the insulin receptor can result in severe hypoglycemia, which is associated with high mortality if left untreated. This disorder is usually a self-limited condition that resolves over months in most cases. Therapy consisting of high-dose glucocorticoid (prednisone, 60 mg/d) prevents hypoglycemia by inhibiting the insulinomimetic effect of the antireceptor antibody but does not hasten its disappearance from plasma.

Summary

Under physiologic conditions, glucose plays a critical role in providing energy to the CNS. A precipitous drop in the availability of this substrate results in dramatic symptoms that signal a medical emergency and warrant immediate therapy aimed at restoring plasma glucose to normal levels. A systemic approach to the differential diagnosis is useful in identifying the cause of hypoglycemia. Once established, a specific and/or definitive intervention that addresses that underlying problem can be implemented. In most cases, this systemic approach to diagnosis and therapy is rewarded with a good outcome for the patient.

References

[1] Merimee TJ, Tyson JE. Stabilization of plasma glucose during fasting; normal variations in two separate studies. N Engl J Med 1974;291(24):1275–8.
[2] Whipple AO. The surgical therapy of hyperinsulinism. J Int Chir 1938;3:237–76.
[3] Hepburn DA, Deary IJ, Frier BM, et al. Symptoms of acute insulin-induced hypoglycemia in humans with and without IDDM. Factor-analysis approach. Diabetes Care 1991;14(11): 949–57.
[4] Towler DA, Havlin CE, Craft S, et al. Mechanism of awareness of hypoglycemia. Perception of neurogenic (predominantly cholinergic) rather than neuroglycopenic symptoms. Diabetes 1993;42(12):1791–8.
[5] Fischer KF, Lees JA, Newman JH. Hypoglycemia in hospitalized patients. Causes and outcomes. N Engl J Med 1986;315(20):1245–50.
[6] Holstein A, Plaschke A, Egberts EH. Incidence and costs of severe hypoglycemia. Diabetes Care 2002;25(11):2109–10.
[7] Johnson ES, Koepsell TD, Reiber G, et al. Increasing incidence of serious hypoglycemia in insulin users. J Clin Epidemiol 2002;55(3):253–9.
[8] Hart SP, Frier BM. Causes, management and morbidity of acute hypoglycaemia in adults requiring hospital admission. QJM 1998;91(7):505–10.

[9] Vriesendorp TM, van Santen S, DeVries JH, et al. Predisposing factors for hypoglycemia in the intensive care unit. Crit Care Med 2006;34(1):96–101.
[10] Su CC. Etiologies of acute hypoglycemia in a Taiwanese hospital emergency department. J Emerg Med 2006;30(3):259–61.
[11] Malouf R, Brust JC. Hypoglycemia: causes, neurological manifestations, and outcome. Ann Neurol 1985;17(5):421–30.
[12] The Diabetes Control and Complications Trial Research Group. Hypoglycemia in the Diabetes Control and Complications Trial. Diabetes 1997;46(2):271–86.
[13] UK Prospective Diabetes Study (UKPDS) Group. Intensive blood-glucose control with sulphonylureas or insulin compared with conventional treatment and risk of complications in patients with type 2 diabetes (UKPDS 33). Lancet 1998;352(9131):837–53.
[14] Leese GP, Wang J, Broomhall J, et al. Frequency of severe hypoglycemia requiring emergency treatment in type 1 and type 2 diabetes: a population-based study of health service resource use. Diabetes Care 2003;26(4):1176–80.
[15] Shorr RI, Ray WA, Daugherty JR, et al. Incidence and risk factors for serious hypoglycemia in older persons using insulin or sulfonylureas. Arch Intern Med 1997;157(15):1681–6.
[16] Service FJ. Hypoglycemic disorders. N Engl J Med 1995;332(17):1144–52.
[17] Shilo S, Berezovsky S, Friedlander Y, et al. Hypoglycemia in hospitalized nondiabetic older patients. J Am Geriatr Soc 1998;46(8):978–82.
[18] Gerich J, Davis J, Lorenzi M, et al. Hormonal mechanisms of recovery from insulin-induced hypoglycemia in man. Am J Physiol 1979;236(4):E380–5.
[19] Cryer PE. Glucose counterregulation: prevention and correction of hypoglycemia in humans. Am J Physiol 1993;264(2 Pt 1):E149–55.
[20] Amiel SA, Sherwin RS, Simonson DC, et al. Effect of intensive insulin therapy on glycemic thresholds for counterregulatory hormone release. Diabetes 1988;37(7):901–7.
[21] Mitrakou A, Fanelli C, Veneman T, et al. Reversibility of unawareness of hypoglycemia in patients with insulinomas. N Engl J Med 1993;329(12):834–9.
[22] Cryer PE. Diverse causes of hypoglycemia-associated autonomic failure in diabetes. N Engl J Med 2004;350(22):2272–9.
[23] Charles MA, Hofeldt F, Shackelford A, et al. Comparison of oral glucose tolerance tests and mixed meals in patients with apparent idiopathic postabsorptive hypoglycemia: absence of hypoglycemia after meals. Diabetes 1981;30(6):465–70.
[24] Palardy J, Havrankova J, Lepage R, et al. Blood glucose measurements during symptomatic episodes in patients with suspected postprandial hypoglycemia. N Engl J Med 1989; 321(21):1421–5.
[25] Fariss BL. Prevalence of post-glucose-load glycosuria and hypoglycemia in a group of healthy young men. Diabetes 1974;23(3):189–91.
[26] Hofeldt FD. Reactive hypoglycemia. Metabolism 1975;24(10):1193–208.
[27] Lev-Ran A, Anderson RW. The diagnosis of postprandial hypoglycemia. Diabetes 1981; 30(12):996–9.
[28] Hofeldt FD. Reactive hypoglycemia. Endocrinol Metab Clin North Am 1989;18(1): 185–201.
[29] Service GJ, Thompson GB, Service FJ, et al. Hyperinsulinemic hypoglycemia with nesidioblastosis after gastric-bypass surgery. N Engl J Med 2005;353(3):249–54.
[30] Patti ME, McMahon G, Mun EC, et al. Severe hypoglycaemia post-gastric bypass requiring partial pancreatectomy: evidence for inappropriate insulin secretion and pancreatic islet hyperplasia. Diabetologia 2005;48(11):2236–40.
[31] Meier JJ, Butler AE, Galasso R, et al. Hyperinsulinemic hypoglycemia after gastric bypass surgery is not accompanied by islet hyperplasia or increased β-cell turnover. Diabetes Care 2006;29(7):1554–9.
[32] Grunberger G, Weiner JL, Silverman R, et al. Factitious hypoglycemia due to surreptitious administration of insulin. Diagnosis, treatment, and long-term follow-up. Ann Intern Med 1988;108(2):252–7.

[33] van Staa T, Abenhaim L, Monette J. Rates of hypoglycemia in users of sulfonylureas. J Clin Epidemiol 1997;50(6):735–41.
[34] Duncan GG, Jenson W, Eberly RJ. Factitious hypoglycemia due to chlorpropamide. Report of a case, with clinical similarity to an islet cell tumor of the pancreas. JAMA 1961; 175:904–6.
[35] Jordan RM, Kammer H, Riddle MR. Sulfonylurea-induced factitious hypoglycemia. A growing problem. Arch Intern Med 1977;137(3):390–3.
[36] Fernando R. Homicidal poisoning with glibenclamide. Med Sci Law 1999;39(4):354–8.
[37] Manning PJ, Espiner EA, Yoon K, et al. An unusual cause of hyperinsulinaemic hypoglycaemia syndrome. Diabet Med 2003;20(9):772–6.
[38] Sketris I, Wheeler D, York S. Hypoglycemic coma induced by inadvertent administration of glyburide. Drug Intell Clin Pharm 1984;18(2):142–3.
[39] Scala-Barnett DM, Donoghue ER. Dispensing error causing fatal chlorpropamide intoxication in a nondiabetic. J Forensic Sci 1986;31(1):293–5.
[40] Field JB, Williams HE, Mortimore GE. Studies on the mechanism of ethanol-induced hypoglycemia. J Clin Invest 1963;42:497–506.
[41] Lumeng L, Davis EJ. Mechanism of ethanol suppression of gluconeogenesis. Inhibition of phosphoenolpyruvate synthesis from glutamate and alphaketaglutarate. J Biol Chem 1970; 245(12):3179–85.
[42] Zaleski J, Bryla J. Ethanol-induced impairment of gluconeogenesis from lactate in rabbit hepatocytes: correlation with an increased reduction of mitochondrial NAD pool. Int J Biochem 1980;11(3–4):237–42.
[43] Madison LL, Lochner A, Wulff J. Ethanol-induced hypoglycemia. II. Mechanism of suppression of hepatic gluconeogenesis. Diabetes 1967;16(4):252–8.
[44] Arena FP, Dugowson C, Saudek CD. Salicylate-induced hypoglycemia and ketoacidosis in a nondiabetic adult. Arch Intern Med 1978;138(7):1153–4.
[45] Raschke R, Arnold-Capell PA, Richeson R, et al. Refractory hypoglycemia secondary to topical salicylate intoxication. Arch Intern Med 1991;151(3):591–3.
[46] Hirsch IB, Boyle PJ, Craft S, et al. Higher glycemic thresholds for symptoms during beta-adrenergic blockade in IDDM. Diabetes 1991;40(9):1177–86.
[47] Poretsky L, Moses AC. Hypoglycemia associated with trimethoprim/sulfamethoxazole therapy. Diabetes Care 1984;7(5):508–9.
[48] Waskin H, Stehr-Green JK, Helmick CG, et al. Risk factors for hypoglycemia associated with pentamidine therapy for Pneumocystis pneumonia. JAMA 1988;260(3):345–7.
[49] Taylor TE, Molyneux ME, Wirima JJ, et al. Blood glucose levels in Malawian children before and during the administration of intravenous quinine for severe falciparum malaria. N Engl J Med 1988;319(16):1040–7.
[50] Limburg PJ, Katz H, Grant CS, et al. Quinine-induced hypoglycemia. Ann Intern Med 1993;119(3):218–9.
[51] Barbato M. Another problem with Kinidin. Med J Aust 1984;141(10):685.
[52] Goldberg IJ, Brown LK, Rayfield EJ. Disopyramide (Norpace)-induced hypoglycemia. Am J Med 1980;69(3):463–6.
[53] Graumlich JF, Habis S, Avelino RR, et al. Hypoglycemia in inpatients after gatifloxacin or levofloxacin therapy: nested case-control study. Pharmacotherapy 2005;25(10): 1296–302.
[54] Park-Wyllie LY, Juurlink DN, Kopp A, et al. Outpatient gatifloxacin therapy and dysglycemia in older adults. N Engl J Med 2006;354(13):1352–61.
[55] Chiolero R, Tappy L, Gillet M, et al. Effect of major hepatectomy on glucose and lactate metabolism. Ann Surg 1999;229(4):505–13.
[56] Luo JC, Hwang SJ, Wu JC, et al. Paraneoplastic syndromes in patients with hepatocellular carcinoma in Taiwan. Cancer 1999;86(5):799–804.
[57] Felig P, Brown WV, Levine RA, et al. Glucose homeostasis in viral hepatitis. N Engl J Med 1970;283(26):1436–40.

[58] Gerich JE, Meyer C, Woerle HJ, et al. Renal gluconeogenesis: its importance in human glucose homeostasis. Diabetes Care 2001;24(2):382–91.
[59] Sovik O, Oseid S, Vidnes J. Ketotic hypoglycemia in a four-year-old boy with adrenal cortical insufficiency. Acta Paediatr Scand 1972;61(4):465–9.
[60] Artavia-Loria E, Chaussain JL, Bougneres PF, et al. Frequency of hypoglycemia in children with adrenal insufficiency. Acta Endocrinol Suppl (Copenh) 1986;279:275–8.
[61] Pia A, Piovesan A, Tassone F, et al. A rare case of adulthood-onset growth hormone deficiency presenting as sporadic, symptomatic hypoglycemia. J Endocrinol Invest 2004; 27(11):1060–4.
[62] Nadler HL, Neumann LL, Gershberg H. Hypoglycemia, growth retardation, and probable isolated growth hormone deficiency in a 1-year-old child. J Pediatr 1963;63:977–83.
[63] LaFranchi S, Buist NR, Jhaveri B, et al. Amino acids as substrates in children with growth hormone deficiency and hypoglycemia. Pediatrics 1981;68(2):260–4.
[64] Wolfsdorf JI, Sadeghi-Nejad A, Senior B. Hypoketonemia and age-related fasting hypoglycemia in growth hormone deficiency. Metabolism 1983;32(5):457–62.
[65] De Feo P, Perriello G, Torlone E, et al. Demonstration of a role for growth hormone in glucose counterregulation. Am J Physiol 1989;256(6 Pt 1):E835–43.
[66] De Feo P, Perriello G, Torlone E, et al. Contribution of cortisol to glucose counterregulation in humans. Am J Physiol 1989;257(1 Pt 1):E35–42.
[67] Khani S, Tayek JA. Cortisol increases gluconeogenesis in humans: its role in the metabolic syndrome. Clin Sci (Lond) 2001;101(6):739–47.
[68] Boyle PJ, Cryer PE. Growth hormone, cortisol, or both are involved in defense against, but are not critical to recovery from, hypoglycemia. Am J Physiol 1991;260(3 Pt 1):E395–402.
[69] Megyesi K, Kahn CR, Roth J, et al. Hypoglycemia in association with extrapancreatic tumors: demonstration of elevated plasma NSILA-s by a new radioreceptor assay. J Clin Endocrinol Metab 1974;38(5):931–4.
[70] Gorden P, Hendricks CM, Kahn CR, et al. Hypoglycemia associated with non-islet-cell tumor and insulin-like growth factors. N Engl J Med 1981;305(24):1452–5.
[71] Daughaday WH, Emanuele MA, Brooks MH, et al. Synthesis and secretion of insulin-like growth factor II by a leiomyosarcoma with associated hypoglycemia. N Engl J Med 1988; 319(22):1434–40.
[72] Daughaday WH, Kapadia M. Significance of abnormal serum binding of insulinlike growth factor II in the development of hypoglycemia in patients with nonislet- cell tumors. Proc Natl Acad Sci USA 1989;86(17):6778–82.
[73] Daughaday WH, Trivedi B. Measurement of derivatives of proinsulin-like growth factor-II in serum by a radioimmunoassay directed against the E-domain in normal subjects and patients with nonislet cell tumor hypoglycemia. J Clin Endocrinol Metab 1992;75(1):110–5.
[74] Wu JC, Daughaday WH, Lee SD, et al. Radioimmunoassay of serum IGF-I and IGF-II in patients with chronic liver diseases and hepatocellular carcinoma with or without hypoglycemia. J Lab Clin Med 1988;112(5):589–94.
[75] Ishida S, Noda M, Kuzuya N, et al. Big insulin-like growth factor II-producing hepatocellular carcinoma associated with hypoglycemia. Intern Med 1995;34(12):1201–6.
[76] Todd JF, Stanley SA, Roufosse CA, et al. A tumour that secretes glucagon-like peptide-1 and somatostatin in a patient with reactive hypoglycaemia and diabetes. Lancet 2003; 361(9353):228–30.
[77] Shetty MR, Boghossian HM, Duffell D, et al. Tumor-induced hypoglycemia: a result of ectopic insulin production. Cancer 1982;49(9):1920–3.
[78] Morgello S, Schwartz E, Horwith M, et al. Ectopic insulin production by a primary ovarian carcinoid. Cancer 1988;61(4):800–5.
[79] Seckl MJ, Mulholland PJ, Bishop AE, et al. Hypoglycemia due to an insulin-secreting small-cell carcinoma of the cervix. N Engl J Med 1999;341(10):733–6.
[80] Service FJ, Dale AJ, Elveback LR, et al. Insulinoma: clinical and diagnostic features of 60 consecutive cases. Mayo Clin Proc 1976;51(7):417–29.

[81] Service FJ, McMahon MM, O'Brien PC, et al. Functioning insulinoma—incidence, recurrence, and long-term survival of patients: a 60-year study. Mayo Clin Proc 1991;66(7): 711–9.
[82] Hirshberg B, Livi A, Bartlett DL, et al. Forty-eight-hour fast: the diagnostic test for insulinoma. J Clin Endocrinol Metab 2000;85(9):3222–6.
[83] Service FJ, Natt N, Thompson GB, et al. Noninsulinoma pancreatogenous hypoglycemia: a novel syndrome of hyperinsulinemic hypoglycemia in adults independent of mutations in Kir6.2 and SUR1 genes. J Clin Endocrinol Metab 1999;84(5):1582–9.
[84] Thompson GB, Service FJ, Andrews JC, et al. Noninsulinoma pancreatogenous hypoglycemia syndrome: an update in 10 surgically treated patients. Surgery 2000;128(6):937–44 [discussion: 944–5].
[85] Kane C, Shepherd RM, Squires PE, et al. Loss of functional KATP channels in pancreatic beta-cells causes persistent hyperinsulinemic hypoglycemia of infancy. Nat Med 1996;2(12): 1344–7.
[86] Nestorowicz A, Wilson BA, Schoor KP, et al. Mutations in the sulonylurea receptor gene are associated with familial hyperinsulinism in Ashkenazi Jews. Hum Mol Genet 1996; 5(11):1813–22.
[87] Thomas P, Ye Y, Lightner E. Mutation of the pancreatic islet inward rectifier Kir6.2 also leads to familial persistent hyperinsulinemic hypoglycemia of infancy. Hum Mol Genet 1996;5(11):1809–12.
[88] Nestorowicz A, Inagaki N, Gonoi T, et al. A nonsense mutation in the inward rectifier potassium channel gene, Kir6.2, is associated with familial hyperinsulinism. Diabetes 1997; 46(11):1743–8.
[89] Glaser B, Kesavan P, Heyman M, et al. Familial hyperinsulinism caused by an activating glucokinase mutation. N Engl J Med 1998;338(4):226–30.
[90] Stanley CA, Lieu YK, Hsu BY, et al. Hyperinsulinism and hyperammonemia in infants with regulatory mutations of the glutamate dehydrogenase gene. N Engl J Med 1998; 338(19):1352–7.
[91] Khokher MA, Avasthy N, Taylor AM, et al. Insulin-receptor antibody and hypoglycaemia associated with Hodgkin's disease. Lancet 1987;1(8534):693–4.
[92] Moller DE, Ratner RE, Borenstein DG, et al. Autoantibodies to the insulin receptor as a cause of autoimmune hypoglycemia in systemic lupus erythematosus. Am J Med 1988; 84(2):334–8.
[93] Arioglu E, Andewelt A, Diabo C, et al. Clinical course of the syndrome of autoantibodies to the insulin receptor (type B insulin resistance): a 28-year perspective. Medicine (Baltimore) 2002;81(2):87–100.
[94] Taylor SI, Barbetti F, Accili D, et al. Syndromes of autoimmunity and hypoglycemia. Autoantibodies directed against insulin and its receptor. Endocrinol Metab Clin North Am 1989;18(1):123–43.
[95] Hirata Y, Tominaga M, Ito JI, et al. Spontaneous hypoglycemia with insulin autoimmunity in Graves' disease. Ann Intern Med 1974;81(2):214–8.
[96] Redmon B, Pyzdrowski KL, Elson MK, et al. Hypoglycemia due to an insulin-binding monoclonal antibody in multiple myeloma. N Engl J Med 1992;326(15):994–8.
[97] Blackshear PJ, Rotner HE, Kriauciunas KA, et al. Reactive hypoglycemia and insulin autoantibodies in drug-induced lupus erythematosus. Ann Intern Med 1983;99(2):182–4.
[98] Gorden P, Skarulis MC, Roach P, et al. Plasma proinsulin-like component in insulinoma: a 25-year experience. J Clin Endocrinol Metab 1995;80(10):2884–7.
[99] Gruppuso PA, Gorden P, Kahn CR, et al. Familial hyperproinsulinemia due to a proposed defect in conversion of proinsulin to insulin. N Engl J Med 1984;311(10):629–34.
[100] Hirshberg B, Cochran C, Skarulis MC, et al. Malignant insulinoma: spectrum of unusual clinical features. Cancer 2005;104(2):264–72.

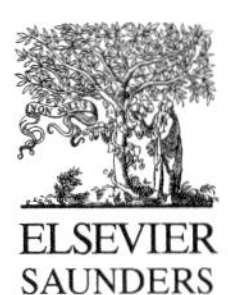

ELSEVIER
SAUNDERS

Endocrinol Metab Clin N Am
35 (2006) 767–775

ENDOCRINOLOGY
AND METABOLISM
CLINICS
OF NORTH AMERICA

Acute Adrenal Insufficiency

Roger Bouillon, MD, PhD, FRCP

Clinic and Laboratory of Endocrinology, University Hospital Gasthuisberg, Herestraat 49, B-3000 Leuven, Belgium

The adrenal gland is a mixture of the steroid hormone–producing adrenal cortex and the adrenal medulla, which is responsible for the secretion of catecholamines. Although both parts of the adrenal gland largely function independently of each other, the congenital absence of a functional adrenal cortex (because of glucocorticoid receptor mutations) causes a developmental absence of the adrenal medulla. After a bilateral adrenalectomy catecholamines can still be produced by the autonomic nervous system, but there is a total inability to synthesize and secrete glucocorticoid and mineralocorticoid hormones (cortisol and aldosterone), indicating the unique role of the adrenal cortex. The secretion of cortisol and aldosterone is controlled by different mechanisms, whereby the pituitary axis (corticotropin-releasing hormone [CRH] or corticotropin) is vital for cortisol secretion and the renin-angiotensin system is vital for aldosterone secretion. Cytokines, ion concentrations, and many other factors can directly or mostly indirectly influence cortisol or aldosterone secretion, however.

Cortisol regulates a wide variety of genes involved in energy metabolism (eg, glucose-protein–fatty acid metabolism), mineral homeostasis, and immune function and influences many more cellular functions. Aldosterone has a more focused action on mineral homeostasis [1].

Etiology of adrenal insufficiency

Adrenal insufficiency is a hormone deficiency syndrome attributable to primary adrenal diseases or caused by a wide variety of pituitary-hypothalamic disorders (Box 1). Diseases causing primary adrenal insufficiency usually destroy the total adrenal cortex, causing a combined deficiency of glucocorticoids and mineralocorticoids and adrenal androgens, and such diseases sometimes even cause adrenal medulla deficiency. The clinical

E-mail address: roger.bouillon@med.kuleuven.be

doi:10.1016/j.ecl.2006.09.004

Box 1. Etiology of adrenal insufficiency

Primary adrenal insufficiency

- Autoimmune diseases (isolated or associated with polyglandular insufficiencies)
- Adrenal infections and inflammation (eg, tuberculosis, fungal diseases, AIDS)
- Bilateral metastasis
- After adrenalectomy[a]
- Adrenal enzyme deficiency
- Adrenal hemorrhage or necrosis caused by (meningococcal) sepsis or coagulation disorders[a]
- Idiopathic
- Drug-induced
- Adrenoleukodystrophy and other congenital disorders

Secondary adrenal insufficiency

- Pituitary or hypothalamic tumor (including craniopharyngioma)
- Pituitary irradiation
- Pituitary surgery[a]
- Pituitary/brain trauma[a]
- Infections or inflammatory/autoimmune disorders in pituitary region (eg, sarcoidosis, hypophysitis)
- Pituitary necrosis or bleeding (eg, postpartum Sheehan syndrome)[a]
- Acute interruption of prolonged pharmacologic glucocorticoid therapy[a]
- Causes of adrenal insufficiency with increased risk for presentation as acute adrenal crisis[a]

[a] Adrenal insufficiency with increased risk for presentation as acute adrenal crisis.

symptoms are therefore usually more prominent than in cases of secondary insufficiency and can start as an acute crisis of adrenal insufficiency.

Secondary adrenal insufficiency more selectively impairs glucocorticoid deficiency so that the mineralocorticoid function is better maintained and therefore less likely to cause an acute crisis. If such diseases (see Box 1) evolve gradually over time, they rarely cause an abrupt-onset adrenal insufficiency crisis, whereas acute destruction of the adrenal or pituitary gland or acute interruption of glucocorticoid therapy is more likely to cause an acute-onset adrenal failure crisis.

Apart from this classic presentation of an endocrine deficiency as the cause of generalized chronic or acute disease (adrenal crisis) [1–5], there is increasing attention to relative adrenal insufficiency in patients with acute (nonadrenal or pituitary) critical illness. Such patients still secrete cortisol (and corticotropin in the early phases of critical illness) but less than expected during acute stress, and the survival of such patients can be improved by pharmacologic doses of glucocorticoids [1,3,4,6,7]. The adrenal (dys)function of such patients with critical illness is described separately in this issue in the article by Schütz and Müller and has been reviewed recently [6].

Although adrenal insufficiency has been known as a clinical syndrome for a long time, new risk groups have been identified, because as many as 20% of AIDS patients eventually develop adrenal insufficiency [8,9]. Moreover, patients with head trauma develop pituitary insufficiency much more frequently than previously recognized [10].

The hypothalamic-pituitary-adrenal axis is vital to the body's ability to cope with severe stress, such as that induced by natural or iatrogenic trauma or infection, and such function has been amply demonstrated in human patients and experimental animals, including animal models of engineered adrenal insufficiency [11,12].

Cortisol replacement therapy is usually highly effective when started before secondary organ failure compromises survival. Therefore, early recognition, correct diagnosis, and treatment save lives.

Symptoms of adrenal insufficiency

Primary and secondary adrenal insufficiency (excluding critical illness adrenal insufficiency and adrenal insufficiency secondary to acute interruption of chronic glucocorticoid therapy) are rare diseases, affecting less than 0.1% of the population [1], and usually present slowly over time with nonspecific symptoms of chronic fatigue, weakness and lethargy, anorexia and weight loss, postural hypotension, abdominal complaints (eg, nausea, vomiting, diffuse abdominal pain), and loss of libido as well as loss of axillary and pubic hair in women. Hyperpigmentation (attributable to excess proopiomelanocortin and melanocyte-stimulating hormone), especially of non–sunlight-exposed skin areas, is an imported clinical hallmark for the attentive and suspicious physician. Abnormal serum electrolytes—low sodium, high potassium, and, occasionally, hypercalcemia and fasting hypoglycemia, and especially this combination—are highly suspicious for adrenal insufficiency.

Acute adrenal insufficiency (adrenal crisis) is mainly attributable to mineralocorticoid deficiency; thus, the clinical presentation is dominated by hypotension or hypotensive shock. This shock is mainly caused by sodium and plasma volume depletion, but the associated prostaglandin excess (prostacyclin) and decreased responsiveness to norepinephrine and angiotensin II may aggravate the circulatory collapse. The clinical picture may be much more complex because of a mixture of preceding slow-onset symptoms and signs, such as acute abdominal pain, or symptoms attributable to the etiology of the acute adrenal insufficiency (eg, sepsis, pituitary or adrenal hemorrhage or necrosis, surgery or trauma).

Diagnosis of adrenal insufficiency

In view of the wide spectrum of clinical symptoms and signs of chronic adrenal insufficiency, a strategy for screening for such hormone deficiency should be broadly applied, whereby serum cortisol levels are the first choice. In nonacute situations, this should be early morning cortisol levels because of the known diurnal variation; however, in patients with severe illness, cortisol levels should be high anyway, and levels greater than 20 μg/dL in a nonacutely stressed person exclude adrenal insufficiency. Total plasma cortisol levels are still widely used for diagnostic purposes, whereas cortisol is tightly bound to CBG (cortisol binding globulin or transcortin). Because CBG can fluctuate according to (rare) genetic disorders because of exposure to estrogens or because of chronic (liver and kidney) diseases or acute illness (acute critical illness), total cortisol levels may not reflect free cortisol levels. Direct measurement of free cortisol is cumbersome and not amenable in an emergency situation. Free cortisol levels calculated on the basis of the law of mass order using total cortisol and transcortin, as described by our laboratory [14], carefully reflect direct estimation of free cortisol, and this has recently been confirmed even in patients with a wide variety of critical illnesses [15].

Basal corticotropin levels are high in case of primary adrenal disorders (>100 pg/mL) and therefore are equivalent to thyroid-stimulating hormone (TSH) measurements for the screening of primary hypothyroidism. High renin and low aldosterone also argue for primary adrenal insufficiency. Dynamic testing with injection of corticotropin or insulin-induced hypoglycemia is frequently needed to confirm adrenal insufficiency, however (Box 2). Once adrenal insufficiency is confirmed, additional exploration is needed to identify the etiology of the disease (see Box 1).

In acute illness possibly attributable to adrenal insufficiency, a different diagnostic strategy should be applied, because immediate therapeutic intervention is absolutely needed even before the diagnosis is formally confirmed. The first principle is to be highly suspicious of adrenal crisis in case of unexplained hypotension, especially in patients with increased risk (eg, AIDS patients, patients on prior glucocorticoid therapy, patients with known autoimmune diseases or with a history of chronic fatigue and hyperpigmentation) or in those displaying acute symptoms related to the diseases known to cause acute adrenal crisis (see Box 1). Moreover, simple diagnostic screening should be used based on what is rapidly available (plasma concentration of

Box 2. Diagnostic testing for chronic adrenal insufficiency

1. Screening test
   - Early morning basal total/free serum cortisol[a] and plasma corticotropin
   - Plasma aldosterone, and renin activity
   - (Urinary free cortisol excretion)
2. Stimulation test
   - Stimulation of adrenal function (in case of suspicion of primary adrenal insufficiency, stimulation with 1 or 250 μg corticotropin(1-24), followed by cortisol measurements after 30 and 60 minutes[b])
   - Stimulation of pituitary-adrenal axis (in case of suspicion of adrenal insufficiency, especially of hypothalamic-pituitary origin) by insulin-induced hypoglycemia
     - Regular insulin (0.1 U) administered intravenously
     - Basal and 30-60-90 minutes after start of insulin tolerance test of cortisol and corticotropin[c] (and growth hormone in case of suspected multiple pituitary hormone deficiency)
   - Stimulation with CRH is useful for the differential diagnosis between hypothalamic and pituitary origin of adrenal insufficiency and can also be used to replace the "gold standard" test when ITT is contraindicated (eg, epilepsy)
   - Metyrapone test is rather outdated

[a] Normal morning total cortisol levels are between 10 and 20 μg/dL (6:00–8:00 AM) if CBG is normal. Values less than 3 μg/dL (80 nmol/L) are highly suggestive of adrenal insufficiency, and values less than 10 μg/dL (275 nmol/L) certainly require further adrenal evaluation.

[b] Total cortisol levels greater than 20 μg/dL (presuming normal CBG) exclude primary but not always secondary adrenal deficiency. The minimal cortisol threshold after 1 μg of corticotropin is approximately the same as after 250 μg of corticotropin(1–24).

[c] Total cortisol levels after adequate hypoglycemia during ITT should exceed 20 μg/dL (550 nmol/L). Simultaneous measurement of corticotropin may help to define the origin (hypothalamic-pituitary or adrenal) of the disease.

sodium, potassium, and cortisol), followed by a short corticotropin stimulation test (Box 3), and then immediately associated with or followed by therapeutic substitution or intervention until laboratory results are available (Box 4). This diagnostic strategy should include cortisol precursors and metabolites in blood and/or urine when acute adrenal insufficiency is suspected in pediatric patients so as to exclude congenital adrenal hyperplasia [16].

Box 3. Diagnostic procedures in case of suspected acute adrenal insufficiency crisis

A. Serum analysis of
- Sodium, potassium, and HCO_3
- Plasma cortisol[a]
- Plasma sample for corticotropin, renin, and aldosterone

B. Corticotropin stimulation test
- 250 μg administered intravenously with additional cortisol measurement 30 minutes later[a]

Interpretation

Adrenal insufficiency crisis is highly unlikely if
1. Basal total cortisol is greater than 20 μg/dL
2. Postcorticotropin cortisol is greater than 20 μg/dL

[a] Normal morning total cortisol levels are between 10 and 20 μg/dL (6:00–8:00 AM) if CBG is normal. Values less than 3 μg/dL (80 nmol/L) are highly suggestive of adrenal insufficiency, and values less than 10 μg/dL (275 nmol/L) certainly require further adrenal evaluation.

Data from Oelkers W. Adrenal insufficiency. N Engl J Med 1996;335(16):1206–12; and Grinspoon SK, Biller BMK. Laboratory assessment of adrenal insufficiency. J Clin Endocrinol Metab 1994;79(4):923–31; and Grinspoon SK, Biller BMK. Laboratory assessment of adrenal insufficiency. J Clin Endocrinol Metab 1994;79(4):923–31.

Treatment of adrenal insufficiency

The acute treatment of an Addison disease crisis is relatively straightforward, because electrolyte and fluid replacement and hydrocortisone replacement (see Box 4) should be started as soon as the initial diagnostic sampling is complete.

If adrenal insufficiency is confirmed or highly likely based on the acute screening results, replacement therapy should be continued by the intravenous or intramuscular route (at 150–300 mg/d for 2 to 3 days) until full clinical recovery. As such, high cortisol replacement has major mineralocorticoid effects, but because of direct activation of the mineralocorticoid receptor, no additional mineralocorticoid therapy is needed in the acute phase. Indeed, cortisol normally only activates its own receptor, glucocorticoid receptor, and not the mineralocorticoid receptor (MR), although it has the same affinity for the MR as aldosterone because of rapid intrarenal inactivation of cortisol to cortisone. In case of Cushing syndrome or when cortisol replacement therapy far exceeds normal replacement doses, cortisol is not totally inactivated by the 11-β-steroid dehydrogenase, and thus activates the MR and displays

Box 4. Therapeutic strategy in case of suspected acute adrenal insufficiency crisis

1. Diagnostic screening as in Box 3A
2. Start therapeutic intervention with
   - Infusion of sodium chloride 9% and glucose 5% (>>indicating in 6 hours)
   - Diagnostic corticotropin test as in Box 3B
   - Followed by hydrocortisol, 100 mg, administered intravenously or intramuscularly every 8 hours or until results of diagnostic screening are available
3. If diagnostic screening, demonstrate
   - Basal or postcorticotropin cortisol greater than 20 μg/dL, stop further hydrocortisone therapy unless the patient is still critically ill (other criteria apply)
   - Basal and postcorticotropin cortisol levels indicate a likelihood of Addison disease: continue intravenous/intramuscular hydrocortisone, followed by oral substitution
   - Final confirmation of Addison disease and evaluation of its etiology may be appropriate after resolution of acute crisis

major mineralocorticoid effects. This 150- to 300-mg/d replacement dose of hydrocortisone is frequently considered to be a physiologic stress dosage. Serum cortisol levels measured after such so-called "acute replacement" dosages exceed several times the maximal stress cortisol levels found in healthy or even critically ill patients [8,15], however, thereby questioning the need for maintaining such high acute emergency replacement dosages. No clinical studies are yet available allowing us to conclude that a much lower hydrocortisone dose in acute adrenal crisis would generate equivalent or better acute survival, however. Therefore, most centers prefer to start with hydrocortisone at a dose of approximately 200 to 300 mg/d. The mineralocorticoid effect of such doses of hydrocortisone is an additional motivation to maintain this dosage for a few days. Thereafter, the dosage can be rapidly tapered down.

Normal replacement therapy should be given orally (hydrocortisone, ±20 mg/d, in two or three oral doses for adults, and fludrocortisone, 50–200 μg/d). Of course, full exploration of the etiology of the disease and, if applicable or possible, adequate therapy of the primary disease are needed. Detailed information about and education of the patient and of his or her family and a medical emergency alert card as well as appropriate follow-up should be initiated.

There is no general consensus with regard to the fine tuning of glucocorticoid replacement therapy, because posttherapeutic cortisol or corticotropin measurements cannot be easily used for monitoring drug dosage, as for thyroxine (T4) replacement therapy. Generally, the lowest replacement dosage is to be preferred, avoiding clinical symptoms of adrenal insufficiency and monitoring signs of overdosage [13,17]. Because the daily production rate of cortisol is approximately 8 mg/m^2/d based on well-established isotope dilution methodology, the replacement dose of cortisol has been gradually decreased from 30 mg/d or more to 15 to 25 mg/d for patients with stable chronic adrenal insufficiency. This could still be considered as slightly supraphysiologic but is probably needed to compensate for cortisol inactivation into cortisone before it reaches the blood circulation after oral intake. The gradual reduction in the chronic replacement dosage has not markedly increased the frequency of acute adrenal crises, probably because of the simultaneous emphasis on preventive dosage adjustments (50%–100%) during acute diseases (eg, trauma, infection) in patients with chronic adrenal insufficiency.

The mineralocorticoid dosage can be more easily monitored on the basis of blood pressure and plasma renin activity. Dehydroepiandrosterone replacement in women with primary adrenal insufficiency should be considered, because there are an increasing number of studies indicating additional beneficial effects of this drug in patients who cannot otherwise produce androgens.

Summary

Adrenal insufficiency is a rare disorder, usually with gradually evolving clinical symptoms and signs. Occasionally, an acute adrenal insufficiency crisis can become a life-threatening condition because of acute interruption of a normal or hyperfunctioning adrenal or pituitary gland or sudden interruption of adrenal replacement therapy. Acute stress situations (eg, trauma, infection, surgery) can aggravate the symptomatology, dominated by hypotension and shock and sometimes associated with abdominal pain and complicated by symptoms related to the disease causing the adrenal insufficiency.

A simple strategy of diagnostic screening and early intervention with sodium chloride–containing fluids and hydrocortisone, at least until the emergency basal and postcorticotropin cortisol values are available, should be widely implemented for cases with suspicion of an acute Addison disease crisis. Recently recognized risk groups include patients with AIDS or severe head trauma.

In contrast to the rather generous replacement dosage used in emergency situations, the chronic replacement dosage for patients with adrenal insufficiency should be as low as possible with clear instructions for dosage adjustments in case of stress or acute emergencies.

Relative adrenal insufficiency is increasingly recognized in patients with critical illness, especially when associated with sepsis or circulatory failure. The diagnostic criteria and optimal treatment strategy differ from those when the adrenal insufficiency itself is causing the disease.

References

[1] Stewart PM, Quinkler MO. Mineralocorticoid deficiency. In: Degroot LJ, Jameson JL, editors. Endocrinology. Philadelphia: WB Saunders; 2005. p. 2491–9.
[2] de Herder WW, van der Lely AJ. Addisonian crisis and relative adrenal failure. Rev Endocr Metab Disord 2003;4(2):143–7.
[3] Torrey SP. Recognition and management of adrenal emergencies. Emerg Med Clin North Am 2005;23(3):687–702.
[4] Vallotton MB. Endocrine emergencies. Disorders of the adrenal cortex. Baillieres Clin Endocrinol Metab 1992;6(1):41–56.
[5] Salvatori R. Adrenal insufficiency. JAMA 2005;294(19):2481–8.
[6] Arafah BM. Hypothalamic pituitary adrenal function during critical illness: limitations of current assessment methods. J Clin Endocrinol Metab 2006;91(10):3725–45.
[7] Van den Berghe G, de Zegher F, Bouillon R. Clinical review 95: acute and prolonged critical illness as different neuroendocrine paradigms. J Clin Endocrinol Metab 1998;83(6):1827–34.
[8] Cooper MS, Stewart PM. Current concepts—corticosteroid insufficiency in acutely ill patients. N Engl J Med 2003;348(8):727–34.
[9] Freda PU, Bilezikian JP. The hypothalamus-pituitary-adrenal axis in HIV disease. AIDS Read 1999;9(1):43–50.
[10] Urban RJ. Hypopituitarism after acute brain injury. Growth Horm IGF Res 2006;16(Suppl A):S25–9.
[11] Cole TJ, Blendy JA, Monaghan AP, et al. Targeted disruption of the glucocorticoid receptor gene blocks adrenergic chromaffin cell development and severely retards lung maturation. Genes Dev 1995;9:1608–21.
[12] Cole TJ, Myles K, Purton JF, et al. GRKO mice express an aberrant dexamethasone-binding glucocorticoid receptor, but are profoundly glucocorticoid resistant. Mol Cell Endocrinol 2001;173:193–202.
[13] Oelkers W. Adrenal insufficiency. N Engl J Med 1996;335(16):1206–12.
[14] Coolens JL, Van Baelen H, Heyns W. Clinical use of unbound plasma cortisol as calculated from total cortisol and corticosteroid-binding globulin. J Steroid Biochem 1987;26:197–202.
[15] Vanhorebeek I, Peeters RP, Vander Perre S, et al. Cortisol response to critical illness: effect of intensive insulin therapy. J Clin Endocrinol Metab 2006;91(10):3803–13.
[16] Van Vliet G, Czernichow P. Screening for neonatal endocrinopathies: rationale, methods and results. Semin Neonatol 2004;9(1):75–85.
[17] Lukert BP. Editorial: glucocorticoid replacement—how much is enough? J Clin Endocrinol Metab 2006;91(3):793–4.

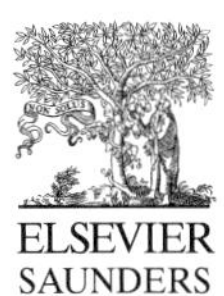
ELSEVIER
SAUNDERS

Endocrinol Metab Clin N Am
35 (2006) 777–791

ENDOCRINOLOGY
AND METABOLISM
CLINICS
OF NORTH AMERICA

The Dynamic Neuroendocrine Response to Critical Illness

Lies Langouche, PhD,
Greet Van den Berghe, MD, PhD*

Department of Intensive Care Medicine, Katholieke Universiteit Leuven, Herestraat 49, B-300 Leuven, Belgium

Sophisticated mechanical devices, a wide array of drugs, and high-technologic monitoring systems have increased tremendously the immediate, short-term survival of critically ill patients suffering from acute, previously lethal, insults. Most of these patients are discharged from an ICU within a few days. At least 30% of the patients, however, enter a chronic phase of critical illness during which they remain dependent on vital organ support and face a more than 20% risk for death. This high mortality usually is ascribed to nonresolving failure of multiple organ systems and vulnerability to infectious complications, rather than determined by the type or severity of the initial disease for which they were admitted to an ICU. Prolonged critical illness is accompanied further by ongoing hypercatabolism, despite artificial feeding, resulting in a profound decrease of lean body mass in the presence of relative preservation of adipose tissue. This induces weakness and prolongs convalescence. Patients become susceptible to infectious complications resulting from acquired impairment of innate immunity, and at the same time, they are at risk for developing excessive systemic inflammation and coagulation disorders, all increasing morbidity and risk for death.

Critical illness is characterized by a uniform dysregulation of all hypothalamic–anterior pituitary axes, long known to contribute to the high risk for morbidity and mortality. Erroneously extrapolating the changes observed in the acute-disease state to the chronic phase of critical illness has misled investigators to use certain endocrine treatments that unexpectedly increased rather than decreased mortality [1,2]. Therefore, a thorough understanding of the pathophysiology underlying these neuroendocrine changes is vital. It is now clear that the neuroendocrine responses to acute and prolonged

* Corresponding author.
E-mail address: greta.vandenberghe@med.kuleuven.be (G. Van den Berghe).

0889-8529/06/$ - see front matter
doi:10.1016/j.ecl.2006.09.007
endo.theclinics.com

critical illness are substantially different [3,4]. Another reason for the misjudgment was that results from early studies on this topic were confounded by side effects of many drugs, such as dopamine, which profoundly affect the circulating concentrations of most anterior pituitary–dependent hormones [5]. This review discusses the updated knowledge on the biphasic alterations occurring within the neuroendocrine system (Table 1) observed during the two phases of critical illness and summarizes the therapeutic implications of these novel insights.

The somatotropic axis

Growth hormone (GH) is secreted by the somatotropes in the pituitary and is essential for linear growth during childhood but serves many more important functions throughout life [6]. The regulation of the physiologic pulsatile release of GH, consisting of peak serum GH levels alternating with virtually undetectable troughs, is important for its metabolic effects [7]. Hypothalamic GH-releasing hormone (GHRH) stimulates, and somatostatin inhibits, the secretion of GH. Several synthetic GH-releasing peptides (GHRPs) and nonpeptide analogs with potent GH-releasing activity have been developed [8]. These GHRPs act via a G-protein–coupled receptor located in the hypothalamus and the pituitary [9]. Ghrelin is a highly conserved endogenous ligand for this receptor and seems to be a third key

Table 1
Overview of the neuroendocrine changes in the acute and in the prolonged phase of critical illness

Hormone	Acute phase	Prolonged phase
1. Somatotropic axis		
Pulsatile GH release	↑	↓
IGF-I	↓	↓↓
ALS	↓	↓↓
IGFBP-3	↓	↓↓
2. Thyroid axis		
Pulsatile TRH release	↑≡	↓
T_4	↑≡	↓
T_3	↓	↓↓
rT_3	↑	↑≡
3. Gonadal and lactotropic axis		
Pulsatile LH release	↑≡	↓
Testosterone	↓	↓↓
Pulsatile PRL release	↑	↓
4. Adrenal axis		
Corticotropin	↑	↓
Cortisol	↑↑	↑≡↓
CBG	↑	≡

Abbreviations: ↑, increase in circulating levels; ↓, decrease in circulating levels; ≡, recurrence to normal circulating levels.

factor in the physiologic control of GH release [10]. GH exerts direct and indirect effects, the latter mediated by insulin-like growth factor-I (IGF-I), of which the bioactivity in turn is regulated by several IGF-binding proteins (IGFBPs).

The acute phase of critical illness

During the first hours to days after an acute insult, the GH profile changes dramatically. The pulse frequency is increased, peak GH levels are elevated, and interpulse concentrations are high [3,11]. Concomitantly, a state of peripheral GH resistance develops, triggered in part by cytokines, such as tumor necrosis factor α and interleukin 6 [11,12]. Despite the clearly enhanced GH secretion, serum concentrations of IGF-I, GH-dependent IGFBP-3 and acid-labile subunit (ALS) decrease [11,13].

A reduced negative feedback inhibition caused by reduced expression of the GH receptor and, therefore, low circulating IGF-I, is suggested as the primary event driving the abundant release of GH in the acute phase of stress [13,14]. Theoretically, this may enhance the direct lipolytic and insulin-antagonizing effects of GH, resulting in elevated fatty acid and glucose levels in the circulation, whereas indirect, IGF-I–mediated somatotropic effects of GH are attenuated. As a result, costly anabolism, largely mediated by IGF-I and considered less vital at this time, may be postponed, which seems appropriate in the struggle for survival.

The prolonged phase of critical illness

Clinical recovery is preceded by a rapid normalization of theses changes. In contrast, in prolonged critically ill patients, when recovery does not occur within a few days, a different GH secretion pattern arises. The pulsatile release of GH becomes suppressed, whereas the nonpulsatile fraction of GH release remains somewhat elevated [15–17]. A strong positive correlation is found between the pulsatile fraction of GH release and circulating IGF-I, IGFBP-3, and ALS levels, which suggests that the loss of pulsatile GH release contributes to the low levels of IGF-I, IGFBP-3, and ALS in prolonged critical illness [15–17]. Furthermore, the administration of GH secretagogues is shown to increase IGF-I and GH-dependent IGFBP levels [15,16]. This indicates that GH responsiveness at least partially recovers in the chronic phase of critical illness. Because the robust release of GH in response to GH secretagogues excludes a possible inability of the somatotropes to synthesize GH, the origin of the relative hyposomatotropism probably is situated within the hypothalamus. A hypothalamic deficiency or inactivity of endogenous GH secretagogues, not of GHRH, is a plausible mediator, as GH release in response to GHRH injection is less pronounced than to a GHRP-2 injection in prolonged critical illness [7].

This chronic GH deficiency, resulting from lack of pulsatile GH secretion, could contribute to the pathogenesis of the wasting syndrome that characterizes prolonged critical illness. This is suggested from the tight relation between biochemical markers of impaired anabolism, such as low serum osteocalcin and leptin concentrations, and the low serum levels of IGF-I and ternary complex binding proteins [17].

The thyroid axis

Thyrotropin-releasing hormone (TRH), secreted by the hypothalamus, stimulates the pituitary thyrotropes to produce thyrotropin, which in turn regulates the synthesis and secretion of thyroid hormones in the thyroid gland. Thyroid hormones are essential for the regulation of energy metabolism and have profound effects on differentiation and growth [18]. Although the thyroid gland predominantly produces thyroxine (T_4), the biologic activity of thyroid hormones is exerted largely by triiodothyronine (T_3) [18]. Different types of deiodinases are responsible for the peripheral activation of T_4 to either T_3 or to the biologically inactive reverse T_3 (rT_3), processes that inherently require the presence of specific thyroid hormone transporters [19,20]. The thyroid hormones in their turn exert an inhibitory feedback control on TRH and thyrotropin secretion.

The acute phase of critical illness

The early response of the thyroid axis after the onset of severe physical stress consists of a rapid decline in the circulating levels of T_3 and a rise in rT_3 levels, predominantly because of altered peripheral conversion of T_4 [21]. Thyrotropin and T_4 levels are elevated briefly but subsequently normalize, although in those who are more severely ill, T_4 levels also may decrease [22]. Although serum thyrotropin levels measured in a single daytime sample are normal in acute critical illness, the thyrotropin profile already is affected, as the normal nocturnal thyrotropin surge is absent [23]. The low T_3 levels persist beyond thyrotropin normalization, a condition referred to as "the low T_3 syndrome." The decrease in circulating T_3 during the first 24 hours after an insult reflects the severity of illness [24]. Furthermore, T_3 levels correlate inversely with mortality [25,26].

Cytokines might be involved in the pathogenesis of the low T_3 syndrome, because they are capable of mimicking the acute stress response of the thyroid axis [27,28]. Cytokine antagonists fail, however, to restore normal thyroid function after endotoxemic challenge [29,30]. Other potential factors of the low T_3 syndrome at the tissue level include low concentrations of thyroid hormone-binding proteins and inhibition of hormone binding, transport, and metabolism by elevated levels of free fatty acids and bilirubin [31]. The immediate fall in circulating T_3 during starvation is interpreted as an adaptation to reduce energy expenditure, thus not warranting intervention [32]. Whether or not this also applies to the reduced thyroid hormone action in the acute phase of critical illness remains controversial [33].

The prolonged phase of critical illness

Patients who need prolonged intensive care show, in addition to the absent nocturnal thyrotropin surge, a dramatically reduced pulsatile thyrotropin secretion. Furthermore, serum levels of T_4 and T_3 are low, and in particular, the decline in T_3 correlates positively with the diminished pulsatile release of thyrotropin [34]. The prognostic value of the disturbed thyroid axis with regard to mortality is illustrated by lower thyrotropin, T_4, and T_3 and higher rT_3 levels in patients who ultimately die compared with those who survive prolonged critical illness [35].

An impaired capacity of the thyrotropes to synthesize thyrotropin, an alteration in set-point for feedback inhibition, inadequate TRH-induced stimulation of thyrotropin, and elevated somatostatin tone may explain these findings. Reduced TRH gene expression in the hypothalamus is described in chronically ill patients who died, which is in line with a predominantly central origin of the suppressed thyroid axis, similar to changes in the somatotropic axis [36]. In addition, the rise in thyrotropin secretion and in peripheral thyroid hormone levels with an intravenous infusion of TRH in prolonged critically ill patients is consistent with such an interpretation [16,17]. Because only the combined infusion of TRH with GHRP improves the pulsatility of the thyrotropin secretory pattern, the reduced levels of endogenous GH secretagogues also may be involved [16]. Because circulating cytokine levels usually are much lower than in the acute phase, they are less likely to be important at this stage of the disease [37]. But other factors, such as endogenous dopamine and prolonged hypercortisolism, may be important [38,39].

In the chronic phase of critical illness, the peripheral metabolism of thyroid hormone also is disturbed and contributes to the low T_3 syndrome. This is illustrated by a reduced activity of type 1 deiodinase (D1), the enzyme-mediating peripheral conversion of T_4 to T_3, and the induction of type 3 deiodinase (D3) activity, responsible for conversion of T_4 to inactive rT_3 [40]. Serum levels of rT_3 and T_3/rT_3 indeed were demonstrated to correlate with postmortem tissue deiodinase activity [35]. Interestingly, concomitant infusion of TRH and GHRP-2 not only increased thyrotropin, T_4, and T_3 levels but also prevented the rise in rT_3 seen with TRH alone. This suggests that deiodinase activity may be affected by GHRP-2, either directly or indirectly, through its effect on the somatotropic axis. Combined administration of TRH and GHRP-2 to a rabbit model of prolonged critical illness decreased D3 activity, whereas TRH infusion alone augmented D1 activity, showing that D1 suppression in critical illness is related to alterations within the thyroid axis, whereas D3 is increased under joint control of the somatotropic and thyroid axes [41,42]. Regulation of thyroid hormone action at the level of the thyroid hormone receptor also seems to be altered by critical illness, possibly causing an upregulated thyroid hormone sensitivity in response to low T_3 levels [43].

The gonadal and lactotropic axis

Gonadotropin-releasing hormone (GnRH), secreted in a pulsatile pattern by the hypothalamus, stimulates the release of luteinizing hormone (LH) and follicle-stimulating hormone (FSH) from the gonadotropes in the pituitary [44]. In women, LH mediates androgen production by the ovary, whereas FSH stimulates the aromatization of androgens to estrogens in the ovary. In men, LH stimulates androgen production by Leydig's cells in the testes, whereas the combined action of FSH and testosterone on Sertoli's cells supports spermatogenesis. Sex steroids exert a negative feedback on GnRH and gonadotropin secretion. Several other hormones and cytokines also are involved in the complex regulation of the gonadal axis [44].

Prolactin (PRL) is a well-known stress hormone produced by the lactotropes in the pituitary, which is physiologically secreted in a pulsatile and diurnal pattern, and is presumed to have immune-enhancing properties [45]. Physiologic control of PRL secretion largely is under the control of dopamine, but several other PRL-inhibiting and -releasing factors can modulate PRL secretion [46].

The acute phase of critical illness

Acute physical stress, such as surgery or myocardial infarction, brings along an immediate fall in the serum levels of testosterone, even though LH levels are elevated [47–49]. This suggests an immediate suppression of androgen production Leydig's cells, which may be viewed, at least in the short term, as an attempt to reduce energy consumption and conserve substrates for more vital functions. Involvement of cytokines again is possible, as put forward by experimental studies [50,51].

PRL levels rise in response to acute physical or psychologic stress [3,52]. Factors possibly involved are vasoactive intestinal peptide, oxytocin, and dopaminergic pathways, but again cytokines or as yet uncharacterized factors also may play a role. The rise in PRL levels after acute stress is believed to contribute to the vital activation of the immune system early in the disease process, but this remains speculative.

The prolonged phase of critical illness

More dramatic changes develop within the male gonadal axis with prolongation of the disease, and hypogonadotropism ensues [53,54]. The circulating levels of testosterone become extremely low and often even are undetectable, in the presence of suppressed mean LH concentrations and pulsatile LH release [55,56]. Total estradiol levels also are relatively low but the level of bioavailable estradiol probably is maintained in view of the simultaneous decrease in sex-hormone–binding globulin [56]. Alternatively, a remarkable rise in estrogen levels is observed in other studies [44]. Together, these data point to increased aromatization of androgens. Because exogenous GnRH is only partially and transiently effective in correcting these abnormalities, they must result from combined central and peripheral defects within the male gonadal axis [56]. Endogenous dopamine, opiates, and in particular the maintained bioactive estradiol level all could be involved as could prolonged exposure of the brain to increased local levels of cytokines [50,55–57]. As testosterone is the most important endogenous anabolic steroid, the abnormalities in the gonadal axis could be important with regard to the catabolic state of critical illness.

The pulsatile fraction of PRL release becomes suppressed in patients in the prolonged phase of critical illness [3,34]. It is unclear whether or not the blunted PRL secretion contributes to the immune suppression or increased susceptibility to infection associated with prolonged critical illness [58]. Endogenous dopamine may, again hypothetically, play a role because exogenous dopamine, a frequently used inotropic drug, suppresses PRL secretion further and concomitantly aggravates T-lymphocyte dysfunction and disturbed neutrophil chemotaxis [38,59].

The adrenal axis

The hypothalamic corticotropin-releasing hormone (CRH) controls the pituitary corticotropes for release of corticotropin, which stimulates the adrenal cortex to produce cortisol [60]. In stress-free healthy humans, cortisol is secreted according to a diurnal pattern and exerts a negative feedback control on both hormones. More than 90% of circulating cortisol is bound to binding proteins, predominantly corticosteroid-binding globulin (CBG) but also albumin; however, only the free hormone is biologically active [61].

The acute phase of critical illness

In the early phase of critical illness, cortisol levels usually rise in response to an increased release of CRH and corticotropin, but the diurnal variation in cortisol secretion is lost [60]. This rise is caused either directly or via resistance to or inhibition of the negative feedback mechanism exerted by cortisol [60,62]. Moreover, CBG levels are decreased substantially, in part the result of elastase-induced cleavage, resulting in proportionally much higher increases in the free hormone [63–67]. Cortisol production and glucocorticoid receptor number or affinity are modulated by several elevated cytokines in acute illness [68].

An appropriate activation of the hypothalamic-pituitary-adrenal axis and cortisol response to critical illness is essential for survival, because very high and low cortisol levels are associated with increased mortality [69–74]. High cortisol levels reflect more severe stress, whereas low levels point to an inability to respond to stress sufficiently, which is labeled "relative adrenal insuffiency." The vital stress-induced hypercortisolism in critically ill patients fosters the acute provision of energy by shifting carbohydrate, fat, and protein metabolism; protects against excessive inflammation by suppression of the inflammatory response; and improves the hemodynamic status by induction of fluid retention and sensitization of the vasopressor response to catecholamines [3,68].

The prolonged phase of critical illness

Cortisol levels usually remain elevated in the chronic phase of critical illness, which seems to be driven by non–corticotropin-mediated pathways, because corticotropin levels are decreased [75,76]. Cortisol levels slowly decrease, only reaching normal levels in the recovery phase [3]. CBG levels recover in the chronic phase of illness [65,67]. Whether or not the persisting elevation in cortisol is beneficial exclusively in prolonged critical illness remains uncertain. Theoretically, it could contribute to the increased susceptibility to infectious complications. Alternatively, the risk for "relative adrenal failure" may increase in the chronic phase of critical illness and may predispose to adverse outcome [77].

Therapeutic implications

Before considering therapeutic intervention, it is extremely important, although very difficult, to differentiate between beneficial and harmful neuroendocrine responses to critical illness. The endocrine adaptations to the acute phase seem to direct toward reducing energy and substrate consumption, driving the release of substrates for vital tissues, postponing costly anabolism, and modulating the immune responses to improve chances for survival. The hypercatabolic reaction probably is beneficial; thus, at present, there is no supportive evidence to intervene. In the chronic phase of critical illness, however, sustained hypercatabolism, despite feeding, results in substantial loss of lean body mass and often concomitant fatty infiltration of vital organs, which may compromise vital functions, cause weakness, and delay or hamper recovery [78]. Therefore, therapeutic intervention to correct these abnormalities theoretically may offer perspectives to improve survival.

Administration of pharmacologic doses of GH, inspired by the assumption of sustained GH resistance in the prolonged phase of critical illness, unexpectedly increases morbidity and mortality [1]. It is now clear that peripheral GH sensitivity recovers, at least partially, in the chronic phase of critical illness and that the administration of such high doses (up to

20-fold substitution dose) may have exposed the patients to toxic side effects. Infusion of IGF-I in healthy volunteers, however, did inhibit protein breakdown and stimulated protein synthesis, although the efficacy of the intervention was reduced with prolonged administration [79]. Initial trials studying administration of high doses of glucocorticoids clearly show that this strategy is ineffective and perhaps even harmful [2,80]. In contrast, studies using—still supraphysiologic—low-dose glucocorticoid replacement therapy for relative adrenal insufficiency report beneficial effects, at least in patients who have septic shock [73,80]. Administration of hydrocortisone in this so-called "replacement dose," however, resulted in several-fold higher total and free cortisol levels, indicating that re-evaluation of the doses used is warranted [67]. It remains controversial whether or not administration of thyroid hormone to patients who are critically ill is beneficial or harmful; also, there is no conclusive clinical benefit demonstrated for androgen treatment in prolonged critical illness [81–83].

As most hypothalamic–pituitary axes show a decreased activity during prolonged critical illness, treatment with hypothalamic-releasing factors to re-activate the pituitary may be more effective and safer than administration of pituitary or peripheral hormones. Infusions of GH secretagogues, TRH or GnRH, are shown to re-activate the corresponding pituitary axes, resulting in elevated levels of the peripheral effector hormones (vide supra). Furthermore, concomitant infusion of GHRP-2 and TRH re-activates the somatotropic and thyrotropic axes but prevents the rise of inactive rT_3 levels seen with TRH alone [16]. This combined intervention is shown associated with a reduction in hypercatabolism and stimulation of anabolism [17]. Additional coactivation of the gonadal axis by administering GnRH together with GHRP-2 and TRH in prolonged critically ill men restored, at least partially, the three pituitary axes and seemed to induce an even more pronounced anabolic effect [84]. These data underline the interaction among the different endocrine axes and the superiority of jointly correcting all hypothalamic–pituitary defects instead of applying a single hormone treatment. Overstimulation of the respective axes, and, thus, toxic side effects of high peripheral hormone levels, are avoided, because endogenous negative feedback mechanisms and the ability to adaptively change peripheral hormonal metabolism remain intact [16,17,84].

It is crucial to take into account certain side effects of single-hormone treatments when interpreting results of available clinical studies. High doses of either GH or glucocorticoids aggravate insulin resistance and hyperglycemia that usually develop during critical illness (reviewed in [85]). Hence, the glucose counter-regulatory toxic side effects may have surpassed any possible benefits of these therapies [1,2,80]. Although it had long been commonly accepted that stress-induced hyperglycemia is beneficial to organs that largely rely on glucose for energy supply but do not require insulin for glucose uptake, recent data on strict blood glucose control with intensive insulin therapy clearly prove otherwise. In a large group of surgical intensive care patients, this intervention strikingly lowered mortality in patients who had prolonged critical illness and largely prevented several critical illness–associated complications [86]. Moreover, even moderate hyperglycemia seemed to be detrimental to the patients [87,88]. The patients developed critical-illness polyneuropathy, bloodstream infections, acute renal failure, and anemia less frequently and were less dependent on prolonged mechanical ventilation and intensive care. In addition, a protective effect on the central and peripheral nervous system, particularly in brain-injured patients, has been demonstrated [87]. Normoglycemic control also prevented immune dysfunction, reduced systemic inflammation, protected the endothelium and hepatic mitochondrial ultrastructure and function, and lowered total and free cortisol levels [67,89–92]. A second large clinical trial, "now on" medical intensive care patients, again showed beneficial effects of intensive insulin therapy on morbidity and mortality in an ICU [93].

The concomitant administration of TRH and GHRP-2—superimposed on strict glycemic control with intensive insulin therapy—holds promise for the future but needs to be tested in a large-scale clinical outcome study, which awaits the availability of these hormone-releasing factors. Furthermore, in view of the glucose counter-regulatory effects of GH and glucocorticoids and the benefits of preventing hyperglycemia with insulin, it also could be hypothesized that when GH or glucocorticoid therapy is combined with tight blood glucose control, the negative outcome with these interventions could in part be prevented.

Summary

The anterior pituitary responds in two distinct phases to severe stress of illness and trauma (see Table 1). In the acute phase of critical illness, the pituitary is secreting actively, but target organs become resistant and concentrations of most peripheral effector hormones are low. These acute adaptations probably are beneficial in the struggle for short-term survival, for which no need for intervention seems necessary. In contrast, prolonged, intensive care–dependent critical illness is hallmarked by a uniform suppression of the neuroendocrine axes, predominantly of hypothalamic origin, which contributes to the low serum levels of the respective target-organ hormones. These chronic alterations no longer may be beneficial, as they participate in the general wasting syndrome of prolonged critical illness. Attempts to reverse these abnormalities with hormonal therapies demonstrate that the choice of hormone and corresponding dosage are of crucial importance and lack of pathophysiologic insight holds danger. The only interventions that so far have proved to affect outcome of critical illness beneficially are intensive insulin therapy and, perhaps, hydrocortisone therapy for some patients. Alternatively, concomitant reactivation of the somatotropic, thyrotropic, and gonadal axes with hypothalamic releasing factors holds promise as a safe therapy to reverse the neuroendocrine and metabolic abnormalities of prolonged critical illness.

References

[1] Takala J, Ruokonen E, Webster NR, et al. Increased mortality associated with growth hormone treatment in critically ill adults. N Engl J Med 1999;341:785–92.
[2] Roberts I, Yates D, Sandercock P, et al. Effect of intravenous corticosteroids on death within 14 days in 10008 adults with clinically significant head injury (MRC CRASH trial): randomised placebo-controlled trial. Lancet 2004;364:1321–8.
[3] Van den Berghe G, de Zegher F, et al. Clinical review 95: acute and prolonged critical illness as different neuroendocrine paradigms. J Clin Endocrinol Metab 1998;83:1827–34.
[4] Weekers F, Van Herck E, Coopmans W, et al. A novel in vivo rabbit model of hypercatabolic critical illness reveals a biphasic neuroendocrine stress response. Endocrinology 2002;143: 764–74.
[5] Debaveye Y, Van den Berghe G. Is there still a place for dopamine in the modern intensive care unit? Anesth Analg 2004;98:461–8.
[6] Cummings DE, Merriam GR. Growth hormone therapy in adults. Annu Rev Med 2003;54: 513–33.
[7] Van den Berghe G, Baxter RC, Weekers F, et al. A paradoxical gender dissociation within the growth hormone/insulin-like growth factor I axis during protracted critical illness. J Clin Endocrinol Metab 2000;85:183–92.
[8] Bowers CY, Momany FA, Reynolds GA, et al. On the in vitro and in vivo activity of a new synthetic hexapeptide that acts on the pituitary to specifically release growth hormone. Endocrinology 1984;114:1537–45.
[9] Howard AD, Feighner SD, Cully DF, et al. A receptor in pituitary and hypothalamus that functions in growth hormone release. Science 1996;273:974–7.
[10] Kojima M, Hosoda H, Date Y, et al. Ghrelin is a growth-hormone-releasing acylated peptide from stomach. Nature 1999;402:656–60.
[11] Ross R, Miell J, Freeman E, et al. Critically ill patients have high basal growth hormone levels with attenuated oscillatory activity associated with low levels of insulin-like growth factor-I. Clin Endocrinol (Oxf) 1991;35:47–54.
[12] Baxter RC, Hawker FH, To C, et al. Thirty-day monitoring of insulin-like growth factors and their binding proteins in intensive care unit patients. Growth Horm IGF Res 1998;8: 455–63.
[13] Hermansson M, Wickelgren RB, Hammarqvist F, et al. Measurement of human growth hormone receptor messenger ribonucleic acid by a quantitative polymerase chain reaction-based assay: demonstration of reduced expression after elective surgery. J Clin Endocrinol Metab 1997;82:421–8.
[14] Defalque D, Brandt N, Ketelslegers JM, et al. GH insensitivity induced by endotoxin injection is associated with decreased liver GH receptors. Am J Physiol 1999;276:E565–72.
[15] Van den Berghe G, de Zegher F, Veldhuis JD, et al. The somatotropic axis in critical illness: effect of continuous growth hormone (GH)-releasing hormone and GH-releasing peptide-2 infusion. J Clin Endocrinol Metab 1997;82:590–9.
[16] Van den Berghe G, de Zegher F, Baxter RC, et al. Neuroendocrinology of prolonged critical illness: effects of exogenous thyrotropin-releasing hormone and its combination with growth hormone secretagogues. J Clin Endocrinol Metab 1998;83:309–19.
[17] Van den Berghe G, Wouters P, Weekers F, et al. Reactivation of pituitary hormone release and metabolic improvement by infusion of growth hormone-releasing peptide and thyrotropin-releasing hormone in patients with protracted critical illness. J Clin Endocrinol Metab 1999;84:1311–23.
[18] Yen PM. Physiological and molecular basis of thyroid hormone action. Physiol Rev 2001;81: 1097–142.

[19] Bianco AC, Salvatore D, Gereben B, et al. Biochemistry, cellular and molecular biology, and physiological roles of the iodothyronine selenodeiodinases. Endocr Rev 2002;23:38–89.

[20] Friesema EC, Jansen J, Visser TJ. Thyroid hormone transporters. Biochem Soc Trans 2005; 33:228–32.

[21] Michalaki M, Vagenakis AG, Makri M, et al. Dissociation of the early decline in serum T(3) concentration and serum IL-6 rise and TNFalpha in nonthyroidal illness syndrome induced by abdominal surgery. J Clin Endocrinol Metab 2001;86:4198–205.

[22] Van den Berghe G. Novel insights into the neuroendocrinology of critical illness. Eur J Endocrinol 2000;143:1–13.

[23] Romijn JA, Wiersinga WM. Decreased nocturnal surge of thyrotropin in nonthyroidal illness. J Clin Endocrinol Metab 1990;70:35–42.

[24] McIver B, Gorman CA. Euthyroid sick syndrome: an overview. Thyroid 1997;7:125–32.

[25] Rothwell PM, Lawler PG. Prediction of outcome in intensive care patients using endocrine parameters. Crit Care Med 1995;23:78–83.

[26] Rothwell PM, Udwadia ZF, Lawler PG. Thyrotropin concentration predicts outcome in critical illness. Anaesthesia 1993;48:373–6.

[27] Boelen A, Platvoet-ter Schiphorst MC, Bakker O, et al. The role of cytokines in the lipopolysaccharide-induced sick euthyroid syndrome in mice. J Endocrinol 1995;146: 475–83.

[28] Van der Poll T, Romijn JA, Wiersinga WM, et al. Tumor necrosis factor: a putative mediator of the sick euthyroid syndrome in man. J Clin Endocrinol Metab 1990;71:1567–72.

[29] Van der Poll T, Van Zee KJ, Endert E, et al. Interleukin-1 receptor blockade does not affect endotoxin-induced changes in plasma thyroid hormone and thyrotropin concentrations in man. J Clin Endocrinol Metab 1995;80:1341–6.

[30] Van der Poll T, Endert E, Coyle SM, et al. Neutralization of TNF does not influence endotoxininduced changes in thyroid hormone metabolism in humans. Am J Physiol 1999;276: R357–62.

[31] Lim CF, Docter R, Visser TJ, et al. Inhibition of thyroxine transport into cultured rat hepatocytes by serum of nonuremic critically ill patients: effects of bilirubin and nonesterified fatty acids. J Clin Endocrinol Metab 1993;76:1165–72.

[32] Gardner DF, Kaplan MM, Stanley CA, et al. Effect of tri-iodothyronine replacement on the metabolic and pituitary responses to starvation. N Engl J Med 1979;300:579–84.

[33] De Groot LJ. Dangerous dogmas in medicine: the nonthyroidal illness syndrome. J Clin Endocrinol Metab 1999;84:151–64.

[34] Van den Berghe G, de Zegher F, Veldhuis JD, et al. Thyrotrophin and prolactin release in prolonged critical illness: dynamics of spontaneous secretion and effects of growth hormone-secretagogues. Clin Endocrinol (Oxf) 1997;47:599–612.

[35] Peeters RP, Wouters PJ, van Toor H, et al. Serum rT3 and T3/rT3 are prognostic markers in critically ill patients and are associated with post-mortem tissue deiodinase activities. J Clin Endocrinol Metab 2005;90(8):4559–61.

[36] Fliers E, Guldenaar SE, Wiersinga WM, et al. Decreased hypothalamic thyrotropin-releasing hormone gene expression in patients with nonthyroidal illness. J Clin Endocrinol Metab 1997;82:4032–6.

[37] Damas P, Reuter A, Gysen P, et al. Tumor necrosis factor and interleukin-1 serum levels during severe sepsis in humans. Crit Care Med 1989;17:975–8.

[38] Van den Berghe G, de Zegher F, Lauwers P. Dopamine and the sick euthyroid syndrome in critical illness. Clin Endocrinol (Oxf) 1994;41:731–7.

[39] Faglia G, Ferrari C, Beck-Peccoz P, et al. Reduced plasma thyrotropin response to thyrotropin releasing hormone after dexamethasone administration in normal subjects. Horm Metab Res 1973;5:289–92.

[40] Peeters RP, Wouters PJ, Kaptein E, et al. Reduced activation and increased inactivation of thyroid hormone in tissues of critically ill patients. J Clin Endocrinol Metab 2003;88: 3202–11.

[41] Weekers F, Michalaki M, Coopmans W, et al. Endocrine and metabolic effects of growth hormone (GH) compared with GH-releasing peptide, thyrotropin-releasing hormone, and insulin infusion in a rabbit model of prolonged critical illness. Endocrinology 2004;145: 205–13.
[42] Debaveye Y, Ellger B, Mebis L, et al. Tissue deiodinase activity during prolonged critical illness: effects of exogenous thyrotropin-releasing hormone and its combination with growth hormone-releasing peptide-2. Endocrinology 2005;146:5604–11.
[43] Timmer DC, Peeters RP, Wouters P, et al. Thyroid hormone receptor alpha splice variants in livers of critically ill patients. Thyroid, in press.
[44] Spratt DI. Altered gonadal steroidogenesis in critical illness: is treatment with anabolic steroids indicated? Best Pract Res Clin Endocrinol Metab 2001;15:479–94.
[45] Ben Jonathan N. Dopamine: a prolactin-inhibiting hormone. Endocr Rev 1985;6:564–89.
[46] Samson WK, Taylor MM, Baker JR. Prolactin-releasing peptides. Regul Pept 2003;114:1–5.
[47] Wang C, Chan V, Yeung RT. Effect of surgical stress on pituitary-testicular function. Clin Endocrinol (Oxf) 1978;9:255–66.
[48] Wang C, Chan V, Tse TF, et al. Effect of acute myocardial infarction on pituitary-testicular function. Clin Endocrinol (Oxf) 1978;9:249–53.
[49] Dong Q, Hawker F, McWilliam D, et al. Circulating immunoreactive inhibin and testosterone levels in men with critical illness. Clin Endocrinol (Oxf) 1992;36:399–404.
[50] Rivier C, Vale W, Brown M. In the rat, interleukin-1 alpha and -beta stimulate adrenocorticotropin and catecholamine release. Endocrinology 1989;125:3096–102.
[51] Guo H, Calkins JH, Sigel MM, et al. Interleukin-2 is a potent inhibitor of Leydig cell steroidogenesis. Endocrinology 1990;127:1234–9.
[52] Noel GL, Suh HK, Stone JG, et al. Human prolactin and growth hormone release during surgery and other conditions of stress. J Clin Endocrinol Metab 1972;35:840–51.
[53] Vogel AV, Peake GT, Rada RT. Pituitary-testicular axis dysfunction in burned men. J Clin Endocrinol Metab 1985;60:658–65.
[54] Woolf PD, Hamill RW, McDonald JV, et al. Transient hypogonadotropic hypogonadism caused by critical illness. J Clin Endocrinol Metab 1985;60:444–50.
[55] Van den Berghe G, de Zegher F, Lauwers P, et al. Luteinizing hormone secretion and hypoandrogenaemia in critically ill men: effect of dopamine. Clin Endocrinol (Oxf) 1994;41: 563–9.
[56] Van den Berghe G, Weekers F, Baxter RC, et al. Five-day pulsatile gonadotropin-releasing hormone administration unveils combined hypothalamic-pituitary-gonadal defects underlying profound hypoandrogenism in men with prolonged critical illness. J Clin Endocrinol Metab 2001;86:3217–26.
[57] Cicero TJ, Bell RD, Wiest WG, et al. Function of the male sex organs in heroin and methadone users. N Engl J Med 1975;292:882–7.
[58] Meakins JL, Pietsch JB, Bubenick O, et al. Delayed hypersensitivity: indicator of acquired failure of host defenses in sepsis and trauma. Ann Surg 1977;186:241–50.
[59] Devins SS, Miller A, Herndon BL, et al. Effects of dopamine on T-lymphocyte proliferative responses and serum prolactin concentrations in critically ill patients. Crit Care Med 1992; 20:1644–9.
[60] Cooper MS, Stewart PM. Corticosteroid insufficiency in acutely ill patients. N Engl J Med 2003;348:727–34.
[61] Burchard K. A review of the adrenal cortex and severe inflammation: quest of the "eucorticoid" state. J Trauma 2001;51:800–14.
[62] Rivier C, Vale W. Modulation of stress-induced ACTH release by corticotropin-releasing factor, catecholamines and vasopressin. Nature 1983;305:325–7.
[63] Pemberton PA, Stein PE, Pepys MB, et al. Hormone binding globulins undergo serpin conformational change in inflammation. Nature 1988;336:257–8.
[64] Hammond GL, Smith CL, Paterson NA, et al. A role for corticosteroid-binding globulin in delivery of cortisol to activated neutrophils. J Clin Endocrinol Metab 1990;71:34–9.

[65] Beishuizen A, Thijs LG, Vermes I. Patterns of corticosteroid-binding globulin and the free cortisol index during septic shock and multitrauma. Intensive Care Med 2001;27: 1584–91.
[66] Hamrahian AH, Oseni TS, Arafah BM. Measurements of serum free cortisol in critically ill patients. N Engl J Med 2004;350:1629–38.
[67] Vanhorebeek I, Peeters RP, Vander Perre S, et al. Cortisol response to critical illness: effect of intensive insulin therapy. J Clin Endocrinol Metab 2006;91(10):3803–13.
[68] Marik PE, Zaloga GP. Adrenal insufficiency in the critically ill: a new look at an old problem. Chest 2002;122:1784–96.
[69] Finlay WE, McKee JI. Serum cortisol levels in severely stressed patients. Lancet 1982;1: 1414–5.
[70] Rothwell PM, Udwadia ZF, Lawler PG. Cortisol response to corticotropin and survival in septic shock. Lancet 1991;337:582–3.
[71] Span LF, Hermus AR, Bartelink AK, et al. Adrenocortical function: an indicator of severity of disease and survival in chronic critically ill patients. Intensive Care Med 1992;18:93–6.
[72] Annane D, Sebille V, Troche G, et al. A 3-level prognostic classification in septic shock based on cortisol levels and cortisol response to corticotropin. JAMA 2000;283:1038–45.
[73] Annane D, Sebille V, Charpentier C, et al. Effect of treatment with low doses of hydrocortisone and fludrocortisone on mortality in patients with septic shock. JAMA 2002;288: 862–71.
[74] Sam S, Corbridge TC, Mokhlesi B, et al. Cortisol levels and mortality in severe sepsis. Clin Endocrinol (Oxf) 2004;60:29–35.
[75] Bornstein SR, Chrousos GP. Clinical review 104: adrenocorticotropin (ACTH)- and non-ACTH-mediated regulation of the adrenal cortex: neural and immune inputs. J Clin Endocrinol Metab 1999;84:1729–36.
[76] Vermes I, Beishuizen A. The hypothalamic-pituitary-adrenal response to critical illness. Best Pract Res Clin Endocrinol Metab 2001;15:495–511.
[77] Barquist E, Kirton O. Adrenal insufficiency in the surgical intensive care unit patient. J Trauma 1997;42:27–31.
[78] Streat SJ, Beddoe AH, Hill GL. Aggressive nutritional support does not prevent protein loss despite fat gain in septic intensive care patients. J Trauma 1987;27:262–6.
[79] Russell-Jones DL, Umpleby AM, Hennessy TR, et al. Use of a leucine clamp to demonstrate that IGF-I actively stimulates protein synthesis in normal humans. Am J Physiol 1994;267: E591–8.
[80] Minneci PC, Deans KJ, Banks SM, et al. Meta-analysis: the effect of steroids on survival and shock during sepsis depends on the dose. Ann Intern Med 2004;141:47–56.
[81] Stathatos N, Levetan C, Burman KD, et al. The controversy of the treatment of critically ill patients with thyroid hormone. Best Pract Res Clin Endocrinol Metab 2001;15:465–78.
[82] Ferrando AA, Sheffield-Moore M, Wolf SE, et al. Testosterone administration in severe burns ameliorates muscle catabolism. Crit Care Med 2001;29:1936–42.
[83] Angele MK, Ayala A, Cioffi WG, et al. Testosterone: the culprit for producing splenocyte immune depression after trauma hemorrhage. Am J Physiol 1998;274:C1530–6.
[84] Van den Berghe G, Baxter RC, Weekers F, et al. The combined administration of GH-releasing peptide-2 (GHRP-2), TRH and GnRH to men with prolonged critical illness evokes superior endocrine and metabolic effects compared to treatment with GHRP-2 alone. Clin Endocrinol (Oxf) 2002;56:655–69.
[85] Langouche L, Van den Berghe G. Glucose metabolism and insulin therapy. Crit Care Clin 2006;22:119–29 [vii.].
[86] Van den Berghe G, Wouters P, Weekers F, et al. Intensive insulin therapy in critically ill patients. N Engl J Med 2001;345:1359–67.
[87] Van den Berghe G, Schoonheydt K, Becx P, et al. Insulin therapy protects the central and peripheral nervous system of intensive care patients. Neurology 2005;64:1348–53.

[88] Van den Berghe G, Wouters PJ, Bouillon R, et al. Outcome benefit of intensive insulin therapy in the critically ill: Insulin dose versus glycemic control. Crit Care Med 2003;31:359–66.

[89] Hansen TK, Thiel S, Wouters PJ, et al. Intensive insulin therapy exerts antiinflammatory effects in critically ill patients and counteracts the adverse effect of low mannose-binding lectin levels. J Clin Endocrinol Metab 2003;88:1082–8.

[90] Langouche L, Vanhorebeek I, Vlasselaers D, et al. Intensive insulin therapy protects the endothelium of critically ill patients. J Clin Invest 2005;115:2277–86.

[91] Vanhorebeek I, De Vos R, Mesotten D, et al. Protection of hepatocyte mitochondrial ultrastructure and function by strict blood glucose control with insulin in critically ill patients. Lancet 2005;365:53–9.

[92] Weekers F, Giulietti AP, Michalaki M, et al. Metabolic, endocrine, and immune effects of stress hyperglycemia in a rabbit model of prolonged critical illness. Endocrinology 2003;144:5329–38.

[93] Van den Berghe G, Wilmer A, Hermans G, et al. Intensive insulin therapy in the medical ICU. N Engl J Med 2006;354:449–61.

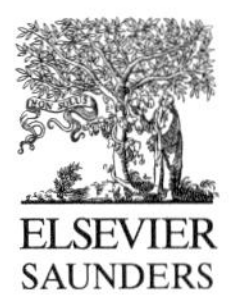

ELSEVIER
SAUNDERS

Endocrinol Metab Clin N Am
35 (2006) 793–805

ENDOCRINOLOGY
AND METABOLISM
CLINICS
OF NORTH AMERICA

Changes Within the Growth Hormone/Insulin-like Growth Factor I/IGF Binding Protein Axis During Critical Illness

Dieter Mesotten, MD, PhD*,
Greet Van den Berghe, MD, PhD

Department of Intensive Care Medicine, University Hospital Gasthuisberg, Catholic University Leuven, B-3000 Leuven, Belgium

Although giants and dwarfs have been around for ages, only a century ago the link between growth disorders and the pituitary was considered. Although transsphenoidal pituitary surgery had already been introduced in 1908 as the preferred treatment for acromegaly, the study of the physiologic properties of growth hormone (GH) had long been marred by the inevitable contamination of the crude pituitary extracts with other pituitary hormones such as thyrotropin and corticotropin [1]. In 1944 and 1970, Li and coworkers [2,3] were the first to isolate and synthesize, respectively, bovine GH. Currently, it is known that GH is released from the somatotrophs of the anterior pituitary gland in a pulsatile fashion [4]. The physiologic stimuli of GH release include stress, exercise, fasting, and sleep.

Classically, two hypothalamic hormones control GH secretion: GH-releasing hormone (GHRH), isolated in 1982 [5,6], which stimulates the production and release of GH, and somatostatin [7], which exerts an inhibitory effect. Since the 1980s, a series of synthetic GH-releasing peptides (GHRPs) and nonpeptide analogues [8], together labeled GH secretagogues, have been designed with potent GH-releasing capacities acting through a specific G-protein–coupled receptor located in the hypothalamus and the pituitary [9]. The endogenous ligand for the GH secretagogue receptor was speculative for a long time until the discovery of ghrelin. This highly

* Corresponding author. Department of Critical Care Medicine, University Hospital Gasthuisberg, B-3000 Leuven, Belgium.

E-mail address: dieter.mesotten@med.kuleuven.be (D. Mesotten).

doi:10.1016/j.ecl.2006.09.010

conserved 28-amino acid peptide originates in the oxyntic cells of the fundus of the stomach and the hypothalamic arcuate nucleus [10]. Ghrelin has emerged as a key factor alongside GHRH and somatostatin, involved in the complex control of GH secretion. These three regulatory factors act in concert, resulting in GH concentrations in the serum that alternate between peaks and virtually undetectable troughs, as observed in healthy humans [4].

Of equal importance in the regulation of GH secretion are several neural and hormonal feedback loops, primarily aimed to maintain a physiologic homeostasis. The GH autofeedback and the feedback of insulin-like growth factor I (IGF-I) stimulate somatostatin and suppress GHRH secretion in the hypothalamus; however, the dominant feedback action of IGF-I occurs directly on the pituitary gland (Fig. 1).

When GH secreted from the pituitary gland reaches the systemic circulation, it exerts its hormonal effects on the peripheral tissues, such as the liver, skeletal muscle, and bone. GH has well-known metabolic effects, such as lipolysis, stimulation of amino acid transport into muscle, and hepatic gluconeogenesis. These effects are mediated through the direct binding of GH to its receptor, with subsequent activation of the Janus kinase 2 (Jak2), signal transducers and activators of transcription 5 (STAT5) and the Shc/Ras/Raf/MAPK signal transduction pathway.

GH affects body growth and metabolism mainly through stimulation of IGF-I production [11]. This indirect pathway was revealed in 1957 by Salmon and Daughaday [12] when they showed that the uptake of inorganic

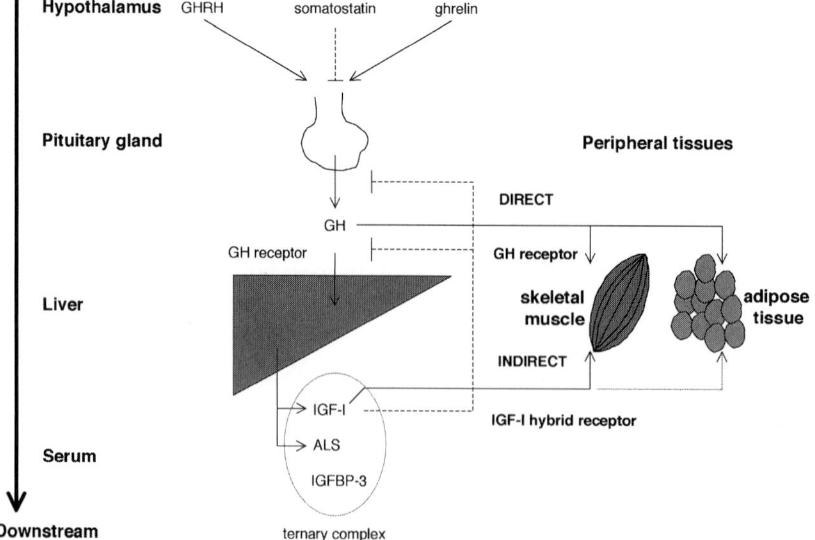

Fig. 1. Schematic overview of the somatotropic axis, where → represents stimulation; ⊥, inhibition; and dashed ⊥, feedback inhibition.

sulfate by cartilage was not affected by GH. This sulfation factor was later renamed somatomedin and, finally, IGF-I.

In the circulation of normal healthy individuals, approximately 90% of IGF-I is bound by IGF-binding protein 3 (IGFBP-3) and acid labile subunit (ALS) to form a large ternary complex, which extends the half-life of IGF-I and regulates its hypoglycemic potential [13,14]. Whereas IGFBP-3 is produced by many cell types, circulating IGF-I and ALS are almost exclusively liver derived [15,16]. The synthesis of the latter proteins is strongly stimulated by GH at the transcriptional level [17]; hence, the circulating components of the ternary complex can be used as markers of peripheral GH effect [18,19], with a better correlation with the pulsatile than the nonpulsatile fraction of the GH secretion [4]. IGFBP-5 can also form an alternative ternary complex with IGF-I and ALS [20].

Under normal circumstances, only a small fraction of IGF-I is bound by the other IGFBPs, notably IGFBP-1, 2, 4, and 6, in binary complexes [21]. IGF-I bound to these "small" IGFBPs may cross the endothelial barrier more easily, increasing its bioavailability [22]. Bioavailability of IGF-I may also be increased by proteolysis of IGFBP-3, such as during pregnancy [23] and non–insulin-dependent diabetes mellitus [24].

The somatotropic axis during critical illness

Critical illness, such as during shock or sepsis, involves a serious metabolic derangement [25]. In the first few days, the net proteolysis in combination with an increased resting energy expenditure depicts a catabolic response. Teleologically, this response may be beneficial as the amino acids, mobilized from peripheral tissues such as skeletal muscle and bone, are used by the central organs. These mobilized amino acids are involved in gluconeogenesis, ureagenesis, the synthesis of acute phase proteins, and oxidation, and are used as substrates for the immune system and wound healing [26]. This reliance on amino acids as an energy source becomes even more pronounced as organ failure progresses [27]. Systemic inflammation, with its cytokines and interleukins, appears to be the main driving force. Other potential contributors to the wasting of muscle mass include immobilization and critical illness polyneuropathy.

Several clinical studies have revealed a link between the catabolic state of critical illness and a suppressed somatotropic GH-IGF-IGFBP axis [28,29]. Additionally, experimental work has shown that lipopolysaccharide injection in animals results in GH receptor downregulation [30], leading to decreased IGF-I production [31]. Through the omission of the feedback inhibition, low IGF-I levels may stimulate GH secretion. The metabolic actions of the somatotropic axis thus undergo an adaptation such that the indirect anabolic actions of GH (through IGF-I) are reduced while the direct effects of the raised basal GH concentrations are enhanced. The latter promote lipolysis and antagonize insulin activity. Fatty acids, released from the lipolysis of triglycerides, may even further inhibit GH receptor gene expression [32].

Recent evidence suggests that the hypothalamic-pituitary response to critical illness follows a biphasic pattern, with an acute and chronic phase [33–35]. The acute phase is characterized by an actively secreting anterior pituitary gland and peripheral resistance to the anabolic hormones. Particularly for the somatotropic axis, acute critical illness results in an elevation in circulating levels of GH [28]. The number of GH bursts released by the somatotrophs is increased, and the peak GH levels, as well as interpulse concentrations, are high [36]. It remains to be elucidated which factor ultimately controls this stimulation of GH release in response to stress; however, it may resemble situations of starvation during which elevated GHRH levels and absence of inhibitory somatostatin result in enhanced circulating GH concentrations [36]. As mentioned earlier, serum concentrations of IGF-I are low during the acute phase of critical illness [37]. The concurrence of elevated GH and low IGF-I levels [38] has been interpreted as resistance to GH, which may be related to decreased expression of the GH receptor [39]. The circulating levels of IGFBPs are also affected. The low serum concentrations of IGF-I are associated with low levels of IGFBP-3 and ALS, which are all regulated by GH at the transcriptional level [37,40]. In addition, serum concentrations of the other small IGF-binding proteins, such as IGFBP-1, 2, 4, and 6, are elevated [37,41]. They normally bind only a small amount of IGF-I compared with IGFBP-3 and are not directly GH regulated. It is difficult to speculate on the consequences of these IGFBP changes during critical illness. The decrease in IGFs in ternary complexes and redistribution into the binary complexes may imply an enhanced IGF transport to the tissues, that is, increased IGF bioavailability. The increased proteolysis of IGFBP-3 during critical illness may further amplify the latter [40,42–44].

Clinical recovery from acute critical illness is preceded by a rapid normalization of these changes: an increase in serum IGF-I and IGFBP-3 levels, a lowering of serum IGFBP-1, and cessation of protease activity [40]. When the patient fails to overcome the critical illness, inevitably, he or she will enter the protracted phase after several days. Despite the fact that the initial inflammatory surge has settled [45], protein hypercatabolism continues and gives rise to functionally important complications such as prolonged immobilization, delayed weaning from mechanical ventilation, impaired tissue repair, and atrophy of the intestinal mucosa, together resulting in prolonged convalescence [46]. This wasting takes place despite adequate nutritional support [47]. Even when the patient manages to recover, the restoration of muscle mass and rehabilitation will require several months.

In the protracted phase of critical illness, the pattern of GH secretion appears to be entirely different from that during the acute phase. It displays a generally reduced pulsatile fraction, a nonpulsatile fraction that is still somewhat elevated, and a pulse frequency that remains high [29,48–50]. The combination of a deficiency of ghrelin, the endogenous ligand for the GH-secretagogue receptor, together with a reduced somatostatin tone and maintenance of some GHRH effect most likely brings about this secretory profile. The result is a mean serum GH concentration that is low to normal. This relative suppression of GH release seems to be dependent more on the length of time than on the type or severity of the critical condition. Intriguingly, a greater loss of pulsatility within the GH secretory pattern and lower IGF-I and ALS levels are observed in male patients when compared with female patients despite an indistinguishable total GH output [51]. It is unclear whether this paradoxical sexual dimorphism is associated with the apparently greater risk of adverse outcome from chronic critical illness in men.

The reduced amount of GH that is released in the pulses correlates positively with low circulating levels of IGF-I, IGFBP-3, and ALS [48–50]. The reduced ratio of GH versus IGF-I compared with that in acute critical illness does not support the notion of prolonged critical illness as a GH-resistant state [52]. The relative hyposomatotropism of essentially hypothalamic origin and preserved GH responsiveness in prolonged critical illness is affirmed by restoration of the pulsatile GH secretory pattern in conjunction with an increase in serum levels of the GH-dependent ternary complex proteins with infusion of GH secretagogues [53]. This relative GH deficiency could contribute to the wasting syndrome because the often low levels of IGF-I and ALS are closely related to biochemical markers of impaired anabolism, such as low serum levels of osteocalcin [50] and leptin [54] during prolonged critical illness.

All other pituitary axes, such as the thyrotropic, gonadotropic, adrenocortical, and lactotropic axis, are characterized by the same biphasic response [34,53]. During acute critical illness, the pituitary is activated with increased (pulsatile) levels of thyroid-stimulating hormone, luteinizing hormone, adrenocorticotropic hormone, and prolactin. During the protracted phase of critical illness, these pituitary-released hormones are decreased. Downstream in the peripheral organs, levels of thyroxine (T4) and triiodothyronine (T3), testosterone, and cortisol further decrease as the patient transcends into the chronic phase of critical illness.

Endocrine strategies for the somatotropic axis during critical illness

Growth hormone

Inspired by the beneficial effects of recombinant human GH (rhGH) in GH-deficient patients on lean body mass and bone remodeling, rhGH has long been considered as a treatment for reversing the feeding-resistant wasting syndrome. Through a wide array of small, often uncontrolled and nonrandomized studies using surrogate markers of outcome, such as the nitrogen balance, muscle glutamine concentrations, muscle strength, and weaning times, administration of high doses of human GH was generally perceived as an effective anabolic therapy in critical illness [55–59].

The first large multi-center prospective, double-blind, randomized, controlled trial on rhGH administration with sufficient power to analyze mortality revealed increased fatalities owing to septic shock or multiple organ failure in the therapeutic arm of the study [60]. In hindsight, several aspects of the study, when combined together, may be at the source of the disastrous outcome. First, the majority of patients included in the trial were ventilated and, consequently, could be deemed truly critically ill. Second, it is crucial that GH administration was started 5 to 8 days from admission and for a maximum of 3 weeks at a dosage of 0.1 mg/kg body weight per day. This regimen may be translated into a supraphysiologic GH dosage in prolonged critically ill patients. In the study, GH therapy increased the markers of GH responsiveness (IGF-I and IGFBP-3) and improved the nitrogen balance, but the reverse side of the medal was an increase of mortality, duration of mechanical ventilation, and hospital stay. The most plausible explanation for the excess mortality is the preponderance of GH counterregulatory effects, inducing insulin resistance, hallmarked by elevated IGFBP-1 and blood glucose levels in the study [61].

Modulation of the immune system by GH was one of the first mechanisms proposed; however, the ambivalent effects of GH on the immune system were reflected in the inability of high-dose GH therapy to alter the proinflammatory cytokine response to surgery or endotoxin [62].

A key could be the prevention of glutamine mobilization and the inhibition of the catabolic rerouting of this amino acid. Glutamine is essential for rapidly dividing cells and for the hepatic production of glutathione [63]. Whether glutamine-enriched total parenteral nutrition in combination with GH will be beneficial remains to be determined [64]. The likely advantages of glutamine supplementation may act through an improved glucose tolerance during critical illness [65].

Additionally, fluid retention, deterioration in the acid-base balance due to increased lipolysis and ketone body production, as well as exacerbation of the cholestatic potential of lipopolysaccharide [66,67] have been suggested as potential mechanisms for the excess mortality associated with GH therapy in long-stay patients in the intensive care unit (ICU) [68]. In the rabbit model of critical illness, rhGH administration resulted in a downregulation of the liver type 3 deiodinase, which inactivates T4 and T3, without causing excess mortality [69].

The use of rhGH in adult chronic critically ill patients should be discouraged [70]; however, specific patient populations, such as convalescing pediatric burn patients, may benefit from GH therapy [71]. The combined administration of GH and IGF-I may not only be additive in their anabolic effects but also safer as they neutralize each other's side effects and act on skeletal muscle through different signaling pathways [72,73].

Growth hormone secretagogues

In light of the catastrophic results of the GH trial, more upstream therapies may be the preferred approach to revive the somatotropic axis in prolonged critically ill patients. In that situation, the goal is restoration of the relative hyposomatotropism of hypothalamic origin by a continuous infusion of GH secretagogues.

Bolus administration of GHRP compared with GHRH resulted in much higher serum GH levels [74], suggesting that the reduced hypothalamic drive may be explained by a deficiency of ghrelin rather than of GHRH. Nevertheless, repeated lipopolysaccharide injections in rats resulted in initially lower ghrelin concentrations, with elevated levels after 2 days [75]. A reduced somatostatin tone may also contribute to the profound response to GH secretagogues, but this cannot be reconciled with the spontaneous dynamics of low GH burst amplitude. The combination of GHRP and GHRH attains the most powerful stimulus of pituitary GH release. This observation shows once again that the attenuated GH production during protracted critical illness is not due to a primary dysfunction in GH synthesis or to a somatostatin-induced suppression of GH secretion. Treatment of prolonged critically ill patients with continuous infusions of GHRP with or without GHRH not only restores the pulsatile GH secretion but also evokes an increase of the GH-dependent ternary complex (IGF-I, IGFBP-3, and ALS), indicating peripheral GH responsiveness [48,49]. The latter was corroborated by the increase in serum GHBP, reflecting GH receptor abundancy, on GH secretagogue administration [51]. The restored IGF-I levels subsequently instigate a feedback inhibition of GH release, preventing overtreatment [50].

To normalize fully the somatotropic axis, stimulation of additional pituitary axes through the administration of thyrotropin-releasing hormone and gonadotropin-releasing hormone seems vital [50,76]. These co-infusions induce anabolism in peripheral lean tissues, reflected by elevated serum insulin, leptin, and osteocalcin levels [50,54].

Intensive insulin therapy

In 2001, a large prospective, randomized, controlled trial in 1548 critically ill patients showed a 40% decrease in mortality and morbidity through strict glycemic control below 6.1 mmol/L (110 mg/dL) with intensive insulin therapy in comparison with the conventional approach, which only recommended insulin therapy when blood glucose levels exceeded 12 mmol/L (220 mg/dL) [77]. The effect occurred particularly in the prolonged critically ill patient population, for whom mortality was reduced from 20.2% to 10.6%.

In a subanalysis of 363 critically ill patients with an ICU stay of more than 7 days, mean GH levels were initially increased before decreasing over time [52]. This observation is in line with the biphasic response during critical illness. Although insulin treatment in diabetes mellitus is known to inhibit GH secretion [78], intensive insulin therapy, when compared with conventional treatment, increases serum GH levels in critically ill patients. Contrary to expectation, intensive insulin therapy also prevented the recovery over time of the circulating levels of IGF-I, IGFBP-3, and ALS. Surprisingly, intensive insulin therapy had no effect on IGFBP-1, the binding protein under direct suppression of insulin [79].

The stimulation of GH secretion in combination with a suppression of the ternary complex proteins suggests an induction of GH resistance by intensive insulin therapy, as can be evidenced by diminished GH-binding protein levels under the latter therapy. Intensive insulin therapy during the chronic phase of critical illness appears to convert prolonged critical illness back into a more acute phenotype. Because patients with a lowered GH response had a better outcome, it can be argued that the maintenance of GH resistance is a "protective" response for survival, which has only been demonstrated in mice models [80–82].

Insulin-like growth factor I

Although no large randomized clinical trials have been performed, IGF-I has been put forward as an anabolic agent for some time [57]. From a theoretical point of view, it comprises several advantages. First, IGF-I is the mediator of the anabolic (indirect) effects of GH. On IGF-I administration, the direct adverse effects of GH, such as lipolysis and sodium retention, could be avoided. At the same time, it has the role of prime feedback inhibitor of GH secretion. Second, IGF-I is able to lower blood glucose levels. This effect has often been regarded as a serious disadvantage, but the latter view should be reversed in light of the Leuven insulin trial and some fascinating animal studies. Mice with a liver-specific IGF-I gene deletion have minimal growth retardation but show significant muscle insulin insensitivity [83]. Conversely, liver-specific IGF-I overexpression improves somatic growth and glucose tolerance [84]. This observation strongly suggests that maintenance of normal serum IGF-I levels is required for normal insulin sensitivity and highlights the link between the somatotropic axis and overall glucose tolerance.

The powerful binding capacity of the IGFBPs has dashed hopes of administering IGF-I on its own [85]. In contrast, the binary complex of IGFBP-3 and IGF-I has been shown to stimulate muscle protein synthesis in patients with burn injuries [86]. IGF-I treatment during acute critical illness may be interesting because it can lower blood glucose levels as well as suppress the increased GH concentrations [87]. In the future, even gene therapy with IGF-I may be available to prevent the wasting of skeletal muscle during critical illness [88].

Summary

Interest in the somatotropic axis, with its complex network of interactions, during critical illness arose only a few decades ago. The distinguished neuroendocrine features of prolonged critical illness were not differentiated from those during the acute phase until the early 1990s. This incomplete understanding of the somatotropic axis has contributed to some disastrous results, such as the multicenter GH trial. Attempts to stimulate the somatotropic axis without a proper preceding neuroendocrine diagnosis should be held obsolete. Moreover, the fascinating link between regulators of carbohydrate metabolism, such as insulin and IGF-I, and the somatotropic axis may lead to future therapeutic possibilities.

References

[1] Lindholm J. Growth hormone: historical notes. Pituitary 2006;9(1):5–10.

[2] Li CH, Evans HM. The isolation of pituitary growth hormone. Science 1944;99:183–4.

[3] Li CH, Dixon JS, Liu WK. Human pituitary growth hormone. XIX. The primary structure of the hormone. Arch Biochem Biophys 1969;133(1):70–91.

[4] Giustina A, Veldhuis JD. Pathophysiology of the neuroregulation of growth hormone secretion in experimental animals and the human. Endocr Rev 1998;19(6):717–97.

[5] Guillemin R, Brazeau P, Bohlen P, et al. Growth hormone-releasing factor from a human pancreatic tumor that caused acromegaly. Science 1982;218(4572):585–7.

[6] Rivier J, Spiess J, Thorner M, et al. Characterization of a growth hormone-releasing factor from a human pancreatic islet tumour. Nature 1982;300(5889):276–8.

[7] Brazeau P, Vale W, Burgus R, et al. Hypothalamic polypeptide that inhibits the secretion of immunoreactive pituitary growth hormone. Science 1973;179(68):77–9.

[8] Bowers CY, Momany FA, Reynolds GA, et al. On the in vitro and in vivo activity of a new synthetic hexapeptide that acts on the pituitary to specifically release growth hormone. Endocrinology 1984;114(5):1537–45.

[9] Howard AD, Feighner SD, Cully DF, et al. A receptor in pituitary and hypothalamus that functions in growth hormone release. Science 1996;273(5277):974–7.

[10] Kojima M, Hosoda H, Date Y, et al. Ghrelin is a growth-hormone-releasing acylated peptide from stomach. Nature 1999;402(6762):656–60.

[11] Berneis K, Keller U. Metabolic actions of growth hormone: direct and indirect. Baillieres Clin Endocrinol Metab 1996;10(3):337–52.

[12] Salmon WD, Daughaday WH. A hormonally controlled serum factor which stimulates sulfate incorporation by cartilage in vitro. J Lab Clin Med 1957;49:825–36.

[13] Baxter RC. Insulin-like growth factor binding proteins as glucoregulators. Metabolism 1995;44(10 Suppl 4):12–7.

[14] Baxter RC. Insulin-like growth factor (IGF)-binding proteins: interactions with IGFs and intrinsic bioactivities. Am J Physiol Endocrinol Metab 2000;278(6):E967–76.

[15] Yakar S, Liu JL, Stannard B, et al. Normal growth and development in the absence of hepatic insulin-like growth factor I. Proc Natl Acad Sci USA 1999;96(13):7324–9.

[16] Boisclair YR, Rhoads RP, Ueki I, et al. The acid-labile subunit (ALS) of the 150 kDa IGF-binding protein complex: an important but forgotten component of the circulating IGF system. J Endocrinol 2001;170(1):63–70.

[17] Ooi GT, Cohen FJ, Tseng LY, et al. Growth hormone stimulates transcription of the gene encoding the acid-labile subunit (ALS) of the circulating insulin-like growth factor-binding protein complex and ALS promoter activity in rat liver. Mol Endocrinol 1997;11(7):997–1007.

[18] Baxter RC. The binding protein's binding protein: clinical applications of acid-labile subunit (ALS) measurement. J Clin Endocrinol Metab 1997;82(12):3941–3.

[19] Brabant G. Insulin-like growth factor-I: marker for diagnosis of acromegaly and monitoring the efficacy of treatment. Eur J Endocrinol 2003;148(Suppl 2):S15–20.

[20] Twigg SM, Baxter RC. Insulin-like growth factor (IGF)-binding protein 5 forms an alternative ternary complex with IGFs and the acid-labile subunit. J Biol Chem 1998;273(11): 6074–9.
[21] Wetterau LA, Moore MG, Lee KW, et al. Novel aspects of the insulin-like growth factor binding proteins. Mol Genet Metab 1999;68(2):161–81.
[22] Baxter RC. The insulin-like growth factor (IGF)-IGF-binding protein axis in critical illness. Growth Horm IGF Res 1999;9(Suppl A):67–9.
[23] Lassarre C, Binoux M. Insulin-like growth factor binding protein-3 is functionally altered in pregnancy plasma. Endocrinology 1994;134(3):1254–62.
[24] Bang P, Brismar K, Rosenfeld RG. Increased proteolysis of insulin-like growth factor-binding protein-3 (IGFBP-3) in noninsulin-dependent diabetes mellitus serum, with elevation of a 29-kilodalton (kDa) glycosylated IGFBP-3 fragment contained in the approximately 130- to 150-kDa ternary complex. J Clin Endocrinol Metab 1994;78(5):1119–27.
[25] Wolfe RR, Martini WZ. Changes in intermediary metabolism in severe surgical illness. World J Surg 2000;24(6):639–47.
[26] Gamrin L, Essen P, Forsberg AM, et al. A descriptive study of skeletal muscle metabolism in critically ill patients: free amino acids, energy-rich phosphates, protein, nucleic acids, fat, water, and electrolytes. Crit Care Med 1996;24(4):575–83.
[27] Cerra FB, Siegel JH, Coleman B, et al. Septic autocannibalism: a failure of exogenous nutritional support. Ann Surg 1980;192(4):570–80.
[28] Ross R, Miell J, Freeman E, et al. Critically ill patients have high basal growth hormone levels with attenuated oscillatory activity associated with low levels of insulin-like growth factor-I. Clin Endocrinol (Oxf) 1991;35(1):47–54.
[29] Van den Berghe G, de Zegher F, Lauwers P, et al. Growth hormone secretion in critical illness: effect of dopamine. J Clin Endocrinol Metab 1994;79(4):1141–6.
[30] Defalque D, Brandt N, Ketelslegers JM, et al. GH insensitivity induced by endotoxin injection is associated with decreased liver GH receptors. Am J Physiol 1999;276(3 Pt 1):E565–72.
[31] Kong SE, Firth SM, Baxter RC, et al. Regulation of the acid-labile subunit in sustained endotoxemia. Am J Physiol Endocrinol Metab 2002;283(4):E692–701.
[32] Thimmarayappa J, Sun J, Schultz LE, et al. Inhibition of growth hormone receptor gene expression by saturated fatty acids: role of kruppel-like zinc finger factor, ZBP-89. Mol Endocrinol 2006;20(1):2747–60.
[33] Van den Berghe G, de Zegher F, Bouillon R. Clinical review 95: acute and prolonged critical illness as different neuroendocrine paradigms. J Clin Endocrinol Metab 1998;83(6):1827–34.
[34] Van den Berghe G. Novel insights into the neuroendocrinology of critical illness. Eur J Endocrinol 2000;143(1):1–13.
[35] Weekers F, Van Herck E, Coopmans W, et al. A novel in vivo rabbit model of hypercatabolic critical illness reveals a biphasic neuroendocrine stress response. Endocrinology 2002;143(3): 764–74.
[36] Hartman ML, Veldhuis JD, Johnson ML, et al. Augmented growth hormone (GH) secretory burst frequency and amplitude mediate enhanced GH secretion during a two-day fast in normal men. J Clin Endocrinol Metab 1992;74(4):757–65.
[37] Baxter RC, Hawker FH, To C, et al. Thirty-day monitoring of insulin-like growth factors and their binding proteins in intensive care unit patients. Growth Horm IGF Res 1998; 8(6):455–63.
[38] Lang CH, Pollard V, Fan J, et al. Acute alterations in growth hormone-insulin-like growth factor axis in humans injected with endotoxin. Am J Physiol 1997;273(1 Pt 2):R371–8.
[39] Hermansson M, Wickelgren RB, Hammarqvist F, et al. Measurement of human growth hormone receptor messenger ribonucleic acid by a quantitative polymerase chain reaction-based assay: demonstration of reduced expression after elective surgery. J Clin Endocrinol Metab 1997;82(2):421–8.
[40] Timmins AC, Cotterill AM, Hughes SC, et al. Critical illness is associated with low circulating concentrations of insulin-like growth factors-I and -II, alterations in insulin-like growth

factor binding proteins, and induction of an insulin-like growth factor binding protein 3 protease. Crit Care Med 1996;24(9):1460–6.
[41] Lang CH, Frost RA. Role of growth hormone, insulin-like growth factor-I, and insulin-like growth factor binding proteins in the catabolic response to injury and infection. Curr Opin Clin Nutr Metab Care 2002;5(3):271–9.
[42] Davies SC, Wass JA, Ross RJ, et al. The induction of a specific protease for insulin-like growth factor binding protein-3 in the circulation during severe illness. J Endocrinol 1991; 130(3):469–73.
[43] Davenport ML, Isley WL, Pucilowska JB, et al. Insulin-like growth factor-binding protein-3 proteolysis is induced after elective surgery. J Clin Endocrinol Metab 1992;75(2):590–5.
[44] Cotterill AM, Mendel P, Holly JM, et al. The differential regulation of the circulating levels of the insulin-like growth factors and their binding proteins (IGFBP) 1, 2 and 3 after elective abdominal surgery. Clin Endocrinol (Oxf) 1996;44(1):91–101.
[45] Damas P, Reuter A, Gysen P, et al. Tumor necrosis factor and interleukin-1 serum levels during severe sepsis in humans. Crit Care Med 1989;17(10):975–8.
[46] Hadley JS, Hinds CJ. Anabolic strategies in critical illness. Curr Opin Pharmacol 2002;2(6): 700–7.
[47] Streat SJ, Beddoe AH, Hill GL. Aggressive nutritional support does not prevent protein loss despite fat gain in septic intensive care patients. J Trauma 1987;27(3):262–6.
[48] Van den Berghe G, de Zegher F, Veldhuis JD, et al. The somatotropic axis in critical illness: effect of continuous growth hormone (GH)-releasing hormone and GH-releasing peptide-2 infusion. J Clin Endocrinol Metab 1997;82(2):590–9.
[49] Van den Berghe G, de Zegher F, Baxter RC, et al. Neuroendocrinology of prolonged critical illness: effects of exogenous thyrotropin-releasing hormone and its combination with growth hormone secretagogues. J Clin Endocrinol Metab 1998;83(2):309–19.
[50] Van den Berghe G, Wouters P, Weekers F, et al. Reactivation of pituitary hormone release and metabolic improvement by infusion of growth hormone-releasing peptide and thyrotropin-releasing hormone in patients with protracted critical illness. J Clin Endocrinol Metab 1999;84(4):1311–23.
[51] Van den Berghe G, Baxter RC, Weekers F, et al. A paradoxical gender dissociation within the growth hormone/insulin-like growth factor I axis during protracted critical illness. J Clin Endocrinol Metab 2000;85(1):183–92.
[52] Mesotten D, Wouters PJ, Peeters RP, et al. Regulation of the somatotropic axis by intensive insulin therapy during protracted critical illness. J Clin Endocrinol Metab 2004;89(7): 3105–13.
[53] Van den Berghe G. Dynamic neuroendocrine responses to critical illness. Front Neuroendocrinol 2002;23(4):370–91.
[54] Van den Berghe G, Wouters P, Carlsson L, et al. Leptin levels in protracted critical illness: effects of growth hormone-secretagogues and thyrotropin-releasing hormone. J Clin Endocrinol Metab 1998;83(9):3062–70.
[55] Gore DC, Honeycutt D, Jahoor F, et al. Effect of exogenous growth hormone on whole-body and isolated-limb protein kinetics in burned patients. Arch Surg 1991;126(1):38–43.
[56] Voerman HJ, van Schijndel RJ, Groeneveld AB, et al. Effects of recombinant human growth hormone in patients with severe sepsis. Ann Surg 1992;216(6):648–55.
[57] Carroll PV. Protein metabolism and the use of growth hormone and insulin-like growth factor-I in the critically ill patient. Growth Horm IGF Res 1999;9(6):400–13.
[58] Wilmore DW. The use of growth hormone in severely ill patients. Adv Surg 1999;33: 261–74.
[59] Raguso CA, Genton L, Kyle U, et al. Management of catabolism in metabolically stressed patients: a literature survey about growth hormone application. Curr Opin Clin Nutr Metab Care 2001;4(4):313–20.
[60] Takala J, Ruokonen E, Webster NR, et al. Increased mortality associated with growth hormone treatment in critically ill adults. N Engl J Med 1999;341(11):785–92.

[61] Van den Berghe G. Increased mortality associated with growth hormone treatment in critically ill adults. N Engl J Med 2000;342(2):135 [author reply: 35–6].
[62] Zarkesh-Esfahani SH, Kolstad O, Metcalfe RA, et al. High-dose growth hormone does not affect proinflammatory cytokine (tumor necrosis factor-α, interleukin-6, and interferon-γ) release from activated peripheral blood mononuclear cells or after minimal to moderate surgical stress. J Clin Endocrinol Metab 2000;85(9):3383–90.
[63] Teng Chung T, Hinds CJ. Treatment with GH and IGF-1 in critical illness. Crit Care Clin 2006;22(1):29–40.
[64] Carroll PV, Jackson NC, Russell-Jones DL, et al. Combined growth hormone/insulin-like growth factor I in addition to glutamine-supplemented TPN results in net protein anabolism in critical illness. Am J Physiol Endocrinol Metab 2004;286(1):E151–7.
[65] Dechelotte P, Hasselmann M, Cynober L, et al. L-alanyl-L-glutamine dipeptide-supplemented total parenteral nutrition reduces infectious complications and glucose intolerance in critically ill patients: the French controlled, randomized, double-blind, multicenter study. Crit Care Med 2006;34(3):598–604.
[66] Liao W, Rudling M, Angelin B. Growth hormone potentiates the in vivo biological activities of endotoxin in the rat. Eur J Clin Invest 1996;26(3):254–8.
[67] Mesotten D, Van den Berghe G, Liddle C, et al. Growth hormone modulation of the rat hepatic bile transporter system in endotoxin-induced cholestasis. Endocrinology 2003; 144(9):4008–17.
[68] Ruokonen E, Takala J. Dangers of growth hormone therapy in critically ill patients. Curr Opin Clin Nutr Metab Care 2002;5(2):199–209.
[69] Weekers F, Michalaki M, Coopmans W, et al. Endocrine and metabolic effects of growth hormone (GH) compared with GH-releasing peptide, thyrotropin-releasing hormone, and insulin infusion in a rabbit model of prolonged critical illness. Endocrinology 2004;145(1): 205–13.
[70] Carroll PV, Van den Berghe G. Safety aspects of pharmacological GH therapy in adults. Growth Horm IGF Res 2001;11(3):166–72.
[71] Przkora R, Herndon DN, Suman OE, et al. Beneficial effects of extended growth hormone treatment after hospital discharge in pediatric burn patients. Ann Surg 2006;243(6):796–801 [discussion: 1–3].
[72] Kupfer SR, Underwood LE, Baxter RC, et al. Enhancement of the anabolic effects of growth hormone and insulin-like growth factor I by use of both agents simultaneously. J Clin Invest 1993;91(2):391–6.
[73] Sotiropoulos A, Ohanna M, Kedzia C, et al. Growth hormone promotes skeletal muscle cell fusion independent of insulin-like growth factor 1 up-regulation. Proc Natl Acad Sci USA 2006;103(19):7315–20.
[74] Van den Berghe G, de Zegher F, Bowers CY, et al. Pituitary responsiveness to GH-releasing hormone, GH-releasing peptide-2 and thyrotrophin-releasing hormone in critical illness. Clin Endocrinol (Oxf) 1996;45(3):341–51.
[75] Hataya Y, Akamizu T, Hosoda H, et al. Alterations of plasma ghrelin levels in rats with lipopolysaccharide-induced wasting syndrome and effects of ghrelin treatment on the syndrome. Endocrinology 2003;144(12):5365–71.
[76] Van den Berghe G, Baxter RC, Weekers F, et al. The combined administration of GH-releasing peptide-2 (GHRP-2), TRH and GnRH to men with prolonged critical illness evokes superior endocrine and metabolic effects compared to treatment with GHRP-2 alone. Clin Endocrinol (Oxf) 2002;56(5):655–69.
[77] Van den Berghe G, Wouters P, Weekers F, et al. Intensive insulin therapy in critically ill patients. N Engl J Med 2001;345(19):1359–67.
[78] Holt RI, Simpson HL, Sonksen PH. The role of the growth hormone-insulin-like growth factor axis in glucose homeostasis. Diabet Med 2003;20(1):3–15.

[79] Mesotten D, Delhanty PJD, Vanderhoydonc F, et al. Regulation of insulin-like growth factor binding protein-1 during protracted critical illness. J Clin Endocrinol Metab 2002; 87(12):5516–23.
[80] Chen NY, Chen WY, Bellush L, et al. Effects of streptozotocin treatment in growth hormone (GH) and GH antagonist transgenic mice. Endocrinology 1995;136(2):660–7.
[81] Flyvbjerg A, Bennett WF, Rasch R, et al. Inhibitory effect of a growth hormone receptor antagonist (G120K-PEG) on renal enlargement, glomerular hypertrophy, and urinary albumin excretion in experimental diabetes in mice. Diabetes 1999;48(2):377–82.
[82] Coschigano KT, Clemmons D, Bellush LL, et al. Assessment of growth parameters and life span of GHR/BP gene-disrupted mice. Endocrinology 2000;141(7):2608–13.
[83] Yakar S, Liu JL, Fernandez AM, et al. Liver-specific igf-1 gene deletion leads to muscle insulin insensitivity. Diabetes 2001;50(5):1110–8.
[84] Liao L, Dearth RK, Zhou S, et al. Liver-specific overexpression of the insulin-like growth factor-I enhances somatic growth and partially prevents the effects of growth hormone deficiency. Endocrinology 2006;147(8):3877–88.
[85] Goeters C, Mertes N, Tacke J, et al. Repeated administration of recombinant human insulin-like growth factor-I in patients after gastric surgery: effect on metabolic and hormonal patterns. Ann Surg 1995;222(5):646–53.
[86] Debroy MA, Wolf SE, Zhang XJ, et al. Anabolic effects of insulin-like growth factor in combination with insulin-like growth factor binding protein-3 in severely burned adults. J Trauma 1999;47(5):904–10 [discussion: 10–1].
[87] Hartman ML, Clayton PE, Johnson ML, et al. A low dose euglycemic infusion of recombinant human insulin-like growth factor I rapidly suppresses fasting-enhanced pulsatile growth hormone secretion in humans. J Clin Invest 1993;91(6):2453–62.
[88] Schakman O, Gilson H, de Coninck V, et al. Insulin-like growth factor-I gene transfer by electroporation prevents skeletal muscle atrophy in glucocorticoid-treated rats. Endocrinology 2005;146(4):1789–97.

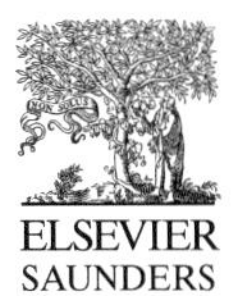

ELSEVIER
SAUNDERS

Endocrinol Metab Clin N Am
35 (2006) 807–821

ENDOCRINOLOGY
AND METABOLISM
CLINICS
OF NORTH AMERICA

Changes Within the Thyroid Axis During the Course of Critical Illness

Liese Mebis, MSc[a], Yves Debaveye, MD[a],
Theo J. Visser, PhD[b],
Greet Van den Berghe, MD, PhD[a,]*

[a]*Department of Intensive Care, Catholic University of Leuven, Leuven, Belgium*
[b]*Department of Internal Medicine, Erasmus University Medical Center, Rotterdam, The Netherlands*

Thyroid hormone acts on virtually all cells of the body and has profound effects on many important physiologic processes, such as differentiation, growth, and metabolism [1,2].

The thyroid axis comprises thyrotropin-releasing hormone (TRH) at the hypothalamic level; thyrotropin at the pituitary level; and thyroxine (T_4), triiodothyronine (T_3), and reverse T_3 (rT_3) at the peripheral level. At the pituitary level, secretion of thyrotropin is stimulated by TRH from the hypothalamus. Thyrotropin is released in secretory bursts superimposed on nonpulsatile secretion and thereby stimulates the thyroid gland to release the prohormone T_4 into the circulation. Peripheral conversion of T_4 produces the metabolic active hormone, T_3, and rT_3, which is believed to be metabolically inactive. T_4 and T_3 in turn exert a negative feedback control on the level of the hypothalamus and the pituitary.

During critical illness, multiple and complex alternations occur in the hypothalamic-pituitary-thyroid (HPT) axis, resulting in what commonly is referred to as the euthyroid sick syndrome. More neutral terms, avoiding the assumption that patients really are euthyroid, are low T_3 syndrome or nonthyroidal illness.

Within 2 hours of the onset of acute stress, such as sepsis, surgery, myocardial infarction, or trauma, circulating T_3 levels drop and rT_3 levels increase. The magnitude of these changes reflects the severity of illness [3–6].

This work was supported by the Fund for Scientific Research–Flanders, Belgium (FWO).

* Corresponding author. Department of Intensive Care Medicine, Catholic University of Leuven, Herestraat 49, B-3000, Leuven, Belgium.

E-mail address: Greta.vandenberghe@med.kuleuven.be (G. Van den Berghe).

doi:10.1016/j.ecl.2006.09.009

endo.theclinics.com

At the same time, circulating levels of T_4 and thyrotropin rise briefly [7] but subsequently normalize. These observed changes in circulating thyroid hormone levels during the acute phase of critical illness are caused largely by disturbances in peripheral thyroid hormone metabolism and binding.

Patients requiring prolonged intensive care therapy enter a chronic phase of illness. In these prolonged critically ill patients, T_4 levels also start to decline and circulating T_3 levels may become very low or even undetectable [8]. Despite the major decreases in serum T_3 and, in severe cases, of T_4, the concentration of thyrotropin, measured in a single sample, typically remains within the normal range [8]. This may indicate that a neuroendocrine dysfunction adds to the pathogenesis of the low T_3 syndrome in the chronic phase of critical illness (Fig. 1).

This article reviews the mechanisms behind the observed changes in thyroid hormone parameters in the acute phase and the chronic phase of critical illness, focusing on the central and the peripheral parts of thyroid hormone metabolism.

Peripheral changes during critical illness

Disturbances in peripheral thyroid hormone metabolism play a major role in the pathogenesis of the low T_3 syndrome during critical illness, particularly during the acute phase of critical illness. These alterations continue to persist in prolonged critical illness, but here a neuroendocrine dysfunction leading to a decline of thyroidal release of T_4 is superimposed on the peripheral adaptations.

Deiodinases

The peripheral metabolism of thyroid hormone involves three deiodinases (D1, D2, and D3) [3]. D1 and D2 have enzymatic outer-ring deiodination activity, which is considered an activating pathway, whereas inner-ring deiodination is an inactivating pathway catalyzed by D3 [9]. D1 is expressed in the thyroid gland, liver, and kidney and generally is considered the main source of circulating T_3 [3,9]. D2 is expressed in the brain, anterior pituitary, thyroid, and skeletal muscle. This enzyme is important for local T_3 production, especially in the brain and pituitary, but skeletal D2 also is believed to contribute to circulating T_3 [10,11]. D3 is present in the brain, skin, placenta, and pregnant uterus and in various fetal tissues. It is the major inactivating enzyme, as it catalyzes the conversion of T_4 into rT_3 and of T_3 into 3,3′-diiodothyronine (3,3′-T2) and thereby is able to protect tissues from excess thyroid hormone [3,9].

During critical illness, multiple alterations occur in the peripheral thyroid hormone metabolism whereby the conversion of T_4 into active T_3 is reduced and, instead, T_4 is metabolized into inactive rT_3. The resulting reciprocal changes in T_3 and rT_3 were observed decades ago and decreased

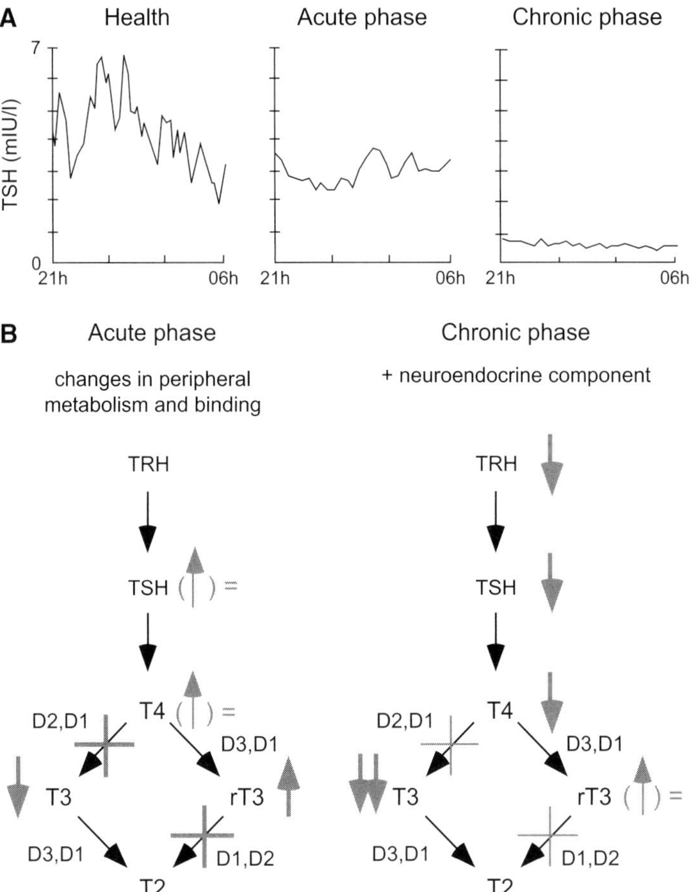

Fig. 1. Response of the thyroid axis to critical illness. (*A*) The nocturnal serum concentration profiles of thyrotropin in critical illness are abnormal and differ markedly between the acute and chronic phase of the disease. (*Modified from* Van den Berghe G, de Zegher F, Bouillon R. Acute and prolonged critical illness as different neuroendocrine paradigms. J Clin Endocrinol Metab 1998;83:1827–34; with permission. © [1998] The Endocrine Society.) (*B*) Simplified overview of the major changes occurring within the thyroid axis during the acute and chronic phase of critical illness. The normal regulation of the thyroid axis is shown in black, whereas the alterations induced by critical illness are indicated in gray. As discussed in the text, for the acute phase of critical illness, thyrotropin and T4 levels are elevated briefly and subsequently return to normal, represented by (↑). T2, diiodothyronine. (*Reproduced from* Van den Berghe G. Novel insights into the neuroendocrinology of critical illness. Eur J Endocrinol 2000;143:1–13; with permission. © [2000] Society of the European Journal of Endocrinology.)

monodeiodination of T_4 was suggested then as a possible mechanism [12,13]. Recently, this premise has been confirmed by Peeters and colleagues, showing that there is a decreased activation and an increased inactivation of thyroid hormone in patients who are critically ill [14]. The role of deiodinases during critical illness has been explored further in a rabbit model of prolonged critical illness [15,16] and in mouse models of acute illness [17,18].

D1 in liver and kidney in general is considered the major source of circulating T_3 and the primary mechanism for rT_3 clearance. D1 activity is stimulated in hyperthyroidism and decreased in hypothyroidism, representing the regulation of D1 activity by T_3 at the transcriptional level [19]. Analysis of postmortem skeletal muscle and liver samples obtained from critically ill patients at the time of death in an ICU indeed showed a marked reduction in liver D1 activity compared with values observed previously in individuals who were healthy [16]. Serum T_3/rT_3 ratio, a marker for the severity of illness, correlated positively with liver D1 activity, being highest in patients who died from severe brain damage and lowest in patients who died from cardiovascular collapse. Furthermore, this has been confirmed in a rabbit model of prolonged critical illness, showing also that the decrease in D1 activity is reversible [15]. Infusion of TRH could restore D1 activity and serum T_4 and T_3 levels back to normal range [15].

D2 is the most recently cloned of the three deiodinases, and new data regarding its properties and function still are accumulating. D2 was known to be important particularly for local T_3 production in the brain [20] but recently it was shown that expression of D2 in the human muscle also may have a significant contribution to circulating T_3 [11,21]. Thyroid status controls D2 activity at the pre- and post-translational levels. T_3 decreases D2 mRNA expression, whereas T_4 and rT_3 facilitates the fast and irreversible degradation of D2 protein [3]. This means that D2 is up-regulated in a hypothyroid state, whereas hyperthyroidism leads to a decrease in D2. Despite low T_3 levels, D2 activity in skeletal muscle of patients who were critically ill was reported to be undetectable [14]. If this is the case, it could be explained by increased levels of rT_3 leading to an increased breakdown of D2 protein [22]. Loss of D2 activity during critical illness thus might contribute to low T_3 levels. From this perspective, decreasing D2 activity may be a cause of the low T_3 syndrome, because it would lead to a decrease in T_3 levels, in turn down-regulating D1 activity. Such a sequence of events during critical illness, however, remains speculative at this time.

D3 is the major thyroid hormone inactivating enzyme. It is expressed mainly in fetal tissues, the pregnant uterus, and the placenta, protecting the fetus against excess T_3 concentrations, which are detrimental to normal development [23]. In adult animals, D3 is expressed in the brain but high levels are restricted to the uteroplacental unit. Because D3 also is found in some tumors and malignant cell lines, D3 has been named an oncofetal protein [24]. These D3-expressing tumors give rise to a condition called consumptive hypothyroidism, wherein circulating thyroid hormone is inactivated massively [25]. The observed alterations in circulating thyroid hormone levels are similar to those during critical illness and induction of D3 activity in liver and skeletal muscle of patients who are critically ill has been documented recently [14]. This finding was confirmed in a rabbit model of prolonged critical illness [15]. Both studies also could show a negative correlation between D3 activity and changes in circulating T_3 and the T_3/rT_3 ratio. By infusing TRH continuously to prolonged ill rabbits, D3 activity and T3 levels were normalized [15]. Addition of a growth hormone (GH) secretagogue to TRH, however, was necessary to prevent the rise in rT_3 observed with TRH alone.

From these data, it can be concluded that in addition to the down-regulation of D1, an induction of D3 activity in liver and muscle is likely to contribute to the low serum T_3 and high serum rT_3 levels seen in acute critically ill patients.

Thyroid hormone transport

To be metabolized by the deiodinases, thyroid hormone first must enter the cell. Until recently, the mechanism of thyroid hormone entry into cells was not clear. The assumption was that the lipophilic nature of thyroid hormones facilitated passive diffusion through the lipid bilayer. In contrast to previous beliefs, it now is known that thyroid hormones need specific transmembrane transporters to cross the plasma membrane. Thyroid hormone uptake in the human liver, for example, is temperature, Na, and energy dependent and rate limiting for subsequent iodothyronine metabolism [26]. In critical illness, T_4 uptake in the liver clearly is decreased and this may contribute to lowered T_3 production [27,28]. Inhibition of liver T_4 uptake during critical illness can be explained by liver adenosine triophosphate (ATP) depletion and increased concentrations of circulating inhibitors, such as indoxyl sulfate, nonesterified fatty acids, and bilirubin [29,30]. Serum of patients who are critically ill is shown to inhibit uptake of T_4 into hepatocytes [29,31,32].

Monocarboxylate transporter 8 (MCT8) is an example of an active and specific thyroid hormone transporter [33]. Expression analysis in liver and muscle tissue of patients who are critically ill, however, suggests that MCT8 is not crucial for transport of iodothyronines, at least not in these tissues [34]. The precise role of MCT8 and of other putative thyroid hormone transporters during acute and chronic critical illness remains to be addressed in future studies.

Tissue levels of thyroid hormone

As discussed previously, circulating thyroid levels are low and tissue uptake of T_4 also is impaired. It would be logical to assume that this results in low thyroid hormone concentrations in the tissue and, thus, a low bioactivity of thyroid hormone. Few data exist, however, on the actual tissue content of T_3 in patients who are critically ill. Arem and colleagues compared tissues from patients who were critically ill with tissues from patients who died acutely [35]. The general finding was a decreased concentration of T_3 in the tissues of patients who were critically ill. Also, in a larger study, circulating T_3 levels are shown to correlate well with skeletal muscle and liver T_3 content in patients who died from critical illness [34]. Consequently, patients who had received thyroid hormone treatment showed higher serum T3 concentrations accompanied by higher levels of muscle T_3.

Thyroid hormone receptors

Once thyroid hormone has entered the cell, it interacts with specific nuclear thyroid hormone receptors (TRs) to exert its functions. TRs are expressed from two separate genes, resulting in two major isoforms, TRα and TRβ. Each gene can be spliced alternately, producing distinct isoforms: TRα-1, TRα-2, TRβ-1, and TRβ-2. The TRα-1 isoform is a bona fide T_3 receptor, whereas TRα-2 acts as a dominant negative isoform. The ratio of these splice variants, therefore, could have a marked influence on T_3-regulated gene expression. An inverse correlation was observed between the T_3/rT_3 ratio and the TRα-1/TRα-2 ratio in liver biopsies of prolonged critically ill patients [36]. Furthermore, higher TRα-1/TRα-2 ratios were present in sicker and older patients as compared with less sick and younger ones. Hence, patients who are critically ill may adapt to decreasing thyroid hormone levels by increasing the expression of the active form of the TR gene. A decline in number and in occupancy of hepatic nuclear T_3 receptors is, however, observed in animal models [37,38].

Sulfation

Recently, the role of sulfation of thyroid hormone in critical illness was investigated. Sulfated iodothyronines do not bind to the TRs, and sulfation mediates a rapid degradation of iodothyronines by D1 [39]. Therefore, the concentrations of sulfated iodothyronines in serum normally are low [40,41]. In prolonged critically ill patients, however, there was a marked elevation of sulfated T_4 (T_4S), which correlated with the severity of illness [42]. The strong negative correlation of hepatic D1 activity with serum T_4S suggests that a decreased liver D1 activity plays an important role in the increase of T_4S levels during critical illness.

Inhibition of thyroid hormone binding

Other factors involved during the acute phase of illness include low concentrations of thyroid binding proteins [43–45] and inhibition of hormone binding [46,47]. It is suggested that a binding inhibitor may be present in the serum or even throughout body tissues. This binding inhibitor can inhibit uptake of hormone by cells or prevent binding to nuclear TRs and, thus, inhibit action of thyroid hormone. This does not, however, explain the reduced generation of T_3 and the low thyrotropin levels. Moreover, the observation of Brent and Hershman that the T_4 pool of prolonged critically ill patients can be replenished easily by exogenous T_4 administration strongly indicates that an inhibitor of binding is not a predominant cause of low serum T_4 [48].

Neuroendocrine changes during critical illness

Central changes play an important role in the pathophysiology of the low T_3 syndrome, especially in the prolonged phase of critical illness where they are superimposed on the peripheral changes (described previously) (see Fig. 1). Subtle changes in the central part of the HPT axis, however, already can be observed in the acute phase of critical illness. In normal physiology, a decrease in circulating thyroid hormone levels results in a fast and robust release of thyrotropin from the pituitary. During acute critical illness, however, levels of thyrotropin rise only briefly (±2 hours) [7] after which they return to normal despite ongoing decline in T_3 concentrations, thus indicating the presence of an altered set-point for feedback inhibition. In addition, the nocturnal thyrotropin surge seen in healthy individuals is absent in acute critically ill patients [7,49].

Prolonged critically ill patients present with a more severe central dysfunction. First, a dramatic reduction in the pulsatile fraction of thyrotropin release is observed. In addition, serum concentrations of T_4 and T_3 are low and correlate positively with the reduced pulsatile thyrotropin release [8,50]. Similar to what is described within the somatotropic axis, this constellation is in line with a predominantly central origin of the suppressed thyroid axis, suggesting reduced TRH availability in the chronic phase of critical illness [51]. Indeed, continuous infusion of TRH in prolonged critically ill patients increases thyrotropin secretion and, concomitantly, increases the low circulating levels of T_4 and T_3 back to normal levels [50]. Further evidence for this concept comes from the work of Fliers and coworkers, who confirmed reduced TRH gene expression in the hypothalamus of patients dying after chronic critical illness as compared with those who died after a road accident or an acute illness [52]. Additionally, a positive correlation of TRH mRNA with serum thyrotropin and T_3 was found. The onset of recovery from severe illness is shown to be preceded by an increase in circulating levels of thyrotropin [53–55].

The neuroendocrine pathophysiology behind these changes is understood incompletely. Injection of cytokines, such as tumor necrosis factor α (TNF-α), interleukin (IL) 1, and IL-6, is able to mimic the acute stress-induced alterations in thyroid status [56,57]. Therefore, it is suggested that these cytokines may play a role in evoking the low-T3 syndrome. Cytokine antagonism studies failed, however, to restore normal thyroid function in humans [58] and in animals [59]. Moreover, in contrast to the acute phase, circulating cytokines usually are low in the chronic phase of severe illness [60] and cytokines were not withheld as independent determinants of the variability in circulating T_3 in a large group of hospitalized patients [61,62], so other mechanisms must be involved. Endogenous dopamine and prolonged hypercortisolism each may play such a role, as exogenous dopamine and corticoids are known to provoke or severely aggravate hypothyroidism in critical illness [63,64].

An up-regulation of D2 in the mediobasal hypothalamus, which is seen in rats and mice after lipopolysacharide (LPS) injection, also may contribute to the suppressed HPT axis by way of an increased local T3 production [17,65,66]. Theoretically, a down-regulation of D3 in the paraventricular nucleus (PVN) also would lead to relatively high hypothalamic T_3 concentrations, thereby suppressing TRH expression [67]. Less then half the concentration of tissue T_3, however, was measured in the hypothalamus of patients who died after chronic severe illness compared with patients who died from an acute trauma [35]. Because LPS injection induces an acute illness rather than a chronic illness, this might explain the contradicting results.

The melanocortin signaling system is another way of controlling TRH neuron function. This system consists of two groups of neurons with opposing functions that synthesize either α–melanocyte-stimulating hormone (α-MSH) or agouti-related protein (AGRP) (for review see Ref. [68]). α-MSH has an activating effect on TRH neurons whereas AGRP suppresses TRH mRNA in the PVN. In addition, neuropeptide Y (NPY) may be involved, as it potentiates the inhibitory effect of AGRP on TRH. The exact role of these neuropeptides in the central pathogenesis of the low T3 syndrome remains puzzling, however, as contradictory results are obtained under different conditions. Although fasting and administration of LPS resulted in an overall suppression of TRH in the PVN, this was accompanied with different patterns of expression of α-MSH and AGRP. During fasting, α-MSH expression decreases and AGRP increases [69], but intriguingly α-MSH expression increases when LPS was administered despite suppression of TRH in the PVN [70]. In addition, NPY expression showed a positive correlation with TRH levels in patients who died from severe illness [71], whereas an inverse correlation is seen during starvation [69]. The precise role of the melanocortin system in critical illness remains to be unraveled.

The human MCT8, a specific thyroid hormone transporter, and the organic anion transporter, OATP1C1, a high-affinity T_4 transporter, are expressed in the hypothalamus, suggesting their regulation also may be important in the altered hypothalamic set-point in critical illness [67,72]. Also, expression TR isoforms are shown to be regulated differentially by thyroid hormone status in different brain regions, including the PVN [73]. All these possibilities need to be addressed in future studies of critical illness.

Should the low triiodothyronine syndrome be treated?

It hitherto has not been clear whether or not the low T_3 syndrome is an adaptive, protective mechanism against hypercatabolism or, alternatively, its cause. It is important to realize the differences between the acute and the chronic phases of critical illness [74–76]. In the acute phase, peripheral changes predominate, and these changes are similar to the ones observed in fasting. Teleologically, the decrease in T3 observed during fasting has been interpreted as an attempt of the body to reduce energy expenditure, to survive, and to prevent severe protein wasting [77,78]. Similarly, the acute changes within the thyroid axis, uniformly present in all types of acute illnesses, could be looked on as a beneficial and adaptive response that does not warrant intervention.

The prolonged phase of critical illness, however, is in a way an unnatural condition. These patients would have died at one time, but with the development of intensive care medicine, they now have a much greater chance of survival. Therefore, the alterations observed during prolonged critical illness cannot be interpreted as selected by evolution; thus, it is unlikely that they represent an adaptive response. In this phase, thyroid hormone levels are correlated inversely with biochemical markers of accelerated catabolism (urea production and bone degradation). These markers of hypercatabolism, however, can be reduced when thyroid hormone is restored to physiologic levels by continuous infusion of TRH in combination with a GH secretagogue (Fig. 2) [79]. This observation may be in favor of low thyroid hormone levels contributing to, rather than protecting from, the hypercatabolism of prolonged critical illness. The negative feedback inhibition, exerted by thyroid hormones on the thyrotrophs to prevent overstimulation of the thyroid axis, was maintained during TRH infusion in prolonged critical illness [50,80]. This self-limitation may be important during critical illness to protect against hyperthyroidism, which inadvertently would aggravate catabolism.

It remains controversial whether or not direct administration of T_3 or T_4 to raise circulating T_3 levels has clinical benefits [35,81]. To date, administration of T_4 has failed to demonstrate a clinical benefit, although the impaired conversion of T_4 to T_3 may be a factor in the lack of success [48,82]. Substitution doses of T_3, however, after correction of congenital cardiac anomaly in dopamine-treated pediatric patients are associated with improvements in postoperative cardiac function [83]. A benefit of T_3 treatment in iatrogenic, dopamine-induced hypothyroidism, however, still does not provide evidence of clinical benefit of treating the noniatrogenic low T_3 levels characteristic of prolonged critical illness [84,85]. The advantage of treatment with hypothalamic-releasing factors is that the body remains capable of using its normal feedback systems to generate the appropriate amount of thyroid hormones in the circulation and at the tissue level. This provides a safer treatment strategy than the direct administration of T_3 [50]. In addition, the response of the peripheral tissue to the normalization of serum levels of insulin-like growth factor I (IGF-I) and binding proteins via GH-releasing peptide (GHRP) infusion seems to depend on the co-infusion of TRH and the resultant normalization of the thyroid axis. Although infusion of GHRP-2 alone is accompanied by increases in GH secretion and in serum

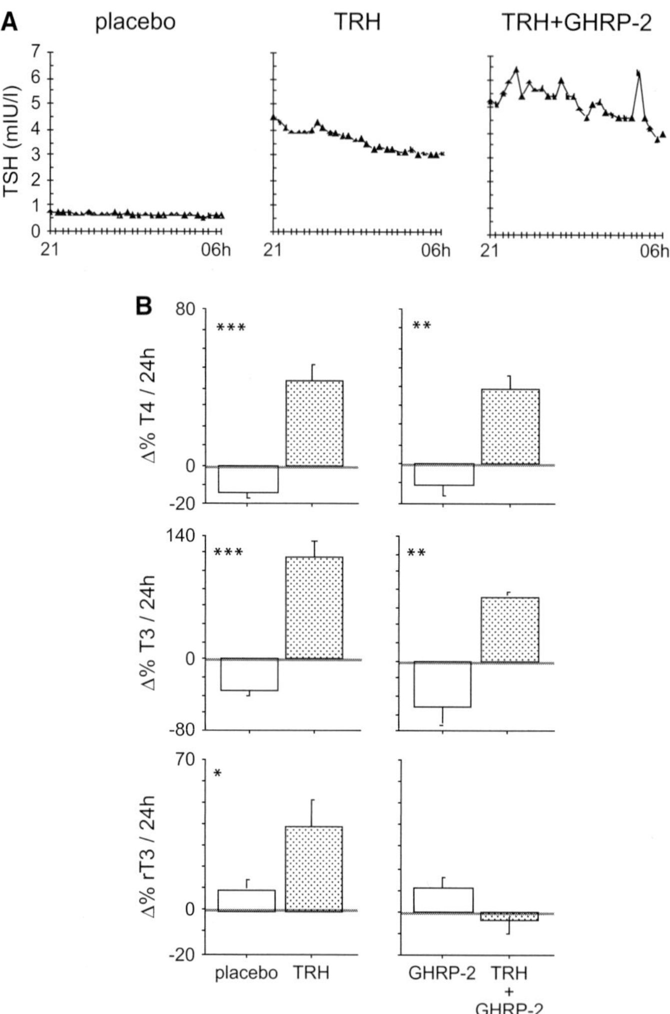

Fig. 2. Effects of TRH and a GH secretagogue on the thyroid axis in prolonged critical illness. (*A*) Nocturnal serum thyrotropin profiles, with continuous infusion of placebo, of TRH (1μg/kg/h) or of TRH plus GHRP-2 (1 + 1 μg/kg/h). The age range of the patients was 68 to 80 years and duration of illness was between 15 and 18 days. Although TRH elevated the thyrotropin secretion, addition of GHRP-2 to the TRH infusion seemed necessary to increase its pulsatile fraction. (*B*) Continuous administration of TRH (1 μg/kg/h), infused alone or together with GHRP-2 (1 + 1 μg/kg/h), induces a significant rise in serum T4 and T3 within 24 hours. Here, rT3 is increased after the infusion of TRH alone, but not if TRH is co-infused with GHRP-2. The patients studied were ill for 12 to 59 days; the age range was 32 to 87 years. (*Reproduced from* Van den Berghe G, de Zegher F, Bouillon R. Acute and prolonged critical illness as different neuroendocrine paradigms. J Clin Endocrinol Metab 1998;83:1827–34; with permission. © [1998] The Endocrine Society.)

concentrations of IGF-I, IGF-binding protein 3, and its acid-labile subunit, none of the anabolic tissue responses, which are evoked by the combined infusion of GHRP and TRH, are present [80]. Further studies need to be undertaken to assess the clinical benefits on morbidity and mortality of TRH infusion alone or in combination with GH secretagogues in prolonged critical illness.

References

[1] Larsen PR, Davies TF, Hay ID. The thyroid gland. In: Wilson JD, Foster DW, Kronenberg HM, et al, editors. Williams textbook of endocrinology. 9th edition. Philadelphia: WB Saunders; 1998. p. 389–515.
[2] Yen PM. Physiological and molecular basis of thyroid hormone action. Physiol Rev 2001;81: 1097–142.
[3] Bianco AC, Salvatore D, Gereben B, et al. Biochemistry, cellular and molecular biology, and physiological roles of the iodothyronine selenodeiodinases. Endocr Rev 2002;23:38–89.
[4] Docter R, Krenning EP, de Jong M, et al. The sick euthyroid syndrome: changes in thyroid hormone serum parameters and hormone metabolism. Clin Endocrinol (Oxf) 1993;39: 499–518.
[5] Rothwell PM, Lawler PG. Prediction of outcome in intensive care patients using endocrine parameters. Crit Care Med 1995;23:78–83.
[6] Wartofsky L, Burman KD. Alterations in thyroid function in patients with systemic illness: the "euthyroid sick syndrome". Endocr Rev 1982;3:164–217.
[7] Michalaki M, Vagenakis AG, Makri M, et al. Dissociation of the early decline in serum T(3) concentration and serum IL-6 rise and TNFalpha in nonthyroidal illness syndrome induced by abdominal surgery. J Clin Endocrinol Metab 2001;86:4198–205.
[8] Van den Berghe G, de Zegher F, Veldhuis JD, et al. Thyrotrophin and prolactin release in prolonged critical illness: dynamics of spontaneous secretion and effects of growth hormone-secretagogues. Clin Endocrinol (Oxf) 1997;47:599–612.
[9] Leonard JL, Koehrle J. Intracellular pathways of iodothyronine metabolism. Philadelphia: Lippincott Williams & Wilkins; 2000.
[10] Bianco AC, Larsen PR. Cellular and structural biology of the deiodinases. Thyroid 2005;15: 777–86.
[11] Luiza Maia A, Kim BW, Huang SA, et al. Type 2 iodothyronine deiodinase is the major source of plasma T3 in euthyroid humans. J Clin Invest 2005;115:2524–33.
[12] Carter JN, Eastmen CJ, Corcoran JM, et al. Inhibition of conversion of thyroxine to triiodothyronine in patients with severe chronic illness. Clin Endocrinol (Oxf) 1976;5:587–94.
[13] Chopra IJ, Chopra U, Smith SR, et al. Reciprocal changes in serum concentrations of 3,3′,5-triiodothyronine (T3) in systemic illnesses. J Clin Endocrinol Metab 1975;41:1043–9.
[14] Peeters RP, Wouters PJ, Kaptein E, et al. Reduced activation and increased inactivation of thyroid hormone in tissues of critically ill patients. J Clin Endocrinol Metab 2003;88: 3202–11.
[15] Debaveye Y, Ellger B, Mebis L, et al. Tissue deiodinase activity during prolonged critical illness: effects of exogenous thyrotropin-releasing hormone and its combination with growth hormone-releasing peptide-2. Endocrinology 2005;146:5604–11.
[16] Weekers F, Van Herck E, Coopmans W, et al. A novel in vivo rabbit model of hypercatabolic critical illness reveals a biphasic neuroendocrine stress response. Endocrinology 2002;143: 764–74.
[17] Boelen A, Kwakkel J, Thijssen-Timmer DC, et al. Simultaneous changes in central and peripheral components of the hypothalamus-pituitary-thyroid axis in lipopolysaccharide-induced acute illness in mice. J Endocrinol 2004;182:315–23.

[18] Boelen A, Kwakkel J, Alkemade A, et al. Induction of type 3 deiodinase activity in inflammatory cells of mice with chronic local inflammation. Endocrinology 2005;146:5128–34.
[19] O'Mara BA, Dittrich W, Lauterio TJ, et al. Pretranslational regulation of type I 5′-deiodinase by thyroid hormones and in fasted and diabetic rats. Endocrinology 1993;133:1715–23.
[20] Crantz FR, Silva JE, Larsen PR. An analysis of the sources and quantity of 3,5,3′-triiodothyronine specifically bound to nuclear receptors in rat cerebral cortex and cerebellum. Endocrinology 1982;110:367–75.
[21] Salvatore D, Bartha T, Harney JW, et al. Molecular biological and biochemical characterization of the human type 2 selenodeiodinase. Endocrinology 1996;137:3308–15.
[22] Gereben B, Goncalves C, Harney JW, et al. Selective proteolysis of human type 2 deiodinase: a novel ubiquitin-proteasomal mediated mechanism for regulation of hormone activation. Mol Endocrinol 2000;14:1697–708.
[23] Zimmerman D. Fetal and neonatal hyperthyroidism. Thyroid 1999;9:727–33.
[24] Richard K, Hume R, Kaptein E, et al. Ontogeny of iodothyronine deiodinases in human liver. J Clin Endocrinol Metab 1998;83:2868–74.
[25] Huang SA, Tu HM, Harney JW, et al. Severe hypothyroidism caused by type 3 iodothyronine deiodinase in infantile hemangiomas. N Engl J Med 2000;343:185–9.
[26] de Jong M, Visser TJ, Bernard BF, et al. Transport and metabolism of iodothyronines in cultured human hepatocytes. J Clin Endocrinol Metab 1993;77:139–43.
[27] Hennemann G, Krenning EP, Polhuys M, et al. Carrier-mediated transport of thyroid hormone into rat hepatocytes is rate-limiting in total cellular uptake and metabolism. Endocrinology 1986;119:1870–2.
[28] Hennemann G, Everts ME, de Jong M, et al. The significance of plasma membrane transport in the bioavailability of thyroid hormone. Clin Endocrinol (Oxf) 1998;48:1–8.
[29] Lim CF, Docter R, Visser TJ, et al. Inhibition of thyroxine transport into cultured rat hepatocytes by serum of nonuremic critically ill patients: effects of bilirubin and nonesterified fatty acids. J Clin Endocrinol Metab 1993;76:1165–72.
[30] Lim CF, Docter R, Krenning EP, et al. Transport of thyroxine into cultured hepatocytes: effects of mild non-thyroidal illness and calorie restriction in obese subjects. Clin Endocrinol (Oxf) 1994;40:79–85.
[31] Sarne DH, Refetoff S. Measurement of thyroxine uptake from serum by cultured human hepatocytes as an index of thyroid status: reduced thyroxine uptake from serum of patients with nonthyroidal illness. J Clin Endocrinol Metab 1985;61:1046–52.
[32] Vos RA, de Jong M, Bernard BF, et al. Impaired thyroxine and 3,5,3′-triiodothyronine handling by rat hepatocytes in the presence of serum of patients with nonthyroidal illness. J Clin Endocrinol Metab 1995;80:2364–70.
[33] Friesema EC, Ganguly S, Abdalla A, et al. Identification of monocarboxylate transporter 8 as a specific thyroid hormone transporter. J Biol Chem 2003;278:40128–35.
[34] Peeters RP, van der Geyten S, Wouters PJ, et al. Tissue thyroid hormone levels in critical illness. J Clin Endocrinol Metab 2005;90:6498–507.
[35] Arem R, Wiener GJ, Kaplan SG, et al. Reduced tissue thyroid hormone levels in fatal illness. Metabolism 1993;42:1102–8.
[36] Timmer DC, Peeters RP, Wouters P, et al. Thyroid hormone receptor alpha splice variants in livers of critically ill patients. Thyroid, in press.
[37] Carr FE, Seelig S, Mariash CN, et al. Starvation and hypothyroidism exert an overlapping influence on rat hepatic messenger RNA activity profiles. J Clin Invest 1983;72:154–63.
[38] Thompson P Jr, Burman KD, Lukes YG, et al. Uremia decreases nuclear 3,5,3′-triiodothyronine receptors in rats. Endocrinology 1980;107:1081–4.
[39] Visser TJ, Kaptein E, Glatt H, et al. Characterization of thyroid hormone sulfotransferases. Chem Biol Interact 1998;109:279–91.
[40] Chopra IJ, Wu SY, Teco GN, et al. A radioimmunoassay for measurement of 3,5,3′-triiodothyronine sulfate: studies in thyroidal and nonthyroidal diseases, pregnancy, and neonatal life. J Clin Endocrinol Metab 1992;75:189–94.

[41] Eelkman Rooda SJ, Kaptein E, Visser TJ. Serum triiodothyronine sulfate in man measured by radioimmunoassay. J Clin Endocrinol Metab 1989;69:552–6.

[42] Peeters RP, Kester MHA, Wouters PJ, et al. Increased T4S levels in critically ill patients due to a decreased hepatic type I deiodinase activity. J Clin Endocrinol Metab 2005;90:6460–5.

[43] Afandi B, Vera R, Schussler GC, et al. Concordant decreases of thyroxine and thyroxine binding protein concentrations during sepsis. Metabolism 2000;49:753–4.

[44] Afandi B, Schussler GC, Arafeh AH, et al. Selective consumption of thyroxine-binding globulin during cardiac bypass surgery. Metabolism 2000;49:270–4.

[45] den Brinker M, Joosten KF, Visser TJ, et al. Euthyroid sick syndrome in meningococcal sepsis: the impact of peripheral thyroid hormone metabolism and binding proteins. J Clin Endocrinol Metab 2005;90:5613–20.

[46] Chopra IJ, Huang TS, Beredo A, et al. Evidence for an inhibitor of extrathyroidal conversion of thyroxine to 3,5,3′-triiodothyronine in sera of patients with nonthyroidal illnesses. J Clin Endocrinol Metab 1985;60:666–72.

[47] Kaptein EM. Thyroid hormone metabolism and thyroid diseases in chronic renal failure. Endocr Rev 1996;17:45–63.

[48] Brent GA, Hershman JM. Thyroxine therapy in patients with severe nonthyroidal illnesses and low serum thyroxine concentration. J Clin Endocrinol Metab 1986;63:1–8.

[49] Wellby ML, Kennedy JA, Barreau PB, et al. Endocrine and cytokine changes during elective surgery. J Clin Pathol 1994;47:1049–51.

[50] Van den Berghe G, de Zegher F, Baxter RC, et al. Neuroendocrinology of prolonged critical illness: effects of exogenous thyrotropin-releasing hormone and its combination with growth hormone secretagogues. J Clin Endocrinol Metab 1998;83:309–19.

[51] Mesotten D, Van den BG. Changes within the GH/IGF-I/IGFBP axis in critical illness. Crit Care Clin 2006;22:17–28 [v].

[52] Fliers E, Guldenaar SE, Wiersinga WM, et al. Decreased hypothalamic thyrotropin-releasing hormone gene expression in patients with nonthyroidal illness. J Clin Endocrinol Metab 1997;82:4032–6.

[53] Bacci V, Schussler GC, Kaplan TB. The relationship between serum triiodothyronine and thyrotropin during systemic illness. J Clin Endocrinol Metab 1982;54:1229–35.

[54] Hamblin PS, Dyer SA, Mohr VS, et al. Relationship between thyrotropin and thyroxine changes during recovery from severe hypothyroxinemia of critical illness. J Clin Endocrinol Metab 1986;62:717–22.

[55] Peeters RP, Wouters PJ, van Toor H, et al. Serum 3,3′,5′-triiodothyronine (rT3) and 3,5,3′-triiodothyronine/rT3 are prognostic markers in critically ill patients and are associated with postmortem tissue deiodinase activities. J Clin Endocrinol Metab 2005;90:4559–65.

[56] Boelen A, Platvoet-ter Schiphorst MC, Bakker O, et al. The role of cytokines in the lipopolysaccharide-induced sick euthyroid syndrome in mice. J Endocrinol 1995;146:475–83.

[57] van der Poll T, Romijn JA, Wiersinga WM, et al. Tumor necrosis factor: a putative mediator of the sick euthyroid syndrome in man. J Clin Endocrinol Metab 1990;71:1567–72.

[58] van der Poll T, Van Zee KJ, Endert E, et al. Interleukin-1 receptor blockade does not affect endotoxin-induced changes in plasma thyroid hormone and thyrotropin concentrations in man. J Clin Endocrinol Metab 1995;80:1341–6.

[59] Boelen A, Platvoet-ter Schiphorst MC, Wiersinga WM. Immunoneutralization of interleukin-1, tumor necrosis factor, interleukin-6 or interferon does not prevent the LPS-induced sick euthyroid syndrome in mice. J Endocrinol 1997;153:115–22.

[60] Damas P, Reuter A, Gysen P, et al. Tumor necrosis factor and interleukin-1 serum levels during severe sepsis in humans. Crit Care Med 1989;17:975–8.

[61] Boelen A, Platvoet-ter Schiphorst MC, Wiersinga WM. Association between serum interleukin-6 and serum 3,5,3′-triiodothyronine in nonthyroidal illness. J Clin Endocrinol Metab 1993;77:1695–9.

[62] Boelen A, Schiphorst MC, Wiersinga WM. Relationship between serum 3,5,3′-triiodothyronine and serum interleukin-8, interleukin-10 or interferon gamma in patients with nonthyroidal illness. J Endocrinol Invest 1996;19:480–3.
[63] Van den Berghe G, de Zegher F, Lauwers P. Dopamine and the sick euthyroid syndrome in critical illness. Clin Endocrinol (Oxf) 1994;41:731–7.
[64] Faglia G, Ferrari C, Beck-Peccoz P, et al. Reduced plasma thyrotropin response to thyrotropin releasing hormone after dexamethasone administration in normal subjects. Horm Metab Res 1973;5:289–92.
[65] Diano S, Naftolin F, Goglia F, et al. Fasting-induced increase in type II iodothyronine deiodinase activity and messenger ribonucleic acid levels is not reversed by thyroxine in the rat hypothalamus. Endocrinology 1998;139:2879–84.
[66] Fekete C, Sarkar S, Christoffolete MA, et al. Bacterial lipopolysaccharide (LPS)-induced type 2 iodothyronine deiodinase (D2) activation in the mediobasal hypothalamus (MBH) is independent of the LPS-induced fall in serum thyroid hormone levels. Brain Res 2005; 1056:97–9.
[67] Alkemade A, Friesema EC, Unmehopa UA, et al. Neuroanatomical pathways for thyroid hormone feedback in the human hypothalamus. J Clin Endocrinol Metab 2005;90:4322–34.
[68] Lechan RM, Fekete C. Role of melanocortin signaling in the regulation of the hypothalamic-pituitary-thyroid (HPT) axis. Peptides 2006;27:310–25.
[69] Ahima RS, Saper CB, Flier JS, et al. Leptin regulation of neuroendocrine systems. Front Neuroendocrinol 2000;21:263–307.
[70] Sergeyev V, Broberger C, Hokfelt T. Effect of LPS administration on the expression of POMC, NPY, galanin, CART and MCH mRNAs in the rat hypothalamus. Brain Res Mol Brain Res 2001;90:93–100.
[71] Fliers E, Unmehopa UA, Manniesing S, et al. Decreased neuropeptide Y (NPY) expression in the infundibular nucleus of patients with nonthyroidal illness. Peptides 2001;22: 459–65.
[72] Pizzagalli F, Hagenbuch B, Stieger B, et al. Identification of a novel human organic anion transporting polypeptide as a high affinity thyroxine transporter. Mol Endocrinol 2002;16: 2283–96.
[73] Clerget-Froidevaux MS, Seugnet I, Demeneix BA. Thyroid status co-regulates thyroid hormone receptor and co-modulator genes specifically in the hypothalamus. FEBS Lett 2004; 569:341–5.
[74] Van den Berghe G, de Zegher F, Bouillon R. Acute and prolonged critical illness as different neuroendocrine paradigms. J Clin Endocrinol Metab 1998;83:1827–34.
[75] Van den Berghe G. Novel insights into the neuroendocrinology of critical illness. Eur J Endocrinol/European Federation Of Endocrine Societies 2000;143:1–13.
[76] Van den Berghe G. Dynamic neuroendocrine responses to critical illness. Front Neuroendocrinol 2002;23:370–91.
[77] Gardner DF, Kaplan MM, Stanley CA, et al. Effect of tri-iodothyronine replacement on the metabolic and pituitary responses to starvation. N Engl J Med 1979;300:579–84.
[78] Utiger RD. Decreased extrathyroidal triiodothyronine production in nonthyroidal illness: benefit or harm? Am J Med 1980;69:807–10.
[79] Van den Berghe G, Wouters P, Weekers F, et al. Reactivation of pituitary hormone release and metabolic improvement by infusion of growth hormone-releasing peptide and thyrotropin-releasing hormone in patients with protracted critical illness. J Clin Endocrinol Metab 1999;84:1311–23.
[80] Van den Berghe G, Baxter RC, Weekers F, et al. The combined administration of GH-releasing peptide-2 (GHRP-2), TRH and GnRH to men with prolonged critical illness evokes superior endocrine and metabolic effects compared to treatment with GHRP-2 alone. Clin Endocrinol (Oxf) 2002;56:655–69.
[81] Vaughan GM, Mason AD Jr, McManus WF, et al. Alterations of mental status and thyroid hormones after thermal injury. J Clin Endocrinol Metab 1985;60:1221–5.

[82] Becker RA, Vaughan GM, Ziegler MG, et al. Hypermetabolic low triiodothyronine syndrome of burn injury. Crit Care Med 1982;10:870–5.
[83] Bettendorf M, Schmidt KG, Grulich-Henn J, et al. Tri-iodothyronine treatment in children after cardiac surgery: a double-blind, randomised, placebo-controlled study. Lancet 2000; 356:529–34.
[84] Debaveye Y, Van den Berghe G. Is there still a place for dopamine in the modern intensive care unit? Anesth Analg 2004;98:461–8.
[85] Van den Berghe G, de Zegher F, Vlasselaers D, et al. Thyrotropin-releasing hormone in critical illness: from a dopamine-dependent test to a strategy for increasing low serum triiodothyronine, prolactin, and growth hormone concentrations. Crit Care Med 1996;24:590–5.

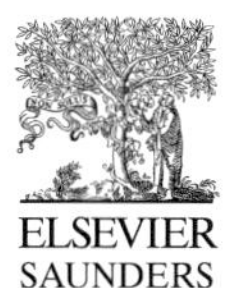

Endocrinol Metab Clin N Am 35 (2006) 823–838

ENDOCRINOLOGY AND METABOLISM CLINICS OF NORTH AMERICA

The Hypothalamic-Pituitary-Adrenal Axis in Critical Illness

Philipp Schuetz, MD, Beat Müller, MD*

Clinic of Endocrinology, Diabetes and Clinical Nutrition, Department of Internal Medicine, University Hospital Basel, Petersgraben 4, Basel CH-4031, Switzerland

Life-threatening disease induces acute adaptive responses specific to the stimulus and generalized responses when the disturbances are more extensive and sustained [1]. An appropriate adaptation of the hypothalamic-pituitary-adrenal (HPA) axis to stress is essential for survival [2,3]. Increasing circulating levels of adrenal steroids (eg, cortisol) are the consequence of an acutely and markedly activated anterior pituitary (ie, adrenocorticotropin hormone [ACTH]) and hypothalamic (eg, corticotropin-releasing hormone [CRH] and vasopressin, also termed *antidiuretic hormone* [ADH]) response [4]. This response happens under the influence of higher cortical functions, spinal and peripheral baroreceptors, among others. The acute stress response adapts throughout the course of critical illness [5]. In addition, disease-related variations in the binding capacities of circulating proteins (ie, cortisol-binding globulin and albumin) result in even more fluctuating levels of free stress hormones during critical illness [6–10]. The tissue and cellular responses to free circulating hormone levels vary substantially based on the receptor and postreceptor levels (eg, by modulation of the number and activity of cellular receptors or the activity of downstream responses, respectively) [11–15]. The half-life of cortisol in the blood is increased during stress owing to a decreased rate of hepatic extraction and renal enzymatic inactivation of cortisol to cortisone by 11β-hydroxysteroid dehydrogenase [16]. The immuno-neuro-endocrine interactions are bidirectional, mutually potentiating and attenuating, and not fortuitous. Several gluco- and mineralocorticoids modulate the immune response distinctively [17]. On the other hand, cytokines (eg, tumor necrosis factor, interleukins, and macrophage-migration inhibitory factor) and bacterial products (eg, endotoxin) are able to modulate the response of the HPA axis at each level [1].

* Corresponding author.
E-mail address: happy.mueller@unibas.ch (B. Müller).

0889-8529/06/$ - see front matter
doi:10.1016/j.ecl.2006.09.013

Of course, "critical illness" is not a simple disease entity, and, when scanning the literature, one cannot evade the impression that this fact is sometimes neglected. Inducers of life-threatening critical stress include trauma, burns, surgery, infections, and multiple other diseases typically associated with variable levels of inflammation [18]. The mediator profile during these distinct diseases varies substantially [19]. For didactic purposes, any attempt to summarize hormonal changes during so-called "critical illness" is oversimplistic and inherently problematic. These caveats need to born in mind before drawing heroic therapeutic implications from allegedly promising hypotheses for a disease syndrome in the absence of unequivocal scientific evidence.

Timing and profile of steroids during critical illness are essential

Cortisol (also called hydrocortisone or compound F) is considered the primary active glucocorticoid and is essential for the adaptation and maintenance of stress homeostasis during critical illness. It is a pluripotent hormone acting on all tissues to regulate pleiotropic and numerous aspects of metabolism, growth, and physiologic functioning, being in this way essential for survival in critical illness [20–22]. Characteristically, any acute insult will result in an augmented release of cortisol and other adrenal steroids, among other factors mediated by a sharp rise of circulating short-lived ACTH, which, in turn, is driven by CRH, vasopressin, cytokines, and an upregulated noradrenergic system, and other factors [5]. The production of cortisol in the adrenocortical cells in response to ACTH occurs within minutes and begins with the enzymatic cleavage of the side chain of cholesterol to generate pregnenolone and, by additional enzyme systems, cortisol (Fig. 1) [23,24]. The normal feedback system might be altered because hypercortisolism is less suppressible by dexamethasone infusion in septic shock [25]. Moreover, the normal circadian rhythm of cortisol secretion, especially the nadir during night time, is disturbed [26,27]. Reported plasma hormone levels vary widely among studies. The persistence of pulsatile secretion may explain the observed variability, and, accordingly, the accuracy of single samples is potentially inadequate, as is true for all hormones [28]. Furthermore, the interindividual and interassay variability of cortisol and other steroid assays measuring free or total hormone concentrations at different sites and centers can be substantial [6,29,30].

Although the renin-angiotensin-aldosterone system is also activated [31], the acute adaptive adrenal response to stress is typically seen as a shift from mineralocorticoid production to a marked increase in glucocorticoid production. In addition, in acute illness, the biologic effects of cortisol increase owing to a decrease in cortisol binding globulin and an increase in receptor sensitivity and number [1,10].

Metabolically, hypercortisolism acutely induces glycogen, fat, and protein breakdown so that energy becomes abundantly available to critical

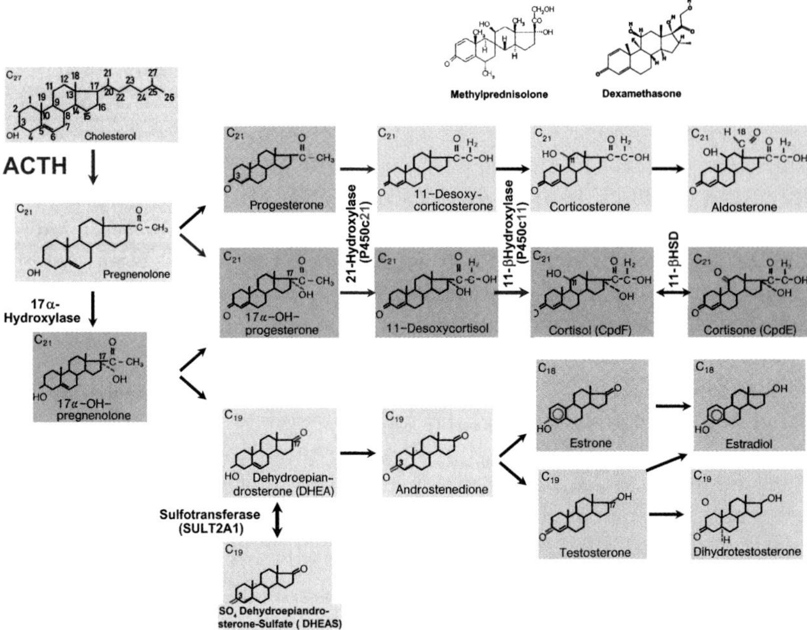

Fig. 1. Adrenal steroidogenesis and commonly used generic steroid drugs. 11-βHSD, 11 beta hydroxysteroid dehydrogenase.

organs. Cortisol-mediated retention of intravascular fluid and an enhanced ionotropic and vasopressor response to catecholamines and angiotensin II offer hemodynamic advantages in the "fight or flight" reflex. The acute steroid excess can be interpreted as an attempt of the organism to mute its own inflammatory cascade to protect against an overresponse of the endogenous "fire brigade" [5].

This acute phase typically lasts for a few hours or days. If death or recovery does not occur within a few days of intensive medical care, the critical illness becomes protracted. Arguably, a protracted severe illness with intensive care has not been critical during the evolution of mankind. Contemporary medical technology through its artificial life support systems has created conditions never before experienced by complex life forms [1]. Accordingly, the neuroendocrine response in this subsequent chronic phase of illness may be considered to be insufficient rather than beneficial for the adaptation to chronic disease.

Hormonally during the prolonged phase of critical illness of weeks to months there is a dissociation between high plasma cortisol and low ACTH levels, suggesting non-ACTH mediated mechanisms for regulation of the adrenal cortex [32]. Cytokines and other circulating factors might suppress ACTH synthesis and secretion. For example, endothelin 1 [33], atrial natriuretic peptides [33,34], and pro-adrenomedullin [35] are elevated at stages when ACTH is suppressed. Moreover, despite an increase in plasma renin activity, paradoxically, a decreased concentration of aldosterone is found in protracted critical illness [36,37]. Upon recovery, normal responses are seen, indicating the reversibility of this phenomenon.

Metabolically, there is a delay and suppression of anabolic processes, resulting in typical features of prolonged critical care cachexia, including breakdown of muscle tissue, loss of lean body mass, polyneuropathy, generalized tissue wasting, and dystrophy [38–41]. These changes resemble the features of Cushing's syndrome, in which a subtle (ie, average cortisol production rate of 36 mg/d) and prolonged (ie, months to years) corticoid excess leads to severe morbidity and, if left untreated, to a mortality rate of more than 50% within 5 years [42].

Dehydroepiandrosterone sulfate (DHEAS) is the most abundant adrenal steroid in the human circulation. The adrenals secrete DHEA and DHEAS, but only DHEA is considered biologically active, mediating its action mainly indirectly via downstream conversion to sex steroids and intermediate steroids with potentially distinct properties (Fig. 1) [43]. The conversion of DHEA sulfotransferase (SULT2A1) is the rate-limiting step regulating the equilibrium between DHEA and DHEAS [44]. SULT2A1 is downregulated in sepsis [45], which suggests that circulating DHEAS levels may not appropriately reflect the biologically active DHEA pool. DHEA administration showed beneficial effects on experimental induced sepsis in rodents [46–51]. Serum cortisol is increased while DHEAS is decreased in septic shock and trauma patients, especially if moribund [52,53]; however, when compared with the level in healthy controls, DHEA is significantly increased in sepsis but decreased after trauma. Most severely ill patients have higher cortisol and lower DHEA and a significantly higher cortisol to DHEA ratio. Similarly, the cortisol to DHEA ratio is significantly increased in nonsurvivors of septic shock whereas the ratio in survivors does not differ from that in controls [52]. In another study [54], lowered DHEAS and androstenedione levels could be measured in chronically ill males but not in ill females. 17α-OH-progesterone and 17α-OH-pregnenolone levels in subgroups of the patients suggested a probable enzymatic block in the δ-5-pathway of androgen biosynthesis in severe illness.

These findings have been interpreted as a shift from adrenal androgen toward glucocorticoid biosynthesis. Accordingly, acute and sustained hypogonadism in both sexes is virtually always observed during any critical illness [55,56]. This constellation suggests a stress-induced intra-adrenal shift of pregnenolone metabolism away from the mineralocorticoid and adrenal androgen pathway toward the glucocorticoid pathway, indicating a resetting between the immunostimulatory (DHEA) and immunosuppressive (cortisol) adrenocortical hormones [1,53,57,58]. This mechanism may ultimately also fail, as indicated by the 20-fold higher incidence of adrenal insufficiency seen in critically ill patients over the age of 50 years who had been treated in the intensive care unit for more than 14 days [59].

The question of a normal or abnormal response

Increased circulating cortisol levels seem to reflect an increasing severity of illness (Fig. 2) [60,61], and mortality associated with untreated adrenal insufficiency increases with the severity of the acute stress [62]. Similarly, peri- and postoperative basal cortisol concentrations reflect the degree of surgical stress [63,64]. Peak cortisol levels are achieved in the immediate postoperative period, around the time of extubation [65,66]. Cortisol levels after major surgery resemble the levels during the acute phase of septic shock [60,67,68]. Although in the acute phase of critical illness, the secretory activity of the HPA axis is essentially maintained or augmented, it starts to diminish during the chronic phase, that is, after a few weeks of protracted critical illness [60,69]. Nonsurvivors of sepsis and patients with relative adrenal insufficiency had the lowest DHEAS values, suggesting that DHEAS might be a prognostic marker and a sign of exhausted adrenal reserve in critical illness [53]. During severe illness, co-morbidities such as head injury or adrenal hemorrhage, pharmacologic agents (eg, etomidate, opioids, ketokonazole), or inflammatory mediators (eg, tumor necrosis factor-α, interleukins) can impair the proper stress response of the HPA axis [70]. The interindividual range of measured serum cortisol in a given stress situation is wide [71,72]. The characteristics and extent of the HPA response also vary in different age

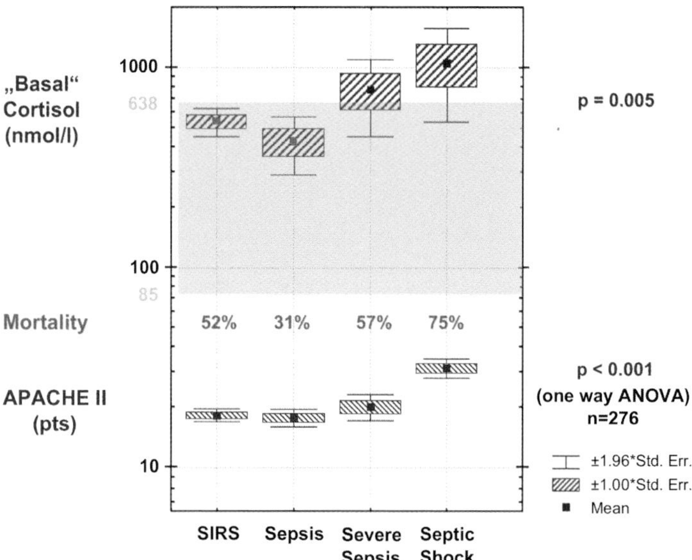

Fig. 2. Circulating cortisol levels in different severities of disease and infection. ANOVA, analysis of variance; APACHE II, acute physiologic and chronic health evaluation II score; SIRS, systemic inflammatory response syndrome. (*Data from* Muller B, Becker KL, Schachinger H, et al. Calcitonin precursors are reliable markers of sepsis in a medical intensive care unit. Crit Care Med 2000;28(4):977–83.)

groups, namely, in children [73]. This dispersion of results complicates the differentiation of a normal from an abnormal adrenal response in the course of acute illness. In addition, critical illness can alter and impair the proper stress response of the HPA axis [70].

The terms *relative* or *functional* adrenal insufficiency have been proposed for hypotensive septic critically ill patients who show hemodynamic improvement upon cortisol administration. In these patients, the cortisol levels, despite being within the normal reference range or even elevated, are still considered inadequate for the severity of stress, and the patient may be unable to respond to any additional or protracted stress [70].

Corticosteroid insufficiency is difficult to discern clinically and must be actively sought by the treating physician. There are no clinical indicators (eg, eosinophilia, vasopressor dependence, or hemodynamic response) with proven diagnostic accuracy, partly because of a lack of a reference standard [74,75]. The life-threatening dangers of stress in untreated absolute adrenal insufficiency are undisputable. In contrast, there is a debate concerning the definition of relative adrenal insufficiency, its treatment, and the identification of patients at risk [1,70,74,76,77].

A simple and widely used test is the stimulation of cortisol with injection of synthetic ACTH (Synacthen) in hypotensive critically ill patients. A basal level of cortisol of greater than 935 nmol/L combined with an increase (Δ) of cortisol less than 250 nmol/L (9 μg/dL) after stimulation with 250 μg of ACTH has been associated with a mortality rate of 80%, arguably pointing to a relative adrenal insufficiency [60]. Nevertheless, circulating ACTH levels after a standard injection of 250 μg of ACTH are extremely high (10,00–60,000 pg/mL) and much higher than the 100 to 300 pg/mL found after stimulation with 1 μg of synthetic ACTH [68,74,78]. Because the 250-μg ACTH stimulation test induces supraphysiologic ACTH concentrations, the 1-μg synthetic ACTH test has been suggested to be more sensitive to diagnose adrenocortical insufficiency [79]. In healthy individuals, 1 μg is the lowest ACTH dose to cause a maximal cortisol response, and there is no diurnal variation of cortisol response to submaximal ACTH stimulation [79]. There is a stress-dependent dissociation of the cortisol response to increasing doses of synthetic ACTH in situations of stress, as shown during strong surgical stress (Fig. 3) [61]. Accordingly, in stressed patients without HPA disease, cortisol concentrations are higher after stimulation with 250 μg as compared with 1 μg of ACTH. The adrenal reserve is not completely used and is not the limiting organ in this model of strong surgical stress.

What is really measured with adrenal stimulation tests [74,80]? Is an additional rise in cortisol upon ACTH stimulation of any clinical significance, namely, the arguably decisive increment (Δ) in serum cortisol concentration of 250 nM (9 μg/dL) from baseline [81]? In the study by Widmer and coworkers, approximately 40% of surgical patients did not achieve this target change in cortisol, yet none of them sustained any adverse clinical consequences from severe surgical stress without glucocorticoid substitution

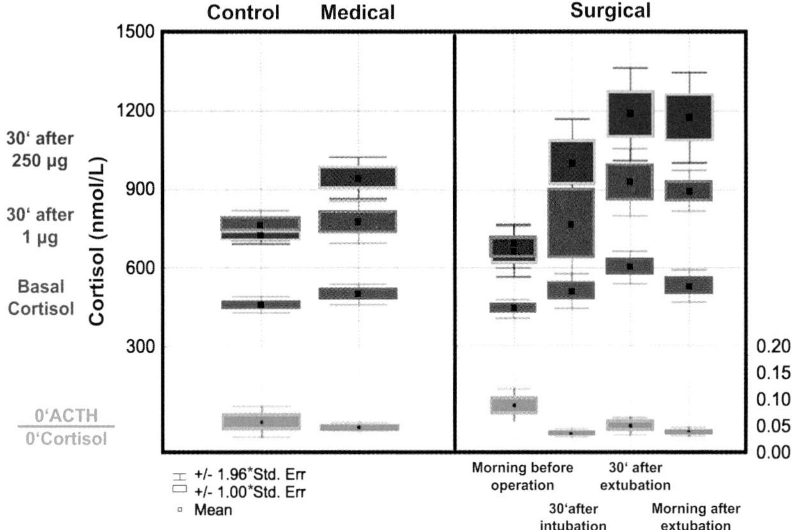

Fig. 3. Variable cortisol response to ACTH. Squares denote mean; boxes denote ± standard error of the mean; and whiskers denote ± 1.96 × standard error of the mean. For subjects in Group A and B, the mean values of each subject over all 4 days is shown. In Group C, basal and peak cortisol concentrations increased, whereas the basal ACTH levels and basal ACTH/basal cortisol ratio decreased during the operation (all $P \leq .001$). Overview shows the basal (purple) and peak cortisol concentrations after stimulation with 1 μg (red) and 250 μg (blue) of ACTH in subjects in Group A, B, and C. Basal ($P < .00001$ for trend) and peak cortisol (after 1 μg ACTH: $P = .07$; after 250 μg ACTH: $P = .02$) concentrations increased in the three stress groups (A, B, C3). To convert cortisol from nmol/L into μg/dL, divide by 27.7. (*Adapted from* Widmer IE, Puder JJ, Konig C, et al. Cortisol response in relation to the severity of stress and illness. J Clin Endocrinol Metab 2005;90(8):4582.)

[61]. Indeed, in the setting of severe illness and stress, the use of the low-dose (1-μg) ACTH stimulation test may increase the number of overdiagnosed patients [82,83]. Because of the circadian rhythm in healthy individuals, basal cortisol levels are lower in the evening than in the morning, yet the stimulated cortisol levels will be similar. This observation is true regardless of whether the stimulation is performed by using ACTH [84], insulin hypoglycemia [85], metyrapone [86], or CRH [87]; therefore, the incremental rise (Δ) of cortisol is inherently negatively correlated with basal cortisol levels and not a useful parameter. Furthermore, the interindividual variability of different cortisol and other steroid hormone assays performed at different sites can be substantial [29]. This variability calls for a complete rethinking of the term *relative adrenal insufficiency* [80].

Treatment

Whether "iatrogenic" hypercortisolism during critical illness is truly needed and beneficial remains uncertain. Even a continuous, intended-to-be-physiologic "low-dose" infusion of hydrocortisone results in several fold higher levels (up to 3000–5000 nM) as compared with maximal endogenous hypercortisolism reached during the severest near-death stress in patients with intact adrenal reserve [88,89]. Concerning the treatment of relative adrenal insufficiency in patients with septic shock, one single large trial found a reduction of mortality; however, this change occurred only post hoc in the subgroup of patients with an impaired rise (Δ) of cortisol less than 250 nM (<9 μg/dL) 30 minutes after the injection of 250 μg of synthetic ACTH [81]. Previously published criteria for the prognostic characterization of critical illness from the same group were not considered [60]. The large confidence interval of pre- and poststimulation cortisol levels in this study reveals that the patients were heterogeneous and clearly included a sizable number of patients with true "absolute" adrenal insufficiency, potentially skewing the results [90]. Furthermore, in contrast to all other studies, in this trial, oral fludrocortisone was added to the intravenous administration of hydrocortisone [81]. The administration of tablets in critically ill patients may be cumbersome; therefore, fludrocortisone is often omitted in routine intensive care. Unfortunately, as the researchers in this study state, there was "no interest in formally demonstrating a deleterious effect of corticosteroids" [81]. Suggesting thereafter that corticosteroids do not have potential for harm in critically ill septic patients is untenable [91]. Despite these limitations, this study had a landslide impact on the management of critically ill patients by affecting not only patients who had vasopressor-refractory septic shock but also and, albeit, unproven, other "therapy-refractory" intensive care unit patients with milder or even without infections. Possibly, the administration of steroids was so welcomed and became fashionable because the time had come to resurrect past rites (Fig. 4). In the context of such controversy, the premature publication of preliminary data from small underpowered studies in high-impact journals is of little help [92]. Some intensivists argued that a hemodynamic improvement can be observed after the administration of "stress doses" (ie, 50 to 200 mg) of hydrocortisone, justifying its administration to reduce the harmful doses of catecholamines needed to maintain blood pressure. In this context, the question was raised whether one should use hydrocortisone as a therapy to improve the charts or the outcome of patients [93].

Multiple studies were performed by opinion leaders from both sides, not surprisingly yielding opposite conclusions, especially with regard to dosing of the steroids and the interpretations of the change in cortisol after ACTH stimulation [71,74,94–98]. The comparison of different studies in systematic reviews and meta-analyses is inherently problematic, because the patient groups included differ widely in terms of underlying diagnosis (eg, patients sustaining infections, acute lung injury, acute respiratory distress syndrome, burns, malaria, and other entities), inclusion criteria (eg, all consecutive patients versus subgroups of selected patients, different severities of infection ranging from sepsis to severe sepsis to refractory septic shock), and

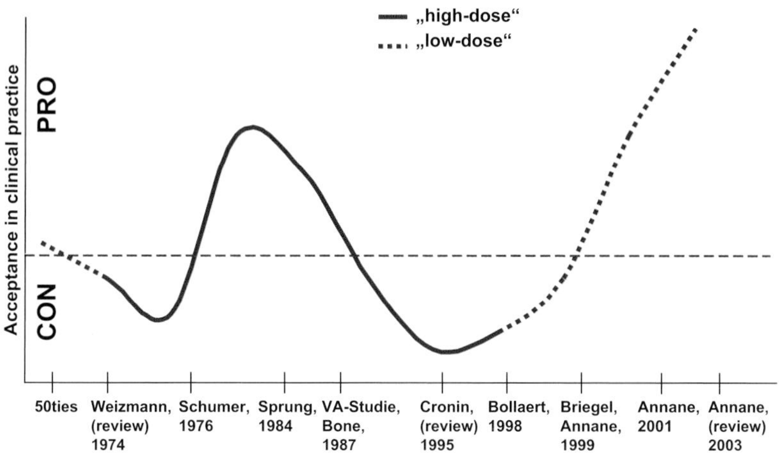

Fig. 4. A historical view of the use of steroids in the treatment of sepsis showing "ups and downs." (*Adapted from* F.M. Brunkhorst, MD, personal communication, 2006.)

the timing of inclusion (on admission, during the early phase of critical illness, and during the course of disease after failing to respond to other supportive interventions such as the administration of fluids and catecholamines). In part, patients were post hoc dichotomized based on an allegedly inadequate response in the ACTH stimulation test [81] or "basal" cortisol levels [90]. The remedies tested were diverse and included hydrocortisone [97], methylprednisolone [99], dexamethasone [100], fludrocortisone [81], and even DHEA [101–103] in part combined and among others. The circulating half-life ($T_{1/2}$), biologic effects, and potency of these drugs vary widely. Similarly, the correlation between a given circulating $T_{1/2}$ of a glucocorticoid and its duration of action is poor [21]. Dosages applied in critically ill patients ranged from so-called "supraphysiological" [97] to "low-dose" [81] to "high dose" [99,100]. The use of these terms is not validated given the fact that one is unable to determine and monitor the true needs for a given individual with a specific critical disease at a certain time point. All of the different steroids administered have markedly distinct biologic effects, which is self-evident based on their variable structure (see Fig. 1). Subtle differences in the biochemistry of steroid hormones can alter the biologic response dramatically. For example, the only difference between the "male" hormone testosterone and the "female" hormone estradiol (see Fig. 1) is the interchangeable oxidation of a hydroxyl side group. Nevertheless, phenotypic differences between both sexes can be impressive. In this context, the differences between the steroids used therapeutically in critical illness, including but not limited to glucocorticoids and mineralocorticoids, are even more important and should not be neglected.

Upon cessation, any short or long-term exposure to "supraphysiological" glucocorticoid dosages will expose the patient subsequently to the risk of "absolute" insufficiency of the HPA axis, that is, Addison's syndrome. This iatrogenic complication can be life threatening in stress situations (eg, recurrence of the critical illness). Rapid restoration of ACTH release with CRH infusion suggests that the suppression of the HPA axis after iatrogenic hypercortisolism is predominantly due to reduced CRH secretion [104]. The extent and duration of this functional deficiency is unpredictable, may last from weeks to years, and is largely independent of the dose and duration of steroid therapy [105,106]. This observation has led to the conservative practice of replacing glucocorticoid before an anticipated stress in any patient who has received supraphysiologic dosages of glucocorticoids within the past year [22,107].

There is little definitive advice to offer concerning the use of pharmacologic doses of glucocorticoids in critical illness in general, especially in critically ill patients who do not meet the criteria for "relative adrenal insufficiency." The alleged benefits should be weighed against the proven dangers of therapy, such as hyperglycemia [108,109] and a suppression of the immune response [96,99,110–112]. In comatose patients with cerebral malaria, high-dose dexamethasone treatment has been proven deleterious [113]. The ebb and flow of attitudes regarding the usefulness of large-dose steroid treatment in spinal cord injured patients, also referred to as "CRASH-landing of steroids" based on the acronym of a seminal study, is a case in point [114–116]. The clinical frustrations of dealing with severe sepsis and its high mortality rate may tempt many clinicians to use corticosteroids; however, our urge to do something should not tempt us to do anything. Adhering to the results of current randomized controlled trials is the best guide to clinical practice. More rigorously controlled multicenter studies are required to further clarify this complex clinical enigma. The results of one such trial, the ongoing CORTICUS study, are anxiously awaited by intensivists [117].

Summary

The interindividual differences in the extent, timing, and modulators of the HPA response during distinct critical illnesses are not trivial. The correct assessment of the adequate individual stress response in severe disease is unresolved. The accurate substitution of the subtle and varying needs of an allegedly disturbed HPA axis is problematic. If we do not learn from previous mistakes regarding the characterization, interpretation, substitution, and suppression of allegedly abnormal endocrine responses in severe and acute diseases, we will continue to repeat them [118,119]. Inappropriate assumptions will lead to inappropriate administrations of potentially life-saving steroids and, ultimately, contradict our principal aim in medicine of "primum non nocere." Further randomized controlled trials are needed to unravel this complex and important clinical problem before widespread therapy can be advocated.

References

[1] Vermes I, Beishuizen A. The hypothalamic-pituitary-adrenal response to critical illness. Best Pract Res Clin Endocrinol Metab 2001;15(4):495–511.

[2] Ledingham IM, Watt I. Influence of sedation on mortality in critically ill multiple trauma patients. Lancet 1983;1(8336):1270.

[3] Absalom A, Pledger D, Kong A. Adrenocortical function in critically ill patients 24 h after a single dose of etomidate. Anaesthesia 1999;54(9):861–7.

[4] Nylen ES, Muller B. Endocrine changes in critical illness. J Intensive Care Med 2004;19(2): 67–82.

[5] Van den Berghe G. The neuroendocrine response to stress is a dynamic process. Best Pract Res Clin Endocrinol Metab 2001;15(4):405–19.

[6] Ho JT, Al-Musalhi H, Chapman MJ, et al. Septic shock and sepsis: a comparison of total and free plasma cortisol levels. J Clin Endocrinol Metab 2006;91(1):105–14.

[7] Polderman KH, van Zanten A, Girbes AR. Free cortisol and critically ill patients. N Engl J Med 2004;351(4):395–7 [author reply: 395–7].

[8] Khan T, Kupfer Y, Tessler S. Free cortisol and critically ill patients. N Engl J Med 2004; 351(4):395–7 [author reply: 395–7].

[9] Hamrahian AH, Oseni TS, Arafah BM. Measurements of serum free cortisol in critically ill patients. N Engl J Med 2004;350(16):1629–38.

[10] Beishuizen A, Thijs LG, Vermes I. Patterns of corticosteroid-binding globulin and the free cortisol index during septic shock and multitrauma. Intensive Care Med 2001;27(10): 1584–91.

[11] Webster JI, Sternberg EM. Role of the hypothalamic-pituitary-adrenal axis, glucocorticoids and glucocorticoid receptors in toxic sequelae of exposure to bacterial and viral products. J Endocrinol 2004;181(2):207–21.

[12] Prigent H, Maxime V, Annane D. Science review: mechanisms of impaired adrenal function in sepsis and molecular actions of glucocorticoids. Crit Care 2004;8(4):243–52.

[13] Silverstein R, Johnson DC. Endogenous versus exogenous glucocorticoid responses to experimental bacterial sepsis. J Leukoc Biol 2003;73(4):417–27.

[14] Briegel J. Cortisol in critically ill patients with sepsis: physiologic functions and therapeutic implications. Wien Klin Wochenschr 2000;112(8):341–52.

[15] Manary MJ, Muglia LJ, Vogt SK, et al. Cortisol and its action on the glucocorticoid receptor in malnutrition and acute infection. Metabolism 2006;55(4):550–4.

[16] Melby JC, Edghal RH, Spink WW. Secretion and metabolism of cortisol after injection of endotoxin. J Lab Clin Med 1960;56:50–62.

[17] Rinaldi S, Adembri C, Grechi S, et al. Low-dose hydrocortisone during severe sepsis: effects on microalbuminuria. Crit Care Med 2006;(Jul):17.

[18] Alarifi AA, van den Berghe GH, Snider RH, et al. Endocrine markers and mediators in critical illness. 3rd edition. Philadelphia: J.B. Lippincott; 2001.

[19] Nylen ES, Alarifi AA. Humoral markers of severity and prognosis of critical illness. Best Pract Res Clin Endocrinol Metab 2001;15(4):553–73.

[20] Munck A, Guyre PM, Holbrook NJ. Physiological functions of glucocorticoids in stress and their relation to pharmacological actions. Endocr Rev 1984;5(1):25–44.

[21] Axelrod L. Corticosteroid therapy. In: Becker KL, editor. Principles and practice of endocrinology and metabolism. 3rd edition. Philadelphia: Lippincott Williams & Wilkins; 2001. p. 751–64.

[22] Lynn LD. Adrenocortical insufficiency. In: Becker KL, editor. Principles and practice of endocrinology and metabolism. 3rd edition. Philadelphia: Lippincott Williams & Wilkins; 2001. p. 739–43.

[23] Manna PR, Dyson MT, Eubank DW, et al. Regulation of steroidogenesis and the steroidogenic acute regulatory protein by a member of the cAMP response-element binding protein family. Mol Endocrinol 2002;16(1):184–99.

[24] Stocco DM, Clark BJ. Regulation of the acute production of steroids in steroidogenic cells. Endocr Rev 1996;17(3):221–44.
[25] Perrot D, Bonneton A, Dechaud H, et al. Hypercortisolism in septic shock is not suppressible by dexamethasone infusion. Crit Care Med 1993;21(3):396–401.
[26] Naito Y, Fukata J, Tamai S, et al. Biphasic changes in hypothalamo-pituitary-adrenal function during the early recovery period after major abdominal surgery. J Clin Endocrinol Metab 1991;73(1):111–7.
[27] Aun F, McIntosh TK, Lee A, et al. The effects of surgery on the circadian rhythms of cortisol. Int Surg 1984;69(2):101–5.
[28] Voerman HJ, Strack van Schijndel RJ, Groeneveld AB, et al. Pulsatile hormone secretion during severe sepsis: accuracy of different blood sampling regimens. Metabolism 1992; 41(9):934–40.
[29] Steele BW, Wang E, Palmer-Toy DE, et al. Total long-term within-laboratory precision of cortisol, ferritin, thyroxine, free thyroxine, and thyroid-stimulating hormone assays based on a College of American Pathologists fresh frozen serum study: do available methods meet medical needs for precision? Arch Pathol Lab Med 2005;129(3):318–22.
[30] Zaloga GP, Marik P. Hypothalamic-pituitary-adrenal insufficiency. Crit Care Clin 2001; 17(1):25–41.
[31] O'Leary E, Hubbard K, Tormey W, et al. Laparoscopic cholecystectomy: haemodynamic and neuroendocrine responses after pneumoperitoneum and changes in position. Br J Anaesth 1996;76(5):640–4.
[32] Hinson JP, Vinson GP, Kapas S, et al. The role of endothelin in the control of adrenocortical function: stimulation of endothelin release by ACTH and the effects of endothelin-1 and endothelin-3 on steroidogenesis in rat and human adrenocortical cells. J Endocrinol 1991;128(2):275–80.
[33] Vermes I, Beishuizen A, Hampsink RM, et al. Dissociation of plasma adrenocorticotropin and cortisol levels in critically ill patients: possible role of endothelin and atrial natriuretic hormone. J Clin Endocrinol Metab 1995;80(4):1238–42.
[34] Morgenthaler NG, Struck J, Christ-Crain M, et al. Pro-atrial natriuretic peptide is a prognostic marker in sepsis, similar to the APACHE II score: an observational study. Crit Care 2005;9(1):R37–45.
[35] Christ-Crain M, Morgenthaler NG, Struck J, et al. Mid-regional pro-adrenomedullin as a prognostic marker in sepsis: an observational study. Crit Care 2005;9(6):R816–24.
[36] Davenport MW, Zipser RD. Association of hypotension with hyperreninemic hypoaldosteronism in the critically ill patient. Arch Intern Med 1983;143(4):735–7.
[37] Zipser RD, Davenport MW, Martin KL, et al. Hyperreninemic hypoaldosteronism in the critically ill: a new entity. J Clin Endocrinol Metab 1981;53(4):867–73.
[38] Wilmore DW. Catabolic illness: strategies for enhancing recovery. N Engl J Med 1991; 325(10):695–702.
[39] Souba WW. Cytokine control of nutrition and metabolism in critical illness. Curr Probl Surg 1994;31(7):577–643.
[40] Weekers F, Van den Berghe G. Endocrine modifications and interventions during critical illness. Proc Nutr Soc 2004;63(3):443–50.
[41] Vanhorebeek I, Van den Berghe G. Hormonal and metabolic strategies to attenuate catabolism in critically ill patients. Curr Opin Pharmacol 2004;4(6):621–8.
[42] Schteingart DE. Cushing syndrome. In: Becker KL, editor. Principles and practice of endocrinology and metabolism. 3rd edition. Philadelphia: Lippincott Williams & Wilkins; 2001. p. 723–38.
[43] Arlt W. Dehydroepiandrosterone replacement therapy. Semin Reprod Med 2004;22(4): 379–88.
[44] Hammer F, Subtil S, Lux P, et al. No evidence for hepatic conversion of dehydroepiandrosterone (DHEA) sulfate to DHEA: in vivo and in vitro studies. J Clin Endocrinol Metab 2005;90(6):3600–5.

[45] Kim MS, Shigenaga J, Moser A, et al. Suppression of DHEA sulfotransferase (Sult2A1) during the acute-phase response. Am J Physiol Endocrinol Metab 2004;287(4):E731–8.
[46] Hildebrand F, Pape HC, Harwood P, et al. Are alterations of lymphocyte subpopulations in polymicrobial sepsis and DHEA treatment mediated by the tumour necrosis factor (TNF)-alpha receptor (TNF-RI)? A study in TNF-RI (TNF-RI(−/−)) knock-out rodents. Clin Exp Immunol 2004;138(2):221–9.
[47] Hildebrand F, Pape HC, Hoevel P, et al. The importance of systemic cytokines in the pathogenesis of polymicrobial sepsis and dehydroepiandrosterone treatment in a rodent model. Shock 2003;20(4):338–46.
[48] Oberbeck R, Dahlweid M, Koch R, et al. Dehydroepiandrosterone decreases mortality rate and improves cellular immune function during polymicrobial sepsis. Crit Care Med 2001; 29(2):380–4.
[49] Ben-Nathan D, Padgett DA, Loria RM. Androstenediol and dehydroepiandrosterone protect mice against lethal bacterial infections and lipopolysaccharide toxicity. J Med Microbiol 1999;48(5):425–31.
[50] Angele MK, Catania RA, Ayala A, et al. Dehydroepiandrosterone: an inexpensive steroid hormone that decreases the mortality due to sepsis following trauma-induced hemorrhage. Arch Surg 1998;133(12):1281–8.
[51] Matsuda A, Furukawa K, Suzuki H, et al. Dehydroepiandrosterone modulates toll-like receptor expression on splenic macrophages of mice after severe polymicrobial sepsis. Shock 2005;24(4):364–9.
[52] Arlt W, Hammer F, Sanning P, et al. Dissociation of serum dehydroepiandrosterone and dehydroepiandrosterone sulfate in septic shock. J Clin Endocrinol Metab 2006;91(7): 2548–54.
[53] Beishuizen A, Thijs LG, Vermes I. Decreased levels of dehydroepiandrosterone sulphate in severe critical illness: a sign of exhausted adrenal reserve? Crit Care 2002;6(5):434–8.
[54] Luppa P, Munker R, Nagel D, et al. Serum androgens in intensive-care patients: correlations with clinical findings. Clin Endocrinol (Oxf) 1991;34(4):305–10.
[55] Nierman DM, Mechanick JI. Hypotestosteronemia in chronically critically ill men. Crit Care Med 1999;27(11):2418–21.
[56] Spratt DI. Altered gonadal steroidogenesis in critical illness: is treatment with anabolic steroids indicated? Best Pract Res Clin Endocrinol Metab 2001;15(4):479–94.
[57] Parker LN, Levin ER, Lifrak ET. Evidence for adrenocortical adaptation to severe illness. J Clin Endocrinol Metab 1985;60(5):947–52.
[58] Reincke M, Lehmann R, Karl M, et al. Severe illness: neuroendocrinology. Ann N Y Acad Sci 1995;771:556–69.
[59] Barquist E, Kirton O. Adrenal insufficiency in the surgical intensive care unit patient. J Trauma 1997;42(1):27–31.
[60] Annane D, Sebille V, Troche G, et al. A 3-level prognostic classification in septic shock based on cortisol levels and cortisol response to corticotropin. JAMA 2000;283(8):1038–45.
[61] Widmer IE, Puder JJ, Konig C, et al. Cortisol response in relation to the severity of stress and illness. J Clin Endocrinol Metab 2005;90(8):4579–86.
[62] Zaloga GP. Sepsis-induced adrenal deficiency syndrome. Crit Care Med 2001;29(3):688–90.
[63] Chernow B, Alexander HR, Smallridge RC, et al. Hormonal responses to graded surgical stress. Arch Intern Med 1987;147(7):1273–8.
[64] Mohler JL, Michael KA, Freedman AM, et al. The serum and urinary cortisol response to operative trauma. Surg Gynecol Obstet 1985;161(5):445–9.
[65] Udelsman R, Norton JA, Jelenich SE, et al. Responses of the hypothalamic-pituitary-adrenal and renin-angiotensin axes and the sympathetic system during controlled surgical and anesthetic stress. J Clin Endocrinol Metab 1987;64(5):986–94.
[66] Donald RA, Perry EG, Wittert GA, et al. The plasma ACTH, AVP, CRH and catecholamine responses to conventional and laparoscopic cholecystectomy. Clin Endocrinol (Oxf) 1993;38(6):609–15.

[67] Rothwell PM, Udwadia ZF, Lawler PG. Cortisol response to corticotropin and survival in septic shock. Lancet 1991;337(8741):582–3.
[68] Marik PE, Zaloga GP. Adrenal insufficiency in the critically ill: a new look at an old problem. Chest 2002;122(5):1784–96.
[69] Van den Berghe G, de Zegher F, Bouillon R. Clinical review 95: acute and prolonged critical illness as different neuroendocrine paradigms. J Clin Endocrinol Metab 1998;83(6): 1827–34.
[70] Cooper MS, Stewart PM. Corticosteroid insufficiency in acutely ill patients. N Engl J Med 2003;348(8):727–34.
[71] Ligtenberg JJ, Zijlstra JG. The relative adrenal insufficiency syndrome revisited: which patients will benefit from low-dose steroids? Curr Opin Crit Care 2004;10(6):456–60.
[72] Rady MY, Johnson DJ, Patel B, et al. Cortisol levels and corticosteroid administration fail to predict mortality in critical illness: the confounding effects of organ dysfunction and sex. Arch Surg 2005;140(7):661–8 [discussion: 669].
[73] Joosten KF, de Kleijn ED, Westerterp M, et al. Endocrine and metabolic responses in children with meningoccocal sepsis: striking differences between survivors and nonsurvivors. J Clin Endocrinol Metab 2000;85(10):3746–53.
[74] Beishuizen A, Thijs LG. Relative adrenal failure in intensive care: an identifiable problem requiring treatment? Best Pract Res Clin Endocrinol Metab 2001;15(4):513–31.
[75] Beishuizen A, Vermes I, Hylkema BS, et al. Relative eosinophilia and functional adrenal insufficiency in critically ill patients. Lancet 1999;353(9165):1675–6.
[76] Ligtenberg JJ, Tulleken JE, van der Werf TS, et al. Unraveling the mystery of adrenal failure in the critically ill. Crit Care Med 2004;32(6):1447–8 [author reply: 1448].
[77] Marik PE. Unraveling the mystery of adrenal failure in the critically ill. Crit Care Med 2004; 32(2):596–7.
[78] Marik PE, Zaloga GP. Adrenal insufficiency during septic shock. Crit Care Med 2003; 31(1):141–5.
[79] Dickstein G, Spigel D, Arad E, et al. One microgram is the lowest ACTH dose to cause a maximal cortisol response: there is no diurnal variation of cortisol response to submaximal ACTH stimulation. Eur J Endocrinol 1997;137(2):172–5.
[80] Dickstein G. On the term "relative adrenal insufficiency" or what do we really measure with adrenal stimulation tests? J Clin Endocrinol Metab 2005;90(8):4973–4.
[81] Annane D, Sebille V, Charpentier C, et al. Effect of treatment with low doses of hydrocortisone and fludrocortisone on mortality in patients with septic shock. JAMA 2002;288(7): 862–71.
[82] Hockings GI, Strakosch CR, Jackson RV. Secondary adrenocortical insufficiency: avoiding potentially fatal pitfalls in diagnosis and treatment. Med J Aust 1997;166(8):400–1.
[83] Nye EJ, Grice JE, Hockings GI, et al. Adrenocorticotropin stimulation tests in patients with hypothalamic-pituitary disease: low dose, standard high dose and 8-h infusion tests. Clin Endocrinol (Oxf) 2001;55(5):625–33.
[84] McGill PE, Greig WR, Browning MC, et al. Plasma cortisol response to synacthen (beta-1–24 Ciba) at different times of the day in patients with rheumatic diseases. Ann Rheum Dis 1967;26(2):123–6.
[85] Nathan RS, Sachar EJ, Langer G, et al. Diurnal variation in the response of plasma prolactin, cortisol, and growth hormone to insulin-induced hypoglycemia in normal men. J Clin Endocrinol Metab 1979;49(2):231–5.
[86] Berneis K, Staub JJ, Gessler A, et al. Combined stimulation of adrenocorticotropin and compound-S by single dose metyrapone test as an outpatient procedure to assess hypothalamic-pituitary-adrenal function. J Clin Endocrinol Metab 2002;87(12):5470–5.
[87] DeCherney GS, DeBold CR, Jackson RV, et al. Diurnal variation in the response of plasma adrenocorticotropin and cortisol to intravenous ovine corticotropin-releasing hormone. J Clin Endocrinol Metab 1985;61(2):273–9.

[88] Keh D, Boehnke T, Weber-Cartens S, et al. Immunologic and hemodynamic effects of "low-dose" hydrocortisone in septic shock: a double-blind, randomized, placebo-controlled, crossover study. Am J Respir Crit Care Med 2003;167(4):512–20.
[89] Oppert M, Reinicke A, Graf KJ, et al. Plasma cortisol levels before and during "low-dose" hydrocortisone therapy and their relationship to hemodynamic improvement in patients with septic shock. Intensive Care Med 2000;26(12):1747–55.
[90] Sessler CN. Steroids for septic shock: back from the dead? (Con). Chest 2003;123(5 Suppl): 482S–9.
[91] Millo J. Corticosteroids for patients with septic shock. JAMA 2003;289(1):41 [author reply: 43–4].
[92] Confalonieri M, Urbino R, Potena A, et al. Hydrocortisone infusion for severe community-acquired pneumonia: a preliminary randomized study. Am J Respir Crit Care Med 2005; 171(3):242–8.
[93] Briegel J. Hydrocortisone and the reduction of vasopressors in septic shock: therapy or only chart cosmetics? Intensive Care Med 2000;26(12):1723–6.
[94] Minneci PC, Deans KJ, Banks SM, et al. Meta-analysis: the effect of steroids on survival and shock during sepsis depends on the dose. Ann Intern Med 2004;141(1):47–56.
[95] Annane D, Bellissant E, Bollaert PE, et al. Corticosteroids for severe sepsis and septic shock: a systematic review and meta-analysis. BMJ 2004;329(7464):480.
[96] Rady MY, Johnson DJ, Patel B, et al. Corticosteroids influence the mortality and morbidity of acute critical illness. Crit Care 2006;10(4):R101.
[97] Bollaert PE, Charpentier C, Levy B, et al. Reversal of late septic shock with supraphysiologic doses of hydrocortisone. Crit Care Med 1998;26(4):645–50.
[98] Annane D, Bellissant E, Bollaert PE, et al. Corticosteroids for treating severe sepsis and septic shock. Cochrane Database Syst Rev 2004;(1):CD002243.
[99] Bone RC, Fisher CJ Jr, Clemmer TP, et al. A controlled clinical trial of high-dose methylprednisolone in the treatment of severe sepsis and septic shock. N Engl J Med 1987;317(11): 653–8.
[100] Sprung CL, Caralis PV, Marcial EH, et al. The effects of high-dose corticosteroids in patients with septic shock: a prospective, controlled study. N Engl J Med 1984;311(18): 1137–43.
[101] Frantz MC, Prix NJ, Wichmann MW, et al. Dehydroepiandrosterone restores depressed peripheral blood mononuclear cell function following major abdominal surgery via the estrogen receptors. Crit Care Med 2005;33(8):1779–86.
[102] Jarrar D, Kuebler JF, Wang P, et al. DHEA: a novel adjunct for the treatment of male trauma patients. Trends Mol Med 2001;7(2):81–5.
[103] Dhatariya KK. Is there a role for dehydroepiandrosterone replacement in the intensive care population? Intensive Care Med 2003;29(11):1877–80.
[104] Gomez MT, Magiakou MA, Mastorakos G, et al. The pituitary corticotroph is not the rate limiting step in the postoperative recovery of the hypothalamic-pituitary-adrenal axis in patients with Cushing syndrome. J Clin Endocrinol Metab 1993;77(1):173–7.
[105] Henzen C, Suter A, Lerch E, et al. Suppression and recovery of adrenal response after short-term, high-dose glucocorticoid treatment. Lancet 2000;355(9203):542–5.
[106] Graber AL, Ney RL, Nicholson WE, et al. Natural history of pituitary-adrenal recovery following long-term suppression with corticosteroids. J Clin Endocrinol Metab 1965;25: 11–6.
[107] Symreng T, Karlberg BE, Kagedal B, et al. Physiological cortisol substitution of long-term steroid-treated patients undergoing major surgery. Br J Anaesth 1981;53(9):949–54.
[108] Van den Berghe G, Wilmer A, Hermans G, et al. Intensive insulin therapy in the medical ICU. N Engl J Med 2006;354(5):449–61.
[109] Van Den Berghe G, Wouters D, Weekers F, et al. Intensive insulin therapy in critically ill patients. N Engl J Med 2001;345:1359–67.

[110] Spencer MT, Bazarian JJ. Evidence-based emergency medicine/systematic review abstract: are corticosteroids effective in traumatic spinal cord injury? Ann Emerg Med 2003;41(3): 410–3.
[111] Galandiuk S, Raque G, Appel S, et al. The two-edged sword of large-dose steroids for spinal cord trauma. Ann Surg 1993;218(4):419–25 [discussion: 425–17].
[112] Muller B, Peri G, Doni A, et al. High circulating levels of the IL-1 type II decoy receptor in critically ill patients with sepsis: association of high decoy receptor levels with glucocorticoid administration. J Leukoc Biol 2002;72(4):643–9.
[113] Warrell DA, Looareesuwan S, Warrell MJ, et al. Dexamethasone proves deleterious in cerebral malaria: a double-blind trial in 100 comatose patients. N Engl J Med 1982;306(6): 313–9.
[114] Roberts I, Yates D, Sandercock P, et al. Effect of intravenous corticosteroids on death within 14 days in 10008 adults with clinically significant head injury (MRC CRASH trial): randomised placebo-controlled trial. Lancet 2004;364(9442):1321–8.
[115] Edwards P, Arango M, Balica L, et al. Final results of MRC CRASH, a randomised placebo-controlled trial of intravenous corticosteroid in adults with head injury—outcomes at 6 months. Lancet 2005;365(9475):1957–9.
[116] Sauerland S, Maegele M. A CRASH landing in severe head injury. Lancet 2004;364(9442): 1291–2.
[117] LaRosa SP. Use of corticosteroids in the sepsis syndrome: what do we know now? Cleve Clin J Med 2005;72(12):1121–7.
[118] Kass EH. High-dose corticosteroids for septic shock. N Engl J Med 1984;311(18):1178–9.
[119] Meduri GU. A historical review of glucocorticoid treatment in sepsis: disease pathophysiology and the design of treatment investigation. Sepsis 1999;312–38.

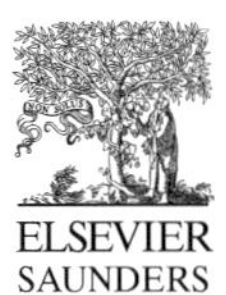
ELSEVIER
SAUNDERS

Endocrinol Metab Clin N Am
35 (2006) 839–857

ENDOCRINOLOGY
AND METABOLISM
CLINICS
OF NORTH AMERICA

Catecholamines and Vasopressin During Critical Illness

Gabriele Bassi, MD[a], Peter Radermacher, MD[b,*], Enrico Calzia, MD[b]

[a]*Istituto di Anestesiologia e Rianimazione dell'Università degli Studi di Milano, Azienda Ospedaliera, Polo Universitario San Paolo, Via Di Rudini 8, Milano 20100, Italy*
[b]*Sektion Anästhesiologische Pathophysiologie und Verfahrensentwicklung, Universitätsklinikum, Parkstrasse 11, Ulm D-89073, Germany*

Systemic hypotension is a life-threatening condition often characterized by an inadequate oxygen delivery to the tissue. Increasing the circulating volume is the first therapeutic approach, but, if fluid therapy is not sufficient to restore an adequate cardiovascular function, vasoactive drugs must be applied. Based on their different pharmacodynamic profiles, vasoactive drugs have been traditionally divided into inotropes, mainly including catecholamines such as epinephrine, dopamine, and dobutamine, and vasopressors such as phenylephrine and vasopressin [1]. As discussed herein, this subdivision may be misleading; in fact, catecholamines often reveal properties of both categories.

This article reviews the rationale of vasoactive drug therapy during shock and discusses their interactions with metabolism and the immune system. Because septic shock is the most frequent type of shock [2] and the most common cause of death in the intensive care unit [3], a special consideration is dedicated to this condition.

Clinical pharmacology of catecholamines

The traditional subdivision of catecholamines into inotropes (ie, mainly acting on β receptors) and vasopressors (ie, mainly acting on α receptors) may be misleading because, to a substantial degree, most of them act on

* Corresponding author. Sektion Anästhesiologische Pathophysiologie und Verfahrensentwicklung, Universitätsklinikum, Parkstrasse 11, Ulm D-89073, Germany.
E-mail address: peter.radermacher@uni-ulm.de (P. Radermacher).

doi:10.1016/j.ecl.2006.09.012 **endo.theclinics.com**

both receptor types. Exceptions are dopexamine and isoproterenol as pure β-adrenergic agonists and phenylephrine, which is the only pure α agonist.

Dobutamine has a weak affinity for α and β_2 receptors and a stronger affinity for β_1-adrenergic receptors. The rationale of using dobutamine is to combine its inotropic and vasodilating effects, considering that the β2 activity can decrease the systemic resistance. This last effect may be useful in septic shock in which dobutamine can be associated with norepinephrine to counterbalance an excessive vasoconstriction [1].

Norepinephrine, in contrast, is a strong nonspecific α agonist with an inotropic effect owing to its affinity for β_1 receptors. Owing to this β_1 action, norepinephrine at least partially compensates for the increased afterload induced by the α–mediated vasoconstriction and maintains or even increases cardiac output.

Epinephrine is the strongest agonist for both α and β receptors. The choice of epinephrine is generally reserved to shock states resistant to dobutamine or norepinephrine treatment. It is not recommended by international guidelines [4,5], although some authorities still debate the use of epinephrine as the first drug in septic shock [6].

Dopamine is the natural agonist for dopaminergic receptors but also has pharmacologically important and dose-dependent effects on the adrenoreceptors. At low doses, the β-adrenergic effects mainly responsible for the inotropic action predominate; at higher dosages, α-mediated vasoconstriction becomes the predominant effect of this drug. Nevertheless, these well-understood specific receptor interactions do not allow one to predict fully the pharmacologic actions of catecholamines in clinical settings. During septic shock, norepinephrine kinetics and dynamics are unpredictable [7], and even the dopamine plasma concentration measured in healthy subjects [8] during a fixed infusion rate differs from the theoretically predicted one. Furthermore, it has become clear that the underlying disease may change receptor densities and binding affinity, and that desensitization may mediate the observed high inter- and intrasubject variability of catecholamine effects [9–11].

In septic shock, the choice of vasoactive drugs mainly relies on empiric experience, because no prospective randomized trials are available. Even a Cochrane Database Review [12] concluded that no evidence supports that any one catecholamine is more effective or safer then any other. Nevertheless, the literature provides useful suggestions for a practical approach to catecholamine therapy. According to the data presented in a review article, norepinephrine seems to be more potent than dopamine for reversing hypotension [5]. Furthermore, a recent multicenter observational study suggests that the use of dopamine, but not that of norepinephrine or dobutamine, is an independent risk factor for intensive care unit mortality in patients with septic shock [13]. An additional observational study supports the benefit of norepinephrine on survival in septic shock when compared with other catecholamines [14]. An ongoing trial is comparing norepinephrine plus dobutamine versus epinephrine [15], and an emerging discussion centers on the use of epinephrine as a first-line drug [16], but, currently, its use is not recommended. Recently, the practical approach for using catecholamines in septic shock was summarized by the Surviving Sepsis Campaign [4].

A major difficulty in validating the efficacy of specific vasoactive drugs in septic shock may arise from the fact that the endpoints of therapy are still undefined. For example, it is still an open issue whether vasoactive drugs should be titrated targeting at a specific arterial pressure threshold [17,18]. Accordingly, because the beneficial effects of increased blood pressure observed in experimental studies have not been confirmed by human studies, recommendations such as titrating norepinephrine to increase mean arterial pressure not above 65 to 70 mm Hg [19] are still not sufficiently supported by scientific data.

The observed correlation between high lactate levels and increased mortality in septic shock [20] may at first glance suggest the usefulness of this variable as a therapeutic guide, but lactate metabolism in septic patients is rather complex to quantify, and an increase may be due to other factors than tissue hypoxia [16,21–23]. In particular, catecholamines, and especially epinephrine, may induce an increase in lactate production derived from direct stimulation of glycolysis while oxygen availability to the cell is not necessary impaired [16,24,25].

Even a supranormal oxygen delivery, which has previously been proposed as a therapeutic goal in septic shock patients, is no longer accepted, because its ineffectiveness has been shown by different studies [4,26].

The strategy for the best vasoactive support in septic patients is still a matter of debate, and an individualized therapy that considers the particular condition of the patient should be the right approach in clinical practice.

Catecholamines and regional perfusion

The net effect of vasoactive drugs on peripheral organ perfusion, especially on the perfusion of the kidney and splanchnic organs, is strongly dependent on many variables, but a general consensus is established around the fact that adequate fluid resuscitation is a prerequisite for any successful vasoactive therapy [4,5]. The specific impact of catecholamines and other vasoactive drugs on the perfusion of these organs is still not fully understood, mainly because observations in healthy subjects cannot be easily translated to pathologic conditions, and the perfusion of the liver and splanchnic region is difficult to study. Definitive evidence is still lacking [27,28].

Dopamine

Theoretically, lower doses of dopamine should increase splanchnic perfusion by acting on the β_2 and dopaminergic receptors, whereas higher doses should be expected to have deleterious effects according to the increasing

α effect [1]. Clinical evidence is ambiguous. Both low and high doses have been considered responsible for the mixed results ranging from increased [29,30] to constant and decreased splanchnic blood flow [31]. When dopamine is compared with epinephrine in septic shock, it seems to grant a better balance between oxygen demand and supply as reflected by the lower gradient between mixed venous and hepatic vein oxygen saturation [32].

A general consensus concerning the methods to assess splanchnic metabolism and flow is still lacking, which has led some investigators to refuse making definitive conclusions regarding the different effects of norepinephrine and dopamine on this vascular region [27]. It is hoped that the results from an ongoing trial comparing norephineprine versus dopamine will add more details on this context.

The effects of dopamine on renal perfusion are clear. Low doses of dopamine result in a combined afferent and efferent arteriolar dilation leading to an increase in renal blood flow. Due to the decrease in intraglomerular pressure, there is only a minor or no increment in glomerular filtration rate. In contrast, at higher concentrations, dopamine causes a marked renal vasoconstriction as expected. Apart from its effects on renal hemodynamics, dopamine takes part in renal sodium regulation by reducing the proximal reabsorption and, at least under physiologic conditions, by contributing to natriuresis as an appropriate response to modest volume expansion. The vasodilator and natriuretic properties of dopamine have previously led to the concept of using low-dose infusions for protecting the kidney against hypoperfusion [33]. Although an increase in urine output has been observed, no clinical study has demonstrated any benefit of low-dose dopamine infusions for preventing or treating acute renal failure [34–39].

Norepinephrine

As is true for dopamine, there is no conclusive evidence on the net effect of norepinephrine on splanchnic hemodynamics. Clinical studies have demonstrated increased [40], unchanged [41,42], or variable effects on splanchnic blood flow [41]. In this context, the evaluation of norepinephrine in comparison with other catecholamines is confused by the frequent addition of dobutamine during septic shock. The addition of dobutamine to norepinephrine resulted in an increased splanchnic perfusion during human septic shock when compared with the use of norepinephrine alone [43], which led to the widely accepted recommendation for combining these two drugs [4,5].

De Backer and colleagues [32] found a higher fractional splanchnic blood flow in septic patients with norepinephrine than with epinephrine, and Guerin and co-workers [28] showed that norepinephrine was superior to dopamine for maintaining fractional splanchnic blood flow in a comparable group of patients.

The effect of norepinephrine on renal hemodynamics is complex. It directly increases afferent arteriolar tone and enhances the efferent arteriolar resistance through a mediation by renin and angiotensin II. As a net effect, it should be expected to decrease renal blood flow, leaving the intraglomerular pressure and the filtration rate unchanged. In the clinical setting, the situation becomes less clear. Although norepinephrine has traditionally been considered detrimental for renal perfusion during septic shock, several studies have reported an improvement in renal blood flow, especially when norepinephrine has been used to restore arterial blood pressure during vasodilatory shock [44]. The question of the dependency of renal perfusion on systemic pressure remains unsolved. One experimental study performed by Bellomo and colleagues [45], which analyzed the effect of norepinephrine infusion in dogs, led to the conclusion that, during endotoxemia, norepinephrine is effective in improving renal blood flow, and this result is not related to an increased perfusion pressure.

With regard to human septic shock, several clinical studies suggest the efficacy and safety of norepinephrine for supporting renal function [46–49]. Furthermore, the only randomized controlled study comparing norepinephrine and dopamine with regard to the renal effects during septic shock suggests that the former is superior not only in reversing hypotension but also for increasing urine output [50]. Interestingly, in a recent review, the same investigators identified norepinephrine as an independent predictor of survival during septic shock [14].

Epinephrine

Although epinephrine is at least as efficient as norepinephrine and even superior to dopamine in restoring hypotension, its effects on regional perfusion limit the utility of this drug to a rescue therapy in severe shock states once other vasoactive drugs have failed [32]. The resulting detrimental effects of epinephrine on the PCO_2 gap, splanchnic blood flow, the difference between mixed venous oxygen and hepatic venous oxygen saturation, and lactate production [51] are the main reasons why epinephrine is considered harmful for the splanchnic region [32,52,53]. Interestingly, an alternative point of view is offered by Levy [16] who argues against the traditional negative consideration of epinephrine during septic shock.

The renal effects of epinephrine have not been specifically addressed by human studies. The detailed role of epinephrine in septic shock is the main focus of an ongoing large randomized trial comparing norepinephrine plus dobutamine versus epinephrine [15]. Until more convincing data are available, the use of epinephrine during shock remains a second-line approach, mainly as a rescue therapy.

Dobutamine

Dobutamine has been tested in septic shock as a unique agent as well as in combination with norepinephrine. The assumption that dobutamine may increase splanchnic blood flow as a consequence of a systemic increase in the cardiac index is widely accepted [54–56], but its presumed selective beneficial effect on splanchnic hemodynamics has not been confirmed [54].

When combined with norepinephrine, dobutamine has proven to be beneficial on splanchnic perfusion; dobutamine was even superior to epinephrine alone [43]. According to these data, dobutamine is recommended in septic shock when combined with norepinephrine as a first-line drug.

No clinical studies have tested the combination of dobutamine and norepinephrine in comparison with dopamine or norepinephrine alone.

Metabolic effects of catecholamines

A re-established perfusion and oxygen delivery do not necessarily imply a functional recovery of the different tissues after a shock state. In fact, the metabolic changes induced by the underlying disease and by the therapeutic actions may potentially influence the outcome. During septic shock, a hypermetabolic condition associated with insulin resistance, hyperlactatemia, and increased oxygen demand may occur simultaneously with mitochondrial dysfunction and decreased organ perfusion [57,58]. In this context, the specific metabolic effects of the different vasoactive drugs, mainly of the catecholamines, must be considered (Fig. 1).

Among the catecholamines, the most prominent metabolic effects are induced by epinephrine. It induces hyperglycemia (by increasing

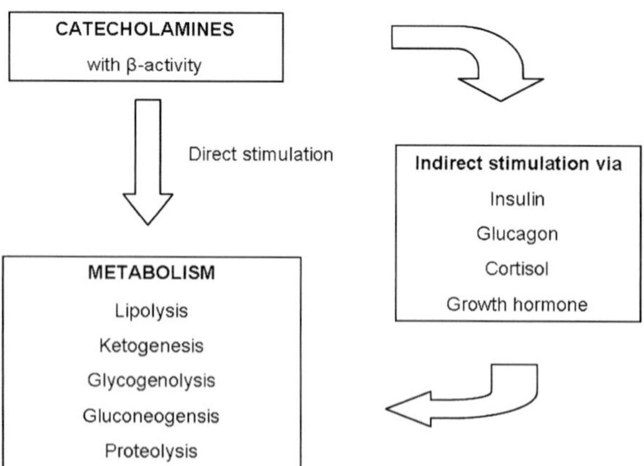

Fig. 1. Direct and indirect effects of catecholamines on cellular metabolism. Mainly mediated via β-adrenoreceptor activity to provide energy substrate in the context of the "flight or fight" response, catecholamines directly stimulate glycogenolysis, gluconeogenesis, lipolysis, and proteolysis. These effects are further enhanced by the pronounced catecholamine-induced stimulation of the anti-anabolic, that is, catabolic hormones, glucagon and cortisol. (*Adapted from* MacDonald IA, Bennet T, Fellows IW, et al. Catecholamines and the control of metabolism in man. Clin Sci 1985;68:613–9; with permission, © Copyright 1985 The Biochemical Society.)

gluconeogenesis and glycogenolysis and by decreasing insulin release through an α_2-mediated action), increases oxygen demand, and enhances plasma lactate concentration [6,59]. These metabolic changes represent a physiologic response to stress conditions and may have an adaptative meaning in a short-term attempt to provide energy. In the long-term clinical setting of septic shock, these changes can be detrimental, because an additional drug-induced increase in gluconeogenesis leads to an increased oxygen demand and, consequently, to an impaired balance between oxygen supply and demand in the liver. Furthermore, because plasma lactate concentration correlates with mortality [20], and because epinephrine has been shown to increase lactate in healthy subjects and septic patients [57], it has been postulated that this drug could lead through an excessive vasoconstriction to a low perfusion–induced cellular hypoxia. These observations and the epinephrine-induced reduction in splanchnic perfusion [52] represent the main arguments against the recommendation of this drug as a first-line agent in septic shock [4,5,60].

The mechanism of the epinephrine-induced increase in lactate levels has recently been discussed by Levy and coworkers [61], who demonstrated that the enhanced lactate concentration during epinephrine infusion was not accompanied by the same increase in the lactate to pyruvate ratio. The same investigators confirmed this experimental observation in a clinical study and provided evidence that, during septic shock treated with epinephrine infusion, lactate production is mainly the result of exaggerated aerobic glycolysis associated with increased activity of Na-K-ATPase [25]. Although these researchers did not demonstrate the link between epinephrine and Na-K- ATPase stimulation in humans, they underscored the need to change the traditional interpretation of increased lactate production as a marker of cellular hypoxia.

Although definitive conclusions with respect to norepinephrine-induced metabolic effects require further investigations, no evidence supports sustained negative effects. In healthy volunteers, except for a slightly increased glycemia without any persisting effects on glucose production and a small increase in lactate concentration [62], no substantial metabolic alterations are described. During septic shock, De Backer and coworkers [32] reported higher glycemia in the norepinephrine group with respect to the dopamine group but did not find adverse metabolic effects.

Limited data are available concerning the metabolic effect of dopamine. Two studies have underscored the supposed negative role of dopamine on liver metabolism. Jakob and coworkers [30] demonstrated a decreased splanchnic oxygen consumption despite an increased splanchnic blood flow induced by dopamine infusion in septic patients. Guerin and colleagues [28], comparing dopamine with norepinephrine, did not find any difference in splanchnic blood flow despite a higher cardiac index and a similar mean arterial pressure in the dopamine group. This hemodynamic difference resulted in a lower splanchnic fractional flow that was associated with lower hepatic lactate uptake and a higher hepatic venous lactate to pyruvate ratio, indicating a detrimental effect on hepatic energy balance in the dopamine group. This hypothesis has not been confirmed by De Backer [32], who reported a similar metabolic profile during dopamine or norepinephrine infusion.

The metabolic effects of dobutamine administration are not completely clear. Although dobutamine is a weak agonist of β_2 receptors, and β_2-receptor activation is known to stimulate gluconeogenesis, dobutamine infusion caused a slight decrease in glucose production in healthy subjects [62] and patients with septic shock [54] or recovering from cardiac surgery [63]. This effect on carbohydrate metabolism was unexpected and led to the hypothesis that dobutamine may not have pronounced β_2 activity and metabolic effects in vivo [62].

Some authorities argue that, theoretically, owing to the absence of major adverse metabolic properties of norepinephrine and dobutamine, the combined administration of these two drugs may be safe with regard to splanchnic perfusion, particularly when compared with epinephrine [52,62,64,65]. This hypothesis has not been tested experimentally.

Catecholamines and immune modulation

An increasing body of evidence supports the role of adrenergic agents in the modulation of immune and inflammatory responses in critically ill patients and experimental models. Almost all inflammatory cells express α and β adrenoreceptors on their surface [66,67], whereas D_1 and D_2 receptors are known to be present on lymphocytes and natural killer cells [68]. Although α_2 adrenoreceptors may also induce the production of a variety of proinflammatory cytokines [69], the immunomodulatory actions of catecholamines are predominantly mediated by β_2 receptors. The definitive and unique effects of catecholamines in the complex network of inflammatory responses are not yet fully elucidated. They can range from modulating T-helper cell migration and maturation [70–72] to controlling cytokine expression [73,74] to promoting apoptosis directly in immune cells [75]. Some researchers have suggested that catecholamines may have an anti-inflammatory action by downregulating the proinflammatory cytokine response. In this context, ephinephrine, but not norepinephrine, mediates the interleukin-6 response of splanchnic reticuloendothelial tissues [76], whereas the ephinephrine-induced increase in interleukin-10 may inhibit TNFα production [77]. Dopamine administration may lead to a functional suppression of neutrophils by attenuation of the chemoattractant effect of interleukin-8 [78].

In addition to its direct effects on the immune system, dopamine can interfere with the response to inflammation through its action on the neuroendocrine system. Dopamine infusion suppresses the release of most of the anterior pituitary dependent hormones and stimulates the synthesis of adrenal glucocorticoids [79]. The concomitant inhibition of growth hormone pulsatile secretion [80], thyroid-stimulating hormone [81], and particularly prolactin, which enhances monocyte and B- and T-cell responses, may aggravate immune dysfunction and the susceptibility to infection. In contrast, dopexamine had minimal effects on pituitary function in high-risk surgical patients [82] but still modulated cellular immune functions during experimental systemic inflammation [83].

Whether these catecholamine-induced alterations of immunologic functions may somehow influence survival in sepsis and septic shock remains to be defined.

Vasopressin

Vasopressin is a natural hormone produced in magnocellular neurons of the hypothalamus and released from the posterior hypophysis. Its secretion is stimulated in response to increases in plasma osmolality and decreases in systemic blood pressure. Under physiologic conditions, vasopressin release is regulated only by changes in osmolality [84], whereas small reductions in arterial pressure have little or no effects. A significant loss in circulating fluid can increase vasopressin levels several fold higher than those usually seen for alterations in osmolality. Two main receptors mediate different effects: V_1 and V_2 receptors. V_1 receptors are located on vascular smooth cells and mediate vasoconstriction and enhancement of prostaglandin release. V_2 receptors are found on the distal convoluted tubules and medullary collecting ducts and mainly mediate an antidiuretic effect. A third receptor, V_3, is located on the anterior hypophysis and pancreatic isles and seems to facilitate the release of corticotropin (ACTH) and intervene in insulin secretion.

Terlipressin is a vasopressin analogue that differs in its pharmacokinetic profile (plasma half-life for terlipressin of 6 hours versus 5 to 15 minutes for vasopressin) and higher affinity for receptor V_1 [85] (V_1/V_2 receptor ratio of 2.2 for terlipressin versus 1 for vasopressin). Vasopressin has been traditionally reserved for the treatment of variceal bleeding [86] and hepatorenal syndrome [87], but its recent introduction as a rescue therapy during cardiac arrest [88,89] and septic shock extends its potential clinical role.

Landry and coworkers [90] documented a vasopressin deficiency in patients with septic shock and observed an improvement in hemodynamic conditions during infusion of vasopressin. This observation led to the conclusion that vasopressin plasma levels are inappropriately low during sepsis and that vasopressin deficiency participates in the pathogenesis of hypotension. Later, Sharshar and colleagues [91] precisely characterized the circulating levels of vasopressin during the different phases of septic shock, concluding that the vasopressin concentration is almost always increased during the early phase of sepsis (first 6 hours), whereas it declines afterward (after 36 hours from the onset of shock). The cause for vasopressin deficiency is still controversial, but because the infusion of vasopressin can reach the expected plasma concentration, it seems unlikely that an increased clearance of this hormone is responsible for the low plasma level during sepsis. An exhaustion of neurohypophysis stores seems to be a more logical conclusion [92]. Sharshar and colleagues [91] even speculated that this fall in vasopressin production may contribute to the development of hypotension. Jochberger and coworkers [93] argued against this latter hypothesis, because they failed to demonstrate any correlation between vasopressin levels and the presence of shock in a mixed critically ill population. They concluded that peripheral hyposensibility rather than deficiency would contribute to hypotension. Although this finding was confirmed during experimental studies, it was not substantiated in humans. Indeed, clinical trials have shown an increased sensitivity to vasopressin during infusion rather than any form of drug tolerance [90,94]. Additionally, vascular vasopressin receptors have been shown to recycle and resensitize rapidly.

Several mechanisms have been proposed to explain hypersensitivity and additional beneficial effects of vasopressin during septic shock. A low plasma vasopressin concentration during the late phase may leave more V_1 receptors available for binding the infused hormone [90] and cause alterations in receptor expression and signal transduction [95], potentiation of vasoconstrictor effects of catecholamines via vasopressin-mediated inactivation of K_{ATP} channels [96], a vasopressin-induced reduction in NO generation [97], and a vasopressin-mediated increase in cortisol levels. All of these observations provide the rationale for the use of vasopressin during vasodilatory and catecholamine-resistant shock states [98].

Effects of vasopressin on systemic hemodynamics during septic shock

According to almost all studies published on this topic, vasopressin [90,94,99–107] and its analogue terlipressin [108–111] have been shown to be as efficient as norepinephrine for maintaining mean arterial pressure in septic shock. Simultaneously, cardiac output is decreased under vasopressin [99–102,104–107]. A decreased cardiac output is also observed under terlipressin [108–111]. A recent experimental study in endotoxic rabbits [112] revealed a marked deterioration of the left ventricular systolic function during vasopressin infusion (assessed by means of systolic aortic blood flow and maximal aortic acceleration). The investigators argued that the myocardial dysfunction was not caused by the increased afterload induced by the vasopressin-mediated vasoconstriction but rather by an impairment of coronary perfusion or a direct effect on cardiac myocytes. By contrast, in clinical trials with vasopressin or terlipressin, no adverse effects on myocardial function or increased incidence of myocardial ischemia or infarction have been observed. In fact, in a mixed population of patients with catecholamine-resistant vasodilatory shock, blood creatin phospokinase activity and troponin concentration decreased [99] when they were treated with vasopressin.

In four studies [100,101,108,109], the decreased cardiac output observed during vasopressin infusion was accompanied by an impaired oxygen delivery, which was only partially compensated by an increase in oxygen extraction, resulting in a condition of oxygen supply dependency. To avoid methodical faults related to the mathematical coupling between oxygen consumption and delivery, in three of these studies [100,101,109], the oxygen consumption was assessed by a metabolic monitor. Albeit, indicating potential deleterious effects at first glance, these data are not uniformly interpreted as harmful. In fact, some authorities [108,109] proposed a beneficial interpretation of the observed decrease in oxygen consumption, assuming that a potential anti-inflammatory role of vasopressin associated with a decreased heart rate would lead to a decrease in metabolic requirements and oxygen demand. Furthermore, in one of these studies [100], a decreased cardiac index was associated with increased fractional splanchnic blood flow despite a systemic impairment of oxygen delivery. In that study, splanchnic oxygen delivery and consumption remained unchanged.

In all of the studies, vasopressin and terlipressin were able to reduce the need for other vasopressors, and, in some cases, a complete weaning from norepinephrine was possible. The ability to increase or restore sensitivity to catecholamines remains the major rationale for supporting the use of vasopressin as a rescue therapy when conventional catecholamines have failed [113].

Two studies [114,115] with different results investigated the effect of vasopressin and terlipressin on sublingual microcirculation during septic shock using an orthogonal polarization spectral imaging technique. Although the infusion of vasopressin at 0.02 U/min did not further impair microcirculation during a distributive shock after cardiopulmonary bypass [114], a single bolus of 1 mg of terlipressin during septic shock caused a complete microflow stop, which was associated with signs of generalized skin vasoconstriction [115]. Despite the limitations of the orthogonal polarization spectral imaging technique and a prudent generalization of case reports, these studies emphasize the potential difference between the two drugs, particularly with respect to the method of administration and the degree of vasoconstriction.

Effects of vasopressin on regional hemodynamics during septic shock

The main rationale for using vasopressin and terlipressin to treat gastrointestinal bleeding is its supposed capacity to induce an intense and selective vasoconstriction in the splanchnic area. Obviously, such an effect may be deleterious in septic shock and has been addressed by different investigations. No definitive conclusions can be drawn with respect to the supposed vascular overconstriction and detrimental effects of vasopressin on splanchnic perfusion during septic shock. Among these studies [99,100,102–104,106,108–110], six supported a negative effect [99,100,102–104,109], one reported no difference when comparing vasopressin with noradrenaline [106], and two observed a beneficial effect [108,110]. A potential confusing factor was represented by the different methods used to study splanchnic perfusion. Although most researchers used gastric tonometry as the main parameter, others analyzed the plasma concentrations of bilirubin or liver enzymes. Only in one study was liver blood flow assessed invasively by means of hepatic vein catheterization [100]. All of these methods may have drawbacks. Although gastric tonometry is a generally well-accepted technique, some authorities argue against its definitive clinical validation [116].

Theoretically, increased plasma levels of bilirubin and liver enzymes may, indeed, reflect liver damage caused by the reduction of hepatic blood flow induced by vasopressin; however, they may also result from a shock-related hepatic dysfunction not specifically related to the administration of vasopressin [99]. Only two studies reported a significant increase in bilirubin and liver enzymes during vasopressin administration in a mixed population of vasodilatory shock [103,104].

Interestingly, replacing noradrenaline by vasopressin, while preserving a constant mean arterial pressure, apparently increases the directly measured splanchnic blood flow despite a simultaneous reduction in the cardiac index as an indicator of an increased fractional splanchnic blood flow [100]. Because no beneficial effects were observed with regard to the gastric mucosal PCO_2 gap, which increased, nor with regard to the splanchnic oxygen delivery or consumption, which remained unchanged, these observations led to the conclusion that, despite the increased hepatosplanchnic blood flow, vasopressin does not necessarily promote an increment of mucosal perfusion.

The net effect of vasopressin on renal function is complex and differs widely between physiologic and pathologic conditions. In physiologic conditions, vasopressin induces water reabsorption by acting on V_2 receptors in response to hyperosmolarity and with a different degree to hypotension. The simultaneous V_1 receptor–mediated renal vascular response increases the efferent arteriolar tone with less or no effect on the afferent one. As a result, the glomerular pressure is increased while the total renal flow is slightly decreased. At the same time, a short negative feedback loop seems to be activated by vasopressin, which enhances local prostaglandin production through the V_1 receptor. Prostaglandins, in particular PGE_2 [117], may minimize the antidiuretic and the vascular response to vasopressin, maintaining renal perfusion.

Paradoxically, different clinical studies performed in septic shock patients to compare norepinephrine and vasopressin, or in which norepinephrine had to be replaced by vasopressin, revealed an increased or unchanged urine production during vasopressin infusion [101,106–110], which was often associated with an increased creatinine clearance [106,108,109]. The exact mechanism of this diuretic effect is poorly understood. Based on experimental evidence, Holmes and colleagues [101] suggested different hypothetical interpretations, such as a role of vasopressin in inducing NO-mediated vasodilation of afferent arteriola [118], a direct action of vasopressin on oxytocin receptors resulting in a natriuretic effect, or a vasopressin-induced release of atrial natriuretic peptide [119]. The same researchers found an increased urine production that lasted for the first 4 hours of vasopressin infusion, whereas no increase in urine flow or creatinine clearance was noted after 48 hours. In a small randomized trial, Patel and coworkers [106] compared 4 hours of noradrenaline infusion with vasopressin titrated to maintain the same mean arterial pressure. They found a significant increase in creatinine clearance and urine output in the vasopressin group, leading to the conclusion that vasopressin may have an antidiuretic role independently from arterial pressure.

Although there is no evidence that vasopressin doses higher than 0.04 U/min may increase urine output, a beneficial effect on renal function has been observed even at low doses of vasopressin (0.02 U/min). Despite these encouraging data, researchers [120] advocate a cautious approach and further investigations before low-dose vasopressin is considered as a "renoprotective" therapy.

Although further studies are accumulating proving potential benefits of vasopressin and terlipressin in septic shock, several concerns remain. Even though no significant adverse effects have been observed, the safety of this therapy remains to be confirmed, because few patients have been treated with vasopressin. Furthermore, a retrospective study of 50 patients noted a mortality rate of 85% when vasopressin was used [101]. These discouraging results may be due to the fact that vasopressin has been used as a second-line drug in catecholamine-refractory cases, particularly severe shock states. Based on the ability of vasopressin to restore catecholamine sensitivity, this seems to be a rationale approach; however, beneficial effects might become evident only if vasopressin is used as a first-line drug. Furthermore, vasopressin may be combined with low-dose catecholamines to prevent the adverse effects of high doses of catecholamines and to add an inotropic effect to the prevalent property of vasopressin as a vasoconstrictor.

Even when considering the potential negative effects of catecholamines on metabolism and the immune system, a different or combined approach could be of interest. No large studies have investigated the effect of vasopressin on metabolism and its impact on the inflammatory response [121]. Many questions regarding the potential clinical role of vasopressin may be answered by the soon to be published results of the ongoing large Canadian randomized trial comparing vasopressin and noradrenaline during septic shock.

Summary

Catecholamines remain fundamental in the treatment of circulatory failure; however, clinicians must focus their attention not only on the hemodynamic effects but also on using a more rationale approach considering the metabolic, endocrinologic, and immunologic consequences of catecholamine administration. Looking at alternative strategies to catecholamines in the treatment of shock, evidence of their beneficial effects on hemodynamic endpoints of vasopressin during septic shock is accumulating. Nevertheless, there are no data demonstrating the superiority of vasopressin to catecholamines in terms of mortality and morbidity, and no definitive conclusion can be drawn with respect to the potential detrimental effects of vasopressin on splanchnic circulation. Furthermore, the metabolic and immunologic consequences of vasopressin remain an open issue. Currently, the use of vasopressin is recommended only in clinical investigation protocols.

References

[1] Kevin TT, Corley BVM. Inotropes and vasopressors in adults and foals. Vet Clin Equine 2004;20:77–106.

[2] Landry DW, Oliver JA. The pathogenesis of vasodilatory shock. N Engl J Med 2001;345(8): 588–95.

[3] Singh S, Evans T. Organ dysfunction during sepsis. Int Care Med 2006;32:349–60.

[4] Dellinger RP, Carlet JM, Masur H, et al. Surviving sepsis campaign guidelines for management of severe sepsis and septic shock. Intensive Care Med 2004;30(4):536–55.

[5] Beale RJ, Hollenberg SM, Vincent JL, et al. Vasopressor and inotropic support in septic shock: an evidence-based review. Crit Care Med 2004;32(11 Suppl):S455–65.

[6] Levy B, Gibot S, Bollaert PE. Is there a place for epinephrine in the management of septic shock? In: Vincent JL, editor. Yearbook of intensive care and emergency medicine. New York: Springer Verlag; 2005. p. 259–68.

[7] Beloeil H, Mazoit X, Benhemou D, et al. Norepinephrine kinetics and dynamics in septic shock and trauma patients. Br J Anaesth 2005;95(6):782–8.

[8] MacGregor DA, Smith TE, Prielipp RC, et al. Pharmacokinetics of dopamine in healthy male subjects. Anesthesiology 2000;92(2):338–46.

[9] MacGregor DA, Prielipp RC, Butterworth JF, et al. Relative efficacy and potency of beta-adrenoceptor agonists for generating cAMP in human lymphocytes. Chest 1996;109(1): 194–200.

[10] Silverman HJ, Penaranda R, Orens JB, et al. Impaired beta-adrenergic receptor stimulation of cyclic adenosine monophosphate in human septic shock: association with myocardial hyporesponsiveness to catecholamines. Crit Care Med 1993;21(1):31–9.

[11] Reinelt H, Radermacher P, Fischer G, et al. Dobutamine and dopexamine and the splanchnic metabolic response in septic shock. Clin Intensive Care 1997;81:38–41.

[12] Müllner M, Urbanek B, Havel C, et al. Vasopressors for shock. Cochrane Database Syst Rev 2004;(3):CD003709.

[13] Sakr Y, Reinhart K, Vincent JL, et al. Does dopamine administration in shock influence outcome? Results of the Sepsis Occurrence in Acutely Ill Patients (SOAP) Study. Crit Care Med 2006;34:589–97.

[14] Martin C, Viviand X, Leone M, et al. Effect of norepinephrine on the outcome of septic shock. Crit Care Med 2000;28(8):2758–65.

[15] Annane D, Mignon P, Bollaert PE, et al. Norepinephrine plus dobutamine versus epinephrine alone for the management of septic shock. Intensive Care Med 2005;31(Suppl 1):S18.

[16] Levy B. Bench to bedside review: is there a place for ephinephrine in septic shock? Crit Care 2005;96:561–5.

[17] Bourgoin A, Leone M, Delmas A, et al. Increasing mean arterial pressure in patients with septic shock: effects on oxygen variables and renal function. Crit Care Med 2005;33(4): 780–6.
[18] De Backer D, Vincent JL. Norepinephrine administration in septic shock: how much is enough? Crit Care Med 2002;30(6):1398–9.
[19] Le Doux D, Astiz ME, Carpati CM, et al. Effects of perfusion pressure on tissue perfusion in septic shock. Crit Care Med 2000;28(8):2729–32.
[20] Bakker J, Coffernils M, Leon M, et al. Blood lactate levels are superior to oxygen derived variables in predicting outcome in human septic shock. Chest 1991;99(4):956–62.
[21] Leverve X. Lactate in the intensive care unit: pyromaniac, sentinel or fireman? Crit Care 2005;9(6):622–3.
[22] Valenza F, Aletti G, Fossali T, et al. Lactate as a marker of energy failure in critically ill patients: hypothesis. Crit Care 2005;9(6):588–93.
[23] Howard J, Luchette F, McCarter F, et al. Lactate is an unreliable indicator of tissue hypoxia in injury or sepsis. Lancet 1999;354(9177):505–8.
[24] Träger K, Radermacher P, De Backer D, et al. Metabolic effects of vasoactive agents. Curr Opin Anaesth 2001;14(2):157–63.
[25] Levy B, Gibot S, Franck P, et al. Relation between muscle Na+ K+ ATPase activity and raised lactate concentrations in septic shock: a prospective study. Lancet 2005;365(9462): 871–5.
[26] Gattinoni L, Brazzi L, Pelosi P, et al. A trial of goal-oriented hemodynamic therapy in critically ill patients. N Engl J Med 1995;333(16):1025–32.
[27] Asfar P, De Backer D, Meier-Hellmann A, et al. Clinical review: influence of vasoactive and other therapies on intestinal and hepatic circulations in patients with septic shock. Crit Care 2004;8(3):170–9.
[28] Guerin JP, Levraut J, Samat-Long C, et al. Effects of dopamine and norepinephrine on systemic and hepatosplanchnic hemodynamics, oxygen exchange, and energy balance in vasoplegic septic patients. Shock 2005;23(1):18–24.
[29] Meier-Hellmann A, Bredle DL, Specht M, et al. The effects of low-dose dopamine on splanchnic blood flow and oxygen uptake in patients with septic shock. Intensive Care Med 1997;23(1):31–7.
[30] Jakob SM, Ruokonen E, Takala J. Effects of dopamine on systemic and regional blood flow and metabolism in septic and cardiac surgery patients. Shock 2002;18(1):8–13.
[31] Gelman S, Mushlin P. Catecholamine-induced changes in the splanchnic circulation affecting systemic hemodynamics. Anesthesiology 2004;100(2):434–9.
[32] De Backer D, Creteur J, Silva E, et al. Effects of dopamine, norepinephrine, and epinephrine on the splanchnic circulation in septic shock: which is best? Crit Care Med 2003;31(6): 1659–67.
[33] Denton MD, Chertow GM, Brady HR. "Renal dose" of dopamine for the treatment of acute renal failure: scientific rationale, experimental studies and clinical trials. Kidney Int 1996;50(1):4–14.
[34] Friedrich JO, Adhikari N, Herridge MS, et al. Meta-analysis: low-dose dopamine increases urine output but does not prevent renal dysfunction or death. Ann Intern Med 2005;142(7): 510–24.
[35] Lassnigg A, Donner E, Grubhofer G, et al. Lack of renoprotective effects of dopamine and furosemide during cardiac surgery. J Am Soc Nephrol 2000;11(1):97–104.
[36] Marik PE, Iglesias J. Low dose dopamine does not prevent acute renal failure in patients with septic shock and oliguria: NORASEPT II Study investigators. Am J Med 1999; 107(4):387.
[37] Hoogenberg K, Smit AJ, Girbes ARJ. Effects of low-dose dopamine on renal and systemic hemodynamics during incremental norepinephrine infusion in healthy volunteers. Crit Care Med 1998;26(2):260–5.

[38] Girbes ARJ, Lieverse AG, Smit AJ, et al. Lack of specific hemodynamic effects of different doses of dopamine after infrarenal aortic surgery. Br J Anaesth 1996;77(6):753–7.
[39] Girbes ARJ, Patten MT, McCloskey BV, et al. The renal and neurohumoral effects of the addition of low-dose dopamine in septic critically ill patients. Intensive Care Med 2000; 26(11):1685–9.
[40] Meier-Hellmann A, Specht M, Hannemann L, et al. Splanchnic blood flow is greater in septic shock treated with norepinephrine than in severe sepsis. Intensive Care Med 1996;22(12): 1354–9.
[41] Ruokonen E, Takala J, Kari A. Regional blood flow and oxygen transport in septic shock. Crit Care Med 1993;21(9):1296–303.
[42] Ruokonen E, Takala J, Uusaro A. Effect of vasoactive treatment on the relationship between mixed venous and regional oxygen saturation. Crit Care Med 1991;19(11):1365–9.
[43] Duranteau J, Sitbon P, Teboul JL. Effects of epinephrine, norepinephrine, or the combination of norepinephrine and dobutamine on gastric mucosa in septic shock. Crit Care Med 1999;28(5):893–900.
[44] Bellomo R, Giantomasso DD. Noradrenaline and the kidney: friends or foes? Crit Care 2001;5(6):294–8.
[45] Bellomo R, Kellum JA, Wisniewski SR, et al. Effects of norepinephrine on the renal vasculature in normal and endotoxemic dogs. Am J Respir Crit Care Med 1999;159(4 pt 1): 1186–92.
[46] Hesselvik JF, Brodin B. Low dose norepinephrine in patients with septic shock and oliguria: effects on afterload, urine flow, and oxygen transport. Crit Care Med 1989;17(2): 179–80.
[47] Meadows D, Edwards JD, Wilkins RG, et al. Reversal of intractable septic shock with norepinephrine therapy. Crit Care Med 1988;16(7):663–6.
[48] Martin C, Eon B, Saux P, et al. Renal effects of norepinephrine used to treat septic shock patients. Crit Care Med 1990;18(3):282–5.
[49] Desjars P, Pinaud M, Bugnon D, et al. Norepinephrine therapy has no deleterious renal effects in human septic shock. Crit Care Med 1990;18(9):1048–9.
[50] Martin C, Papazian L, Perrin G, et al. Norepinephrine or dopamine for the treatment of hyperdynamic septic shock? Chest 1993;103(6):1826–31.
[51] Totaro RJ, Raper RF. Epinephrine-induced lactic acidosis following cardiopulmonary bypass. Crit Care Med 1997;25(10):1693–9.
[52] Meier-Hellmann A, Reinhart K, Bredle DL, et al. Epinephrine impairs splanchnic perfusion in septic shock. Crit Care Med 1997;25(3):399–404.
[53] Levy B, Bollaert PE, Charpentier C, et al. Comparison of norepinephrine and dobutamine to epinephrine for hemodynamics, lactate metabolism, and gastric tonometric variables in septic shock: a prospective randomized study. Intensive Care Med 1997;23(3):282–7.
[54] Reinelt H, Radermacher P, Fischer G, et al. Effects of a dobutamine-induced increase in splanchnic blood flow on hepatic metabolic activity in patients with septic shock. Anesthesiology 1997;86(4):818–24.
[55] Ruokonen E, Uusaro A, Alhava E, et al. The effect of dobutamine infusion on splanchnic blood flow and oxygen transport in patients with acute pancreatitis. Intensive Care Med 1997;23(7):732–7.
[56] Creteur J, De Backer D, Vincent JL. A dobutamine test can disclose hepatosplanchnic hypoperfusion in septic patients. Am J Respir Crit Care Med 1999;160(3):839–45.
[57] Träger K, DeBacker D, Radermacher P. Metabolic alterations in sepsis and vasoactive drug-related metabolic effects. Curr Opin Crit Care 2003;9(4):271–8.
[58] Brealey D, Brand M, Hargreaves I, et al. Association between mitochondrial dysfunction and severity and outcome of septic shock. Lancet 2002;360(9328):219–23.
[59] Ensinger H, Träger K. Metabolic effect of vasoactive drugs. In: Vincent JL, editor. Yearbook of intensive care and emergency medicine. New York: Springer Verlag; 2002. p. 499–509.

[60] Wilson J, Woods I, Fawcett J, et al. Reducing the risk of major elective surgery: randomised controlled trial of preoperative optimisation of oxygen delivery. BMJ 1999;318(7191): 1099–103.
[61] Levy B, Mansart A, Bollaert PE, et al. Effects of epinephrine and norepinephrine on hemodynamics, oxidative metabolism, and organ energetics in endotoxemic rats. Intensive Care Med 2003;29(2):292–300.
[62] Ensinger H, Geisser W, Brinkmann A, et al. Metabolic effects of norepinephrine and dobutamine in healthy volunteers. Shock 2002;18(6):495–500.
[63] Ensinger H, Rantala A, Vogt J, et al. Effect of dobutamine on splanchnic carbohydrate metabolism and amino acid balance after cardiac surgery. Anesthesiology 1999;91(6): 1587–95.
[64] Marik PE, Mohedin M. The contrasting effects of dopamine and norepinephrine on systemic and splanchnic oxygen utilization in hyperdynamic sepsis. JAMA 1994;272(17): 1354–7.
[65] Levy B, Nace L, Bollaert PE, et al. Comparison of systemic and regional effects of dobutamine and dopexamine in norepinephrine-treated septic shock. Intensive Care Med 1999; 25(9):942–8.
[66] Khan MM, Sansoni P, Silverman ED, et al. Beta-adrenergic receptors on human suppressor, helper, and cytolytic lymphocytes. Biochem Pharmacol 1986;35(7):1137–42.
[67] Landmann R. Beta-adrenergic receptors in human leukocyte subpopulations. Eur J Clin Invest 1992;22(Suppl 1):30–6.
[68] Santambrogio L, Lipartiti M, Bruni A, et al. Dopamine receptors on human T- and B-lymphocytes. J Neuroimmunol 1993;45(1–2):113–9.
[69] Bergquist J, Ohlsson B, Tarkowski A. Nuclear factor kappa B is involved in the catecholaminergic suppression of immunocompetent cells. Ann N Y Acad Sci 2000;917:281–9.
[70] Maestroni GJ. Dendritic cell migration controlled by alpha 1b-adrenergic receptors. J Immunol 2000;165(12):6743–7.
[71] Maestroni GJ. Short exposure of maturing, bone marrow-derived dendritic cells to norepinephrine: impact on kinetics of cytokine production and Th development. J Neuroimmunol 2002;129(1–2):106–14.
[72] Sanders VM, Baker RA, Ramer-Quinn DS, et al. Differential expression of the beta 2-adrenergic receptor by Th1 and Th2 clones: implications for cytokine production and B cell help. J Immunol 1997;158(9):4200–10.
[73] Pastores SM, Hasko G, Vizi ES, et al. Cytokine production and its manipulation by vasoactive drugs. New Horiz 1996;4(2):252–64.
[74] Guirao X, Kumar A, Katz J, et al. Catecholamines increase monocyte TNF receptors and inhibit TNF through beta 2-adrenoreceptor activation. Am J Physiol 1997;273(6 Pt 1): E1203–8.
[75] Oberbeck R. Therapeutic implications of immune-endocrine interactions in the critically ill patient. Curr Drug Targets Immune Endocr Metabol Disord 2004;4(2):129–39.
[76] Bergmann M, Gornikiewicz A, Tamandl D, et al. Continuous therapeutic epinephrine but not norepinephrine prolongs splanchnic IL-6 production in porcine endotoxic shock. Shock 2003;20(6):575–81.
[77] van der Poll T, Coyle SM, Barbosa K, et al. Epinephrine inhibits tumor necrosis factor-alpha and potentiates interleukin 10 production during human endotoxemia. J Clin Invest 1996;97(3):713–9.
[78] Sookhai S, Wang JH, Winter D, et al. Dopamine attenuates the chemoattractant effect of interleukin-8: a novel role in the systemic inflammatory response syndrome. Shock 2000; 14(3):295–9.
[79] Van den Berghe G, de Zegher F. Anterior pituitary function during critical illness and dopamine treatment. Crit Care Med 1996;24(9):1580–90.
[80] Van den Berghe G, de Zegher F, Lauwers P, et al. Growth hormone secretion in critical illness: effect of dopamine. J Clin Endocrinol Metab 1994;79(4):1141–6.

[81] Van den Berghe G, de Zegher F, Lauwers P. Dopamine and the sick euthyroid syndrome in critical illness. Clin Endocrinol (Oxf) 1994;41(6):731–7.
[82] Schilling T, Grundling M, Strang CM, et al. Effects of dopexamine, dobutamine or dopamine on prolactin and thyreotropin serum concentrations in high-risk surgical patients. Intensive Care Med 2004;30(6):1127–33.
[83] Oberbeck R. Dopexamine and cellular immune functions during systemic inflammation. Immunobiology 2004;208(5):429–38.
[84] Baylis PH. Osmoregulation and control of vasopressin secretion in healthy humans. Am J Physiol 1987;253(5 pt 2):R671–8.
[85] Bernadich C, Bandi JC, Melin P, et al. Effects of F-180, a new selective vasoconstrictor peptide, compared with terlipressin and vasopressin on systemic and splanchnic hemodynamics in a rat model of portal hypertension. Hepatology 1998;27(2):351–6.
[86] Escorsell A, Ruiz del Arbol L, Planas R, et al. Multicenter randomized controlled trial of terlipressin versus sclerotherapy in the treatment of acute variceal bleeding: the TEST study. Hepatology 2000;32(3):471–6.
[87] Ortega R, Gines P, Uriz J, et al. Terlipressin therapy with and without albumin for patients with hepatorenal syndrome: results of a prospective, nonrandomized study. Hepatology 2002;36(4 pt 1):941–8.
[88] Nolan JP, Deakin CD, Soar J, et al. European Resuscitation Council Guidelines for Resuscitation 2005, Section 4. Adult advanced life support. Resuscitation 2005;67(S1):S39–86.
[89] Wenzel V, Krismer A, Arntz HR, et al. A comparison of vasopressin and epinephrine for out-of-hospital cardiopulmonary resuscitation. N Engl J Med 2004;350(2):105–13.
[90] Landry DW, Levin HR, Gallant EM, et al. Vasopressin deficiency contributes to the vasodilation of septic shock. Circulation 1997;95(5):1122–5.
[91] Sharshar T, Blanchard A, Paillard M, et al. Circulating vasopressin levels in septic shock. Crit Care Med 2003;31(6):1752–8.
[92] Sharshar T, Carlier R, Blanchard A, et al. Depletion of neurohypophyseal content of vasopressin in septic shock. Crit Care Med 2002;30(3):497–500.
[93] Jochberger S, Mayr VD, Luckner G, et al. Serum vasopressin concentrations in critically ill patients. Crit Care Med 2006;34(2):293–9.
[94] Landry DW, Levin HR, Gallant EM, et al. Vasopressin pressor hypersensitivity in vasodilatory septic shock. Crit Care Med 1997;25(8):1279–82.
[95] Patel S, Gaspers LD, Boucherie S, et al. Inducible nitric-oxide synthase attenuates vasopressin-dependent Ca2+ signaling in rat hepatocytes. J Biol Chem 2002;277(37):33776–82.
[96] Wakatsuki T, Nakaya Y, Inoue I. Vasopressin modulates K(+) channel activities of cultured smooth muscle cells from porcine coronary artery. Am J Physiol 1992;263(2 pt 2):H491–6.
[97] Umino T, Kusano E, Muto S, et al. AVP inhibits LPS and IL-1beta-stimulated NO and cGMP via V1 receptor in cultured rat mesangial cells. Am J Physiol 1999;276(3 pt 2):F433–44.
[98] Mutlu GM, Factor P. Role of vasopressin in the management of septic shock. Intensive Care Med 2004;30(7):1276–91.
[99] Dünser MW, Mayr AJ, Ulmer H, et al. The effects of vasopressin on systemic hemodynamics in catecholamine resistant septic and postcardiotomy shock: a retrospective analysis. Anesth Analg 2001;93(1):7–13.
[100] Klinzing S, Simon M, Reinhart K, et al. High-dose vasopressin is not superior to norepinephrine in septic shock. Crit Care Med 2003;31(11):2646–50.
[101] Holmes CL, Walley KR, Chittock DR, et al. The effects of vasopressin on hemodynamics and renal function in severe septic shock: a case series. Intensive Care Med 2001;27(8):1416–21.
[102] van Haren FM, Rozendaal FW, van der Hoeven JG. The effect of vasopressin on gastric perfusion in catecholamine-dependent patients in septic shock. Chest 2003;124(6):2256–60.

[103] Dünser MW, Mayr AJ, Ulmer H, et al. Arginine vasopressin in advanced vasodilatory shock: a prospective, randomized, controlled study. Circulation 2003;107(18):2313–9.
[104] Luckner G, Dünser MW, Jochberger S, et al. Arginine vasopressin in 316 patients with advanced vasodilatory shock. Crit Care Med 2005;33(11):2659–66.
[105] Malay MB, Ashton RC Jr, Landry DW, et al. Low-dose vasopressin in the treatment of vasodilatory septic shock. J Trauma 1999;47(4):699–703.
[106] Patel BM, Chittock DR, Russell JA, et al. Beneficial effects of short-term vasopressin infusion during severe septic shock. Anesthesiology 2002;96(3):576–82.
[107] Tsuneyoshi I, Yamada H, Kakihana Y, et al. Hemodynamic and metabolic effects of low-dose vasopressin infusions in vasodilatory septic shock. Crit Care Med 2001;29(3):487–93.
[108] Morelli A, Rocco M, Conti G, et al. Effects of terlipressin on systemic and regional haemodynamics in catecholamine-treated hyperkinetic septic shock. Intensive Care Med 2004; 30(4):597–604.
[109] Albanese J, Leone M, Del mas A, et al. Terlipressin or norepinephrine in the hyperdynamic septic shock: a prospective, randomized study. Crit Care Med 2005;33(9):1897–902.
[110] O'Brien A, Clapp L, Singer M. Terlipressin for norepinephrine-resistant septic shock. Lancet 2002;359(9313):1209–10.
[111] Leone M, Albanese J, Delmas A, et al. Terlipressin in catecholamine-resistant septic shock patients. Shock 2004;22(4):314–9.
[112] Faivre V, Kaskos H, Callebert J, et al. Cardiac and renal effects of levosimendan, arginine vasopressin, and norepinephrine in lipopolysaccharide treated rabbits. Anesthesiology 2005;103(3):514–21.
[113] Leone M, Martin C. Rescue therapy in septic shock—is terlipressin the last frontier? Crit Care 2006;10(2):131.
[114] Dubois MJ, De Backer D, Creteur J, et al. Effect of vasopressin on sublingual microcirculation in a patient with distributive shock. Intensive Care Med 2003;29(6):1020–3.
[115] Boerma EC, van der Voort PHJ, Ince C. Sublingual microcirculatory flow is impaired by the vasopressin-analogue terlipressin in a patient with catecholamine-resistant septic shock. Acta Anaesthesiol Scand 2005;49(9):1387.
[116] Brinkmann A, Calzia E, Träger K, et al. Monitoring the hepato-splanchnic region in the critically ill patient: measurement techniques and clinical relevance. Intensive Care Med 1998;24(6):542–56.
[117] Hebert RL, Jacobson HR, Breyer MD. PGE_2 inhibits AVP-induced water flow in cortical collecting ducts by protein kinase C activation. Am J Physiol 1990;259(2 pt 2):F318–25.
[118] Rudichenko VM, Beierwaltes WH. Arginine vasopressin induced renal vasodilation mediated by nitric oxide. J Vasc Res 1995;32:100–5.
[119] Gutkowska J, Jankowski M, Lambert C, et al. Oxytocin releases atrial natriuretic peptide by combining with oxytocin receptors in the heart. Proc Natl Acad Sci USA 1997;94(21): 11704–9.
[120] Holmes C. Is low-dose vasopressin the new reno-protective agent? Crit Care Med 2004; 32(9):1972–3.
[121] Asfar P, Hauser B, Iványi Z, et al. Low dose terlipressin during long-term hyperdynamic porcine endotoxemia: effects on hepatosplanchninc perfusion, oxygen exchange, and metabolism. Crit Care Med 2005;33(2):373–80.

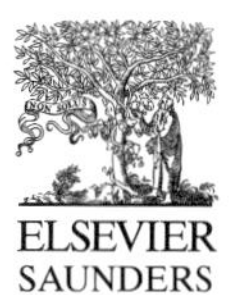
ELSEVIER
SAUNDERS

Endocrinol Metab Clin N Am
35 (2006) 859–872

ENDOCRINOLOGY
AND METABOLISM
CLINICS
OF NORTH AMERICA

Diabetes of Injury: Novel Insights

Ilse Vanhorebeek, PhD,
Greet Van den Berghe, MD, PhD*

Department of Intensive Care Medicine, Katholieke Universiteit Leuven, Herestraat 49, B-300 Leuven, Belgium

In normal individuals, blood glucose levels are tightly regulated within the narrow range of 60 to 140 mg/dL. Glucose levels usually rise during critical illness, however, independent of previously diagnosed diabetes. This condition of dysregulated glucose homeostasis in critically ill patients has been labeled "stress diabetes" or "diabetes of injury" [1,2].

In the acute phase of critical illness, glucose production by the liver is enhanced by upregulation of gluconeogenesis and glycogenolysis. The hyperinsulinemia developing after a transient fall in insulin levels normally suppresses both pathways but is unable to maintain normoglycemia in critical illness. Increased levels of glucagon, cortisol, growth hormone, catecholamines, and cytokines all play a role [3–8]. The hyperglycemic response is maintained during prolonged critical illness, but the mechanism remains relatively unclear. In comparison to the acute phase, cortisol, growth hormone, catecholamine, and cytokine levels usually decrease in the chronic phase of critical illness, whereas glucagon levels are not well documented. Impaired glucose uptake also contributes to the development of hyperglycemia. As the patient is immobilized, the important excercise-stimulated glucose uptake in skeletal muscle is likely abolished. Insulin-stimulated glucose uptake by glucose transporter (GLUT)-4 is compromised [9,10]. Nevertheless, whole-body glucose uptake is increased, accounted for by tissues that are not dependent on insulin for glucose uptake [2,11]. The combined picture of higher levels of insulin, elevated hepatic glucose production, and impaired

This work was supported by research grants from the Katholieke Universiteit Leuven (OT/03/56) and the Fund for Scientific Research (FWO), Flanders, Belgium (G.0278.03). I. Vanhorebeek is a Postdoctoral Fellow of the FWO, Flanders, Belgium. G. Van den Berghe holds an unrestrictive Katholieke Universiteit Leuven Novo Nordisk Chair of Research.

* Corresponding author.
E-mail address: greta.vandenberghe@med.kuleuven.be (G. Van den Berghe).

0889-8529/06/$ - see front matter
doi:10.1016/j.ecl.2006.09.002

peripheral glucose uptake reflects the development of peripheral insulin resistance during critical illness.

Diabetes of injury: how does it affect the outcome of critically ill patients?

The development of hyperglycemia during critical illness has long been considered an adaptive and beneficial stress response. Until recently, it was considered state of the art to tolerate blood glucose levels up to 220 mg/dL in fed critically ill patients [12] and only excessive hyperglycemia exceeding this value was treated. Reasons to treat hyperglycemia greater than this threshold included the occurrence of hyperglycemia-induced osmotic diuresis and fluid shifts at these high levels and the knowledge from the diabetic literature that uncontrolled and pronounced hyperglycemia predisposes to infectious complications [2,13]. Arguments to tolerate glucose levels up to 220 mg/dL were the classic dogma that moderate hyperglycemia in critically ill patients is beneficial for organs that largely rely on glucose for their energy supply but do not require insulin for glucose uptake, such as the brain and blood cells, and the fear of occasional hypoglycemia and consequent brain injury with tight glucose management.

Several recent studies clearly identify the development of hyperglycemia as an important risk factor in terms of mortality and morbidity of critically ill patients, however. Elevated glucose levels predicted increased mortality and length of intensive care unit (ICU) and hospital stay of trauma patients and were associated with infectious morbidity and prolonged need of mechanical ventilation [14–17]. Apart from the predictive value of hyperglycemia for worse survival of patients with severe brain injury, a significant relation was found between high blood glucose levels and worse neurologic status, impaired pupil reactivity, intracranial hypertension, and longer hospital length of stay [18,19]. Similarly, hyperglycemia predicted a higher risk of death after stroke and a poor functional recovery in those patients who survived [20]. Hyperglycemia was also associated with an increased risk of death in patients with myocardial infarction and coronary artery disease [21,22]. In addition, a strong link has been described between increased blood glucose levels and the risk of critical illness polyneuropathy in sepsis and the systemic inflammatory response syndrome [23]. Also, hyperglycemia develops in critically ill children and is associated with a worse outcome [24]. Retrospective analysis of a heterogeneous population of critically ill patients revealed that even a modest degree of hyperglycemia was associated with substantially increased hospital mortality [25].

Strict blood glucose control with intensive insulin therapy in critical illness

The first strong evidence against the traditional concept of tolerating glucose levels up to as high as 200 mg/dL came from the landmark prospective, randomized, controlled study on intensive insulin therapy in surgical critically ill patients [26]. A large group of patients admitted to the ICU predominantly after extensive complicated surgery or trauma or after medical complications of major surgical procedures were included in this study. Patients assigned to the conventional approach received insulin only if glucose concentrations exceeded 215 mg/dL, with the aim of keeping concentrations between 180 and 200 mg/dL, resulting in mean blood glucose levels of 150 to 160 mg/dL (hyperglycemia). Insulin was administered to the patients in the intensive insulin therapy group to maintain blood glucose levels between 80 and 110 mg/dL, which resulted in mean blood glucose levels of 90 to 100 mg/dL (normoglycemia). Tight blood glucose control with insulin strikingly lowered ICU mortality from 8.0% to 4.6% (43% reduction). The benefit was particularly attributed to the group of patients who required intensive care for more than 5 days, with a 48% reduction in mortality from 20.2% to 10.6%. In addition to saving lives, intensive insulin therapy largely prevented several complications associated with critical illness. The incidence of critical illness polyneuropathy was reduced by 44%, the development of blood stream infections was reduced by 46%, and the incidence of acute renal failure requiring dialysis or hemofiltration was reduced by 41%. The number of patients who acquired liver dysfunction with hyperbilirubinemia was lowered by 16%. Furthermore, anemia less frequently developed, as illustrated by the 50% reduction in the median number of red blood cell transfusions needed. Finally, patients were also less dependent on prolonged mechanical ventilation and intensive care. For the subgroup of patients who were included in the study after complicated cardiac surgery, a follow-up study showed that intensive insulin therapy also improved the long-term outcome when given for at least a third day in ICU, with maintenance of the survival benefit up to 4 years after randomization [27]. The risk for hospital readmission and dependency on medical care were similar in both groups. The short-term glycemic control with insulin during intensive care did not induce a substantial burden for the patients, their relatives, or society, but the perceived quality of social and family life seemed to be moderately compromised. Particularly in the group of patients with isolated brain injury, intensive insulin therapy protected the central and peripheral nervous system from secondary insults and improved long-term rehabilitation [28]. Finally, a recent post hoc health care resource use analysis also revealed economic advantages of intensive insulin therapy, with substantial cost savings compared with conventional insulin therapy in this surgical patient population [29].

Importantly, the clinical benefits of intensive insulin therapy were recently confirmed with the demonstration, again by a large, randomized, controlled trial, that the Catholic University of Leuven protocol of glycemic control with insulin [26] was similarly effective in a strictly medical adult ICU patient population [30]. In-hospital mortality was reduced from 40.0% to 37.3% in the intention-to-treat population of 1200 patients. The difference did not reach statistical significance; however, this was not surprising, because the study was not powered for this mortality end point. Nevertheless, in the target group of long-stay patients needing at least a third day of intensive care, for which the study had been powered based on the results of the surgical study, tight glycemic control with insulin significantly reduced in-hospital mortality from 52.5% to 43.0%. Morbidity was significantly reduced in the intention-to-treat group of patients receiving intensive insulin therapy. Development of new kidney injury occurred less frequently, the therapy allowed earlier weaning from mechanical ventilation and earlier discharge from the ICU and from the hospital, and the patients less frequently developed hyperbilirubinemia. The reduction in morbidity was even more striking in the target group of patients remaining in the ICU for at least a third day. These patients were discharged from the hospital, on average, 10 days earlier than patients receiving conventional insulin therapy. In contrast to the surgical patients, there was no difference in bacteremia or the requirement for prolonged antibiotic therapy, but the number of long-stay patients with hyperinflammation was also reduced.

To address some remaining concerns regarding benefit versus potential harm by intensive insulin therapy in certain subgroups of patients, the optimal blood glucose level, and the role of parenteral nutrition, the databases of these two trials were pooled [31]. The analyses revealed that intensive insulin therapy significantly reduced morbidity and mortality (Fig. 1) in a mixed medical/surgical ICU in an intention-to-treat analysis, even more so when continued for at least 3 days, independent of parenteral glucose load, and without causing harm to patients treated for less than 3 days. Intensive insulin therapy beneficially affected morbidity and mortality in all large diagnostic subgroups, except in patients with a prior history of diabetes [31]. Maintenance of blood glucose levels at less than 110 mg/dL was more effective than at 110 to 150 mg/dL to achieve better survival (see Fig. 1) and to reduce morbidity.

In "real life" intensive care of a heterogeneous medical/surgical patient population, an observational study [32] evaluated the impact of implementing a tight glucose management protocol by comparison with historical controls as a reference and also largely confirmed the clinical benefits of this intervention [26]. Intravenous insulin was administered only if glucose levels exceeded 200 mg/dL on two successive measurements, and the aim was to lower glycemia to less than 140 mg/dL. Hence, blood glucose control was somewhat less strict and resulted in mean glucose levels of 131 mg/dL in the protocol period compared with 152 mg/dL in the baseline period. In comparison with the historical control group, the implementation of the glucose control protocol resulted in a 29% decrease in hospital mortality, length of ICU stay decreased by 11%, 75% fewer patients developed new renal failure, and 19% fewer patients required red blood cell transfusion. No effect was seen on the occurrence of severe infections, but this complication was not frequently present in the baseline period. Another prospective,

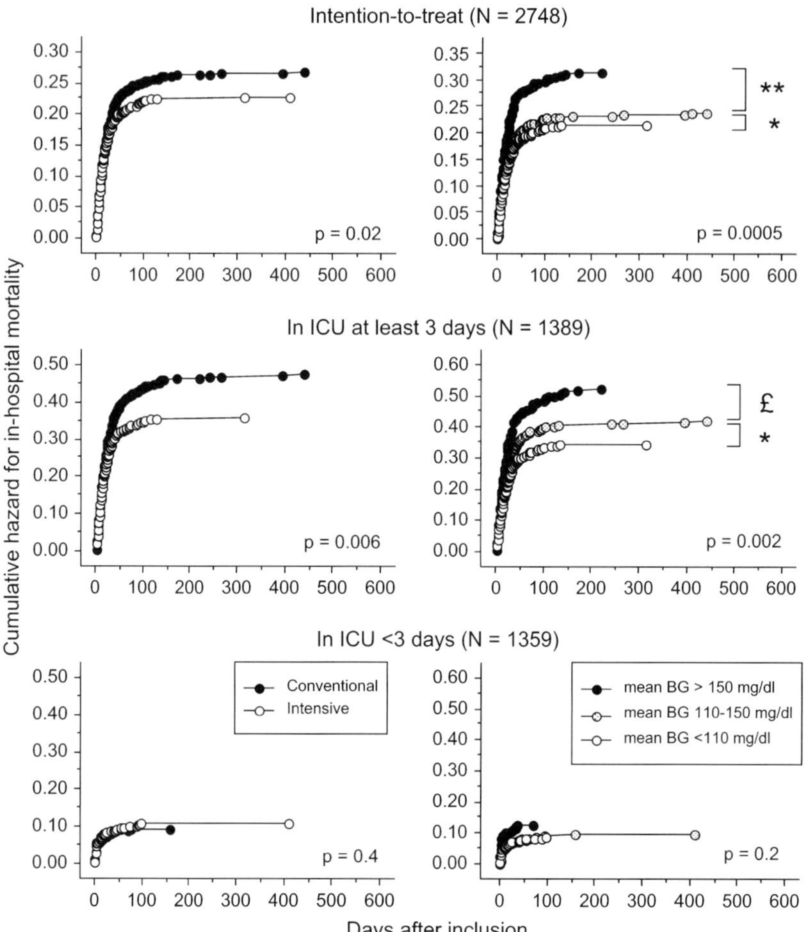

Fig. 1. Impact of intensive insulin therapy (*left panels*) and of the level of blood glucose (BG) control (*right panels*) on hospital mortality among short- and long-stay ICU patients. Numerical probability values were obtained by the log-rank test. Symbols reflect probability values obtained by χ^2 testing for logistic regression analysis per level of BG control. $*P = 0.02$; $**P = 0.007$, $£P = 0.07$. (*Adapted from* Van den Berghe G, Wilmer A, Milants I, et al. Intensive insulin therapy in mixed medical/surgical ICU: benefit versus harm. Diabetes 2006;55(11):3151–9.)

randomized, controlled study in a predominantly general surgical patient population confirmed the findings of a decreased incidence of total nosocomial infections with intensive insulin therapy targeting glucose levels between 80 and 120 mg/dL [33]. This intervention resulted in mean daily glucose levels of 125 mg/dL versus 179 mg/dL in the standard glycemic control group.

Intensive insulin therapy and the risk of hypoglycemia

Severe hypoglycemia (<30 mg/dL) or prolonged hypoglycemia can lead to convulsions, coma, and irreversible brain damage as well as to cardiac arrhythmias. Patients who have an altered mental status, who are intubated, or who are severely ill may be unable to recognize or communicate hypoglycemic symptoms [12]. Moreover, clinical symptoms may be masked by concomitant diseases and by inherent intensive care treatments, such as sedation, analgesia, and mechanical ventilation. Therefore, the risk of hypoglycemia is a major concern when intensive insulin therapy is administered to critically ill patients, and adequate training of the nursing and medical staff is clearly warranted. The best way to achieve blood glucose control during intensive care is by continuous insulin infusion, and the use of oral antidiabetic agents in patients with previously diagnosed diabetes should be discontinued. Specific measures to prevent hypoglycemia include the concomitant administration of insulin and carbohydrates and close monitoring of blood glucose levels initially as well as after stable glucose levels are obtained. Obviously, the insulin dose should be adequately reduced during interruption of enteral feeding.

In both clinical studies performed in Leuven, the risk of hypoglycemia (glucose ≤40 mg/dL) was higher with intensive insulin therapy [26,30]. When both studies were combined, hypoglycemia occurred in 1.8% of the conventionally treated patients and in 11.3% of the patients who received intensive insulin therapy [31]. Importantly, these brief episodes of biochemical hypoglycemia were not associated with obvious clinical problems. Indeed, hypoglycemia did not cause early deaths, only minor immediate and transient morbidity was seen in few patients, and no late neurologic sequelae occurred among hospital survivors. Because the risk of hypoglycemia in the conventional and intensive insulin groups coincided with a higher risk of death, however, it cannot be completely excluded that hypoglycemia counteracted some of the survival benefit of intensive insulin therapy. Because most benefit was gained with the tightest blood glucose control, the risk of hypoglycemia should be weighed against an improved outcome. Clearly, the development of accurate blood glucose monitoring in a continuous way and closed-loop systems for computer-assisted blood glucose control in the ICU should help to avoid any eventual side effect that could be induced by hypoglycemia.

Insights into the mechanisms of an improved outcome with intensive insulin therapy

The blood glucose control and/or other metabolic effects of insulin that accompany tight blood glucose control, and not the insulin dose administered per se, contributed to the improved survival with intensive insulin therapy. Indeed, hyperglycemia and the administration of a high dose of insulin were associated with a high risk of death in surgical critically ill patients, as revealed by multivariate logistic regression analysis [26,34]. The risk of death seemed to be linearly correlated with the degree of hyperglycemia, with no clear cutoff level below which there was no further benefit [34]. The highest risk of death was observed for the conventionally treated patients who developed severe hyperglycemia (150–200 mg/dL), an intermediate risk was seen for patients who received conventional insulin therapy and developed only moderate hyperglycemia (110–150 mg/dL), and the lowest risk was present in the patients whose blood glucose levels were controlled at less than 110 mg/dL with intensive insulin therapy. This was confirmed in the mixed medical/surgical patient population (see Fig. 1) [31]. Other data also suggest that the mortality benefits can be attributed to glycemic control rather than to the absolute insulin doses administered [25,35]. The observed association between high insulin dose and mortality is likely explained by more severe insulin resistance in sicker patients, who have a high risk of death. Glycemic control also accounted for most effects on morbidity [34]. As for mortality, tight glycemic control at less than 110 mg/dL seemed to be of crucial importance for the prevention of critical illness polyneuropathy, bacteremia, anemia, and acute renal failure [31,34]. In particular, a positive linear correlation was observed between glycemia and the risk of developing critical illness polyneuropathy, where multivariate logistic regression analysis also confirmed the crucial role of preventing glucose toxicity to protect the neurons [28].

Mechanisms of glucose toxicity in critical illness and effects of intensive insulin therapy

Normal cells respond to moderate hyperglycemia by downregulation of glucose transporters to protect themselves from deleterious effects [36]. In patients with diabetes, chronic hyperglycemia causes severe complications but in a time frame that is several orders of magnitude longer than the time it took to prevent life-threatening complications with intensive insulin therapy in critical illness. Therefore, it is striking that by avoiding even a moderate degree of hyperglycemia only during the relatively short period the patients needed intensive care, this strategy prevented the most feared complications of critical illness. This indicates that hyperglycemia would be more acutely toxic in critically ill patients than in healthy individuals or diabetic patients. Glucose uptake mediated by the facilitative glucose transporters GLUT-1, GLUT-2, or GLUT-3, which is independent of insulin, may play a role. Several factors induced in critical illness have been shown to upregulate the expression and membrane localization of GLUT-1 and GLUT-3 in different cell types, which may overrule the normal downregulatory protective response against hyperglycemia. These include cytokines, angiotensin II, endothelin-1, vascular endothelial growth factor, and transforming growth factor-β, but hypoxia also seems to be a regulatory factor [37–41]. Furthermore, GLUT-2 and GLUT-3 allow glucose to enter cells directly proportional to the extracellular glucose level over the range of glycemia present in critical illness (Michaelis constant [Km] $\approx$ 9 mmol/L for GLUT-3 and much higher for GLUT-2) [42]. Hence, cellular glucose overload may develop in the central and peripheral nervous system and in endothelial, epithelial, and immune cells as well as in hepatocytes, renal tubules, pancreatic β-cells, and gastrointestinal mucosa. In contrast, cellular systems and tissues that predominantly rely on insulin-dependent glucose transport via GLUT-4, such as skeletal muscle and myocardium, may be relatively protected against hyperglycemia-induced cellular glucose overload and toxicity.

Our recent observation that prevention of hyperglycemia with intensive insulin therapy is protective to the hepatocytic mitochondrial compartment of critically ill patients [43] is consistent with this concept. Whereas ultrastructural abnormalities were virtually absent when blood glucose levels were tightly controlled to normoglycemia, severe alterations were seen in patients in the conventional treatment group, where a large fraction of the hepatocytes contained hypertrophic mitochondria with an increased number of abnormal and irregular cristae and reduced electron density of the matrix. At the functional level, this was associated with higher activities of respiratory chain complex I and complex IV in the patients who received intensive insulin therapy. In contrast, no morphologic abnormalities were detected in skeletal muscle, nor were any of the respiratory chain enzyme complexes affected by insulin therapy. Mitochondrial dysfunction and the associated bioenergetic failure have been regarded as factors contributing to multiple organ failure, the most common cause of death in sepsis and prolonged critical illness, and have indeed been related to a lethal outcome in patients and in a resuscitated long-term rat model of sepsis [44,45]. As such, prevention of hyperglycemia-induced mitochondrial damage to hepatocytes and other cellular systems with passive glucose uptake could theoretically explain some of the protective effects of intensive insulin therapy in severe illness. There is substantial evidence that links diabetes and hyperglycemia to the development of increased oxidative stress, in part attributable to enhanced mitochondrial superoxide production [46]. Cytokine-induced activation of nitric oxide (NO) synthesis increases NO levels in critical illness, whereas hypoxia-reperfusion in patients aggravates superoxide production. Thus, enhanced formation of peroxynitrite may be expected. This reactive nitrogen species is able to induce tyrosine nitration of proteins, and thus to affect their normal function [47], as illustrated by the suppression of mitochondrial complex I activity [48].

High glucose levels compromise all major components of innate immunity [49], including polymorphonuclear neutrophil function and intracellular bactericidal and opsonic activity [50–53]. This may play a role in the increased risk of infections observed for patients who are exposed to such high glucose levels [13,54]. Importantly, intensive insulin therapy largely prevented severe nosocomial infections and lethal sepsis in critically ill patients [26]. In an animal model of prolonged critical illness [55], glucose control with insulin beneficially affected innate immunity by preservation of phagocytosis and the oxidative burst function of monocytes [56].

Thus, it can be concluded that protection from hyperglycemia is crucial in explaining the mechanisms underlying the clinical benefits of intensive insulin therapy. In this regard, studies performed by our group suggest that stimulation of glucose uptake by skeletal muscle mainly explains how intensive insulin therapy lowers circulating glucose levels in critically ill patients rather than by an effect of insulin on hepatic glucose handling [57,58]. This is illustrated by improved responsiveness of insulin-regulated genes in skeletal muscle, whereas it seems that insulin resistance in the liver is not overcome by intensive insulin therapy. Recent data obtained from an animal model of prolonged critical illness, where glucose and insulin levels were independently manipulated, also showed that strict blood glucose control is required to obtain the clinical benefits of intensive insulin therapy [59].

Nonglycemic effects of intensive insulin therapy

Critically ill patients have a severely disturbed serum lipid profile, with an elevated triglyceride level (because of an increase in very-low-density lipoprotein) and low levels of high-density lipoprotein (HDL) and low-density lipoprotein (LDL) cholesterol [60–62]. Intensive insulin therapy prevented the rise in serum triglycerides during full nutritional support and substantially increased circulating HDL and LDL and the level of cholesterol associated with these lipoproteins [57]. Insulin treatment also decreased serum triglycerides and free fatty acids in burned children [63]. Given the important role of triglycerides in energy provision and of lipoproteins in transportation of lipid components and endotoxin scavenging [64–66], a contribution of the (partial) correction of the lipid profile to an improved outcome may be expected. This has indeed been confirmed in multivariate logistic regression analysis, where the effect on dyslipidemia surprisingly even surpassed the effect of glycemic control [57].

The administration of insulin has been put forward as an intervention to attenuate the catabolic syndrome of prolonged critical illness [67,68] because it has well-recognized anabolic properties, including stimulation of muscle protein synthesis and attenuation of protein breakdown [69–71]. This anabolic effect was not obvious from clinical observation in the surgical ICU trial [26], but intensive insulin therapy did result in higher protein content in post-mortem skeletal muscle biopsies of the patients [43] and prevented weight loss in a rabbit model of prolonged critical illness [56]. Altered regulation at the level of the somatotropic axis did not seem to be involved [72].

Intensive insulin therapy lowered serum C-reactive protein (CRP) and mannose-binding lectin levels [73], illustrating a preventive effect on excessive inflammation. This effect was independent of infection prevention. A similar attenuation of the CRP response was seen in a rabbit model of prolonged critical illness [56]. Analysis of an extensive series of pro- and anti-inflammatory cytokines in surgical critically ill patients revealed no major effect of insulin therapy [74]. In burned children, however, the administration of insulin resulted in lower proinflammatory cytokines and proteins and stimulation of the anti-inflammatory cascade, although these effects were largely seen only late after the insult [63]. Similar results were obtained in endotoxemic rats and pigs and thermally injured rats [75–77]. Although the anti-inflammatory effects of insulin therapy may be direct, prevention of hyperglycemia may be crucial as well.

Insulin has also been shown to improve myocardial function and to protect the myocardium during acute myocardial infarction, open-heart surgery, endotoxic shock, and other critical conditions [78,79]. Direct antiapoptotic properties of insulin independent of glucose uptake and involving insulin signaling play a role [78,80,81]. Insulin's cardioprotective action may be at least partly attributable to lowering of glucose levels, however [78]. This likely explains the disappointing results in the absence of adequate glucose control obtained in the recent large randomized Clinical Trial of Reviparin and Metabolic Modulation in Acute Myocardio Infarction Treatment and Evaluation—Estudios Cardiologicas Latin America (CREATE-ECLA) on glucose-insulin-potassium infusion in patients with acute myocardial infarction [82] and in the Diabetes and Insulin-Glucose Infusion in Acute Myocardial Infarction-2 (DIGAMI-2) trial in patients with diabetes and myocardial infarction [83].

As in patients with diabetes, prevention of endothelial dysfunction and hypercoagulation may contribute to the protective effects of insulin therapy in critical illness [84]. Endothelial protection indeed related to prevention of organ failure and death with this intervention [74]. Endothelial activation was reduced, as reflected in lower levels of adhesion molecules. Inhibition of excessive inducible NO synthase–induced NO release is likely involved. Intensive insulin therapy reduced the levels of asymmetric dimethylarginine [85], an endogenous inhibitor of NO synthase activity. The modulation of this arginine derivative by insulin was associated with a better outcome, most likely mediated by reducing the inhibition of the constitutively expressed endothelial NO synthase [86], contributing to preservation of organ blood flow.

Finally, intensive insulin therapy attenuated the cortisol response to critical illness without involvement of altered cortisol-binding activity [87]. This effect was statistically related to an improved outcome.

Summary

More and more evidence argues against the concept that the diabetes of injury is an adaptive beneficial response in the modern ICU era. The development of hyperglycemia is indeed detrimental to the outcome of critically ill patients. Maintenance of normoglycemia with intensive insulin therapy, a simple metabolic intervention, to a large extent prevents morbidity and improves the survival of critically ill patients. Substantial progress has been made in the understanding of the mechanisms underlying these clinical benefits, but more studies are needed to elucidate further the exact pathways involved as well as the relative contribution of the prevention of glucose toxicity and the direct nonglycemic effects of insulin.

References

[1] Thorell A, Nygren J, Ljungqvist O. Insulin resistance: a marker of surgical stress. Curr Opin Clin Nutr Metab Care 1999;2(1):69–78.
[2] McCowen KC, Malhotra A, Bistrian BR. Stress-induced hyperglycaemia. Crit Care Clin 2001;17(1):107–24.
[3] Hill M, McCallum R. Altered transcriptional regulation of phosphoenolpyruvate carboxykinase in rats following endotoxin treatment. J Clin Invest 1991;88(3):811–6.
[4] Khani S, Tayek JA. Cortisol increases gluconeogenesis in humans: its role in the metabolic syndrome. Clin Sci (Lond) 2001;101(6):739–47.
[5] Watt MJ, Howlett KF, Febbraio MA, et al. Adrenalin increases skeletal muscle glycogenolysis, pyruvate dehydrogenase activation and carbohydrate oxidation during moderate exercise in humans. J Physiol 2001;534(Pt 1):269–78.
[6] Flores EA, Istfan N, Pomposelli JJ, et al. Effect of interleukin-1 and tumor necrosis factor/cachectin on glucose turnover in the rat. Metabolism 1990;39(7):738–43.
[7] Sakurai Y, Zhang XJ, Wolfe RR. TNF directly stimulates glucose uptake and leucine oxidation and inhibits FFA flux in conscious dogs. Am J Physiol 1996;270(5 Pt 1):E864–72.
[8] Lang CH, Dobrescu C, Bagby GJ. Tumor necrosis factor impairs insulin action on peripheral glucose disposal and hepatic glucose output. Endocrinology 1992;130(1):43–52.
[9] Wolfe RR, Durkot MJ, Allsop JR, et al. Glucose metabolism in severely burned patients. Metabolism 1979;28(10):1031–9.
[10] Wolfe RR, Herndon DN, Jahoor F, et al. Effect of severe burn injury on substrate cycling by glucose and fatty acids. N Engl J Med 1987;317(7):403–8.
[11] Mizock BA. Alterations in carbohydrate metabolism during stress: a review of the literature. Am J Med 1995;98(1):75–84.
[12] Boord JB, Graber AL, Christman JW, et al. Practical management of diabetes in critically ill patients. Am J Respir Crit Care Med 2001;164(10 Pt 1):1763–7.
[13] Pozzilli P, Leslie RD. Infections and diabetes: mechanisms and prospects for prevention. Diabet Med 1994;11(10):935–41.
[14] Yendamuri S, Fulda GJ, Tinkoff GH. Admission hyperglycemia as a prognostic indicator in trauma. J Trauma 2003;55(1):33–8.
[15] Laird AM, Miller PR, Kilgo PD, et al. Relationship of early hyperglycemia to mortality in trauma patients. J Trauma 2004;56(5):1058–62.
[16] Bochicchio GV, Sung J, Joshi M, et al. Persistent hyperglycemia is predictive of outcome of critically ill trauma patients. J Trauma 2005;58(5):921–4.
[17] Sung J, Bochicchio GV, Joshi M, et al. Admission hyperglycemia is predictive of outcome in critically ill trauma patients. J Trauma 2005;59(1):80–3.
[18] Rovlias A, Kotsou S. The influence of hyperglycemia on neurological outcome in patients with severe head injury. Neurosurgery 2000;46(2):335–42.
[19] Jeremitsky E, Omert LA, Dunham M, et al. The impact of hyperglycemia on patients with severe brain injury. J Trauma 2005;58(1):47–50.
[20] Capes SE, Hunt D, Malmberg K, et al. Stress hyperglycemia and prognosis of stroke in nondiabetic and diabetic patients: a systematic overview. Stroke 2001;32(10):2426–32.
[21] Capes SE, Hunt D, Malmberg K, et al. Stress hyperglycaemia and increased risk of death after myocardial infarction in patients with and without diabetes: a systematic overview. Lancet 2000;355(9206):773–8.

[22] Muhlestein JB, Anderson JL, Horne BD, et al. Effect of fasting glucose levels on mortality rate in patients with and without diabetes mellitus and coronary artery disease undergoing percutaneous coronary intervention. Am Heart J 2003;146(2):351–8.
[23] Bolton CF. Sepsis and the systemic inflammatory response syndrome: neuromuscular manifestations. Crit Care Med 1996;24(8):1408–16.
[24] Faustino EV, Apkon M. Persistent hyperglycemia in critically ill children. J Pediatr 2005; 146(1):30–4.
[25] Krinsley JS. Association between hyperglycemia and increased hospital mortality in a heterogeneous population of critically ill patients. Mayo Clin Proc 2003;78(12):1471–8.
[26] Van den Berghe G, Wouters P, Weekers F, et al. Intensive insulin therapy in critically ill patients. N Engl J Med 2001;345(19):1359–67.
[27] Ingels C, Debaveye Y, Milants I, et al. Strict blood glucose control with insulin during intensive care after cardiac surgery: impact on 4-years survival, dependency on medical care and quality of life. Eur Heart J, in press.
[28] Van den Berghe G, Schoonheydt K, Becx P, et al. Insulin therapy protects the central and peripheral nervous system of intensive care patients. Neurology 2005;64(8): 1348–53.
[29] Van den Berghe G, Wouters PJ, Kesteloot K, et al. Analysis of healthcare resource utilization with intensive insulin therapy in critically ill patients. Crit Care Med 2006;34(3):612–6.
[30] Van den Berghe G, Wilmer A, Hermans G, et al. Intensive insulin therapy in medical intensive care patients. N Engl J Med 2006;354(5):449–61.
[31] Van den Berghe G, Wilmer A, Milants I, et al. Intensive insulin therapy in mixed medical/ surgical ICU: benefit versus harm. Diabetes 2006;55(11):3151–9.
[32] Krinsley JS. Effect of an intensive glucose management protocol on the mortality of critically ill adult patients. Mayo Clin Proc 2004;79(8):992–1000.
[33] Grey NJ, Perdrizet GA. Reduction of nosocomial infections in the surgical intensive-care unit by strict glycemic control. Endocr Pract 2004;10(Suppl 2):46–52.
[34] Van den Berghe G, Wouters PJ, Bouillon R, et al. Outcome benefit of intensive insulin therapy in the critically ill: insulin dose versus glycemic control. Crit Care Med 2003;31(2): 359–66.
[35] Finney SJ, Zekveld C, Elia A, et al. Glucose control and mortality in critically ill patients. JAMA 2003;290(15):2041–7.
[36] Klip A, Tsakiridis T, Marette A, et al. Regulation of expression of glucose transporters by glucose: a review of studies in vivo and in cell cultures. FASEB J 1994; 8(1):43–53.
[37] Pekala P, Marlow M, Heuvelman D, et al. Regulation of hexose transport in aortic endothelial cells by vascular permeability factor and tumor necrosis factor alfa, but not by insulin. J Biol Chem 1990;265(30):18051–4.
[38] Shikhman AR, Brinson DC, Valbracht J, et al. Cytokine regulation of facilitated glucose transport in human articular chondrocytes. J Immunol 2001;167(12):7001–8.
[39] Quinn LA, McCumbee WD. Regulation of glucose transport by angiotensin II and glucose in cultured vascular smooth muscle cells. J Cell Physiol 1998;177(1):94–102.
[40] Clerici C, Matthay MA. Hypoxia regulates gene expression of alveolar epithelial transport proteins. J Appl Physiol 2000;88(5):1890–6.
[41] Sanchez-Alvarez R, Tabernero A, Medina JM. Endothelin-1 stimulates the translocation and upregulation of both glucose transporter and hexokinase in astrocytes: relationship with gap junctional communication. J Neurochem 2004;89(3):703–14.
[42] Tirone TA, Brunicardi C. Overview of glucose regulation. World J Surg 2001;25(4):461–7.
[43] Vanhorebeek I, De Vos R, Mesotten D, et al. Strict blood glucose control with insulin in critically ill patients protects hepatocytic mitochondrial ultrastructure and function. Lancet 2005;365(9453):53–9.
[44] Brealey D, Brand M, Hargreaves I, et al. Association between mitochondrial dysfunction and severity and outcome of septic shock. Lancet 2002;360(9328):219–23.

[45] Brealey D, Karyampudi S, Jacques TS, et al. Mitochondrial dysfunction in a long-term rodent model of sepsis and organ failure. Am J Physiol Regul Integr Comp Physiol 2004; 286(3):R491–7.

[46] Brownlee M. Biochemistry and molecular cell biology of diabetic complications. Nature 2001;414(6865):813–20.

[47] Aulak KS, Koeck T, Crabb JW, et al. Dynamics of protein nitration in cells and mitochondria. Am J Physiol Heart Circ Physiol 2004;286(1):H30–8.

[48] Frost M, Wang Q, Moncada S, et al. Hypoxia accelerates nitric oxide-dependent inhibition of mitochondrial complex I in activated macrophages. Am J Physiol Regul Integr Comp Physiol 2005;288(2):R394–400.

[49] Turina M, Fry DE, Polk HC Jr. Acute hyperglycemia and the innate immune system: clinical, cellular, and molecular aspects. Crit Care Med 2005;33(7):1624–33.

[50] Rassias AJ, Marrin CA, Arruda J, et al. Insulin infusion improves neutrophil function in diabetic cardiac surgery patients. Anesth Analg 1999;88(5):1011–6.

[51] Nielson CP, Hindson DA. Inhibition of polymorphonuclear leukocyte respiratory burst by elevated glucose concentrations in vitro. Diabetes 1989;38(8):1031–5.

[52] Perner A, Nielsen SE, Rask-Madsen J. High glucose impairs superoxide production from isolated blood neutrophils. Intensive Care Med 2003;29(4):642–5.

[53] Rayfield EJ, Ault MJ, Keusch GT, et al. Infection and diabetes: the case for glucose control. Am J Med 1982;72(3):439–50.

[54] Furnary AP, Zerr KJ, Grunkemeier GL, et al. Continuous intravenous insulin infusion reduces the incidence of deep sternal wound infection in diabetic patients after cardiac surgical procedures. Ann Thorac Surg 1999;67(2):352–60.

[55] Weekers F, Van Herck E, Coopmans W, et al. A novel in vivo rabbit model of hypercatabolic critical illness reveals a bi-phasic neuroendocrine stress response. Endocrinology 2002; 143(3):764–74.

[56] Weekers F, Giuletti A-P, Michalaki M, et al. Endocrine and immune effects of stress hyperglycemia in a rabbit model of prolonged critical illness. Endocrinology 2003;144(12): 5329–38.

[57] Mesotten D, Swinnen JV, Vanderhoydonc F, et al. Contribution of circulating lipids to the improved outcome of critical illness by glycemic control with intensive insulin therapy. J Clin Endocrinol Metab 2004;89(1):219–26.

[58] Mesotten D, Delhanty PJ, Vanderhoydonc F, et al. Regulation of insulin-like growth factor binding protein-1 during protracted critical illness. J Clin Endocrinol Metab 2002;87(12): 5516–23.

[59] Ellger B, Debaveye Y, Vanhorebeek I, et al. Survival benefits of intensive insulin therapy in critical illness. Impact of normoglycemia versus glycemia-independent actions of insulin. Diabetes 2006;55(4):1096–105.

[60] Lanza-Jacoby S, Wong SH, Tabares A, et al. Disturbances in the composition of plasma lipoproteins during gram-negative sepsis in the rat. Biochim Biophys Acta 1992;1124(3): 233–40.

[61] Khovidhunkit W, Memon RA, Feingold KR, et al. Infection and inflammation-induced proatherogenic changes of lipoproteins. J Infect Dis 2000;181(Suppl 3):S462–72.

[62] Carpentier YA, Scruel O. Changes in the concentration and composition of plasma lipoproteins during the acute phase response. Curr Opin Clin Nutr Metab Care 2002;5(2):153–8.

[63] Jeschke MG, Klein D, Herndon DN. Insulin treatment improves the systemic inflammatory reaction to severe trauma. Ann Surg 2004;239(4):553–60.

[64] Tulenko TN, Sumner AE. The physiology of lipoproteins. J Nucl Cardiol 2002;9(6): 638–49.

[65] Harris HW, Grunfeld C, Feingold KR, et al. Human very low density lipoproteins and chylomicrons can protect against endotoxin-induced death in mice. J Clin Invest 1990;86(3): 696–702.

[66] Harris HW, Grunfeld C, Feingold KR, et al. Chylomicrons alter the fate of endotoxin, decreasing tumor necrosis factor release and preventing death. J Clin Invest 1993;91(3): 1028–34.
[67] Vanhorebeek I, Van den Berghe G. Hormonal and metabolic strategies to attenuate catabolism in critically ill patients. Curr Opin Pharmacol 2004;4(6):621–8.
[68] Vanhorebeek I, Langouche L, Van den Berghe G. Endocrine aspects of acute and prolonged critical illness. Nature Clin Pract Endocrinol Metab 2006;2(1):20–31.
[69] Gore DC, Wolf SE, Sanford AP, et al. Extremity hyperinsulinemia stimulates muscle protein synthesis in severely injured patients. Am J Physiol Endocrinol Metab 2004;286(4):E529–34.
[70] Agus MSD, Javid PJ, Ryan DP, et al. Intravenous insulin decreases protein breakdown in infants on extracorporeal membrane oxygenation. J Pediatr Surg 2004;39(6):839–44.
[71] Zhang XJ, Chinkes DL, Irtun O, et al. Anabolic action of insulin on skin wound protein is augmented by exogenous amino acids. Am J Physiol Endocrinol Metab 2002;282(6): E1308–15.
[72] Mesotten D, Wouters PJ, Peeters RP, et al. Regulation of the somatotropic axis by intensive insulin therapy during protracted critical illness. J Clin Endocrinol Metab 2004;89(7): 3105–13.
[73] Hansen TK, Thiel S, Wouters PJ, et al. Intensive insulin therapy exerts anti-inflammatory effects in critically ill patients, as indicated by circulating mannose-binding lectin and C-reactive protein levels. J Clin Endocrinol Metab 2003;88(3):1082–8.
[74] Langouche L, Vanhorebeek I, Vlasselaers D, et al. Intensive insulin therapy protects the endothelium of critically ill patients. J Clin Invest 2005;115(8):2277–86.
[75] Jeschke MG, Klein D, Bolder U, et al. Insulin attenuates the systemic inflammatory response in endotoxemic rats. Endocrinology 2004;145(9):4084–93.
[76] Brix-Christensen V, Andersen SK, Andersen R, et al. Acute hyperinsulinemia restrains endotoxin-induced systemic inflammatory response: an experimental study in a porcine model. Anesthesiology 2004;100(4):861–70.
[77] Klein D, Schubert T, Horch RE, et al. Insulin treatment improves hepatic morphology and function through modulation of hepatic signals after severe trauma. Ann Surg 2004;240(2):340–9.
[78] Das UN. Insulin: an endogenous cardioprotector. Curr Opin Crit Care 2003;9(5):375–83.
[79] Jonassen A, Aasum E, Riemersma R, et al. Glucose-insulin-potassium reduces infarct size when administered during reperfusion. Cardiovasc Drugs Ther 2000;14(6):615–23.
[80] Gao F, Gao E, Yue T, et al. Nitric oxide mediates the antiapoptotic effect of insulin in myocardial ischemia-reperfusion: the role of PI3-kinase, Akt and eNOS phosphorylation. Circulation 2002;105(12):1497–502.
[81] Jonassen A, Sack M, Mjos O, et al. Myocardial protection by insulin at reperfusion requires early administration and is mediated via Akt and p70s6 kinase cell-survival signalling. Circ Res 2001;89(12):1191–8.
[82] The CREATE-ECLA Trial Group Investigators. Effect of glucose-insulin-potassium infusion on mortality in patients with acute ST-segment elevation myocardial infarction. The CREATE-ECLA randomized controlled trial. JAMA 2005;293(4):437–46.
[83] Malmberg K, Ryden L, Wedel H, et al. Intense metabolic control by means of insulin in patients with diabetes mellitus and acute myocardial infarction (DIGAMI-2): effects on mortality and morbidity. Eur Heart J 2005;26(7):650–61.
[84] Van den Berghe G. How does blood glucose control with insulin save lives in intensive care? J Clin Invest 2004;114(9):1187–95.
[85] Siroen MPC, van Leeuwen PAM, Nijveldt RJ, et al. Modulation of asymmetric dimethylarginine in critically ill patients receiving intensive insulin treatment: a possible explanation of reduced morbidity and mortality? Crit Care Med 2005;33(3):504–10.
[86] Nijveldt RJ, Teerlink T, van Leeuwen PA. The asymmetric dimethylarginine (ADMA)-multiple organ failure hypothesis. Clin Nutr 2003;22(1):99–104.
[87] Vanhorebeek I, Peeters RP, Vander Perre S, et al. Cortisol response to critical illness: effect of intensive insulin therapy. J Clin Endocrinol Metab 2006;91(10):3803–13.

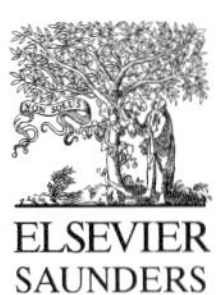

ELSEVIER
SAUNDERS

Endocrinol Metab Clin N Am
35 (2006) 873–894

ENDOCRINOLOGY
AND METABOLISM
CLINICS
OF NORTH AMERICA

Disorders of Body Water Homeostasis in Critical Illness

Suzanne Myers Adler, MD, Joseph G. Verbalis, MD*

Division of Endocrinology and Metabolism and Department of Medicine, Georgetown University School of Medicine, Building D, Suite 232, 4000 Reservoir Road NW, Washington, DC 20007, USA

Disorders of sodium and water homeostasis are among the most commonly encountered disturbances in the critical care setting, because many disease states cause defects in the complex mechanisms that control the intake and output of water and solute. Because body water is the primary determinant of extracellular fluid osmolality, disorders of body water balance can be categorized into hypoosmolar and hyperosmolar disorders depending on the presence of an excess or a deficiency of body water relative to body solute. Because the main constituent of plasma osmolality is sodium, hypoosmolar and hyperosmolar disease states are generally characterized by hyponatremia and hypernatremia, respectively. Both of these disturbances, as well as their overly rapid correction, can cause considerable morbidity and mortality [1–4]. After a brief review of normal water metabolism, this article focuses on the diagnosis and treatment of hyponatremia and hypernatremia in the critical care setting.

Overview of normal water metabolism

Whereas sodium metabolism is predominately regulated by the renin-angiotensin-aldosterone system (RAAS), water metabolism is controlled primarily by arginine vasopressin (AVP). AVP is a nine-amino acid peptide produced by the cell bodies of magnocellular neurons located in the hypothalamic supraoptic and paraventricular nuclei and secreted into the bloodstream from axon terminals located in the posterior pituitary. The primary inputs to these hypothalamic neurons are via hypothalamic osmoreceptors

* Corresponding author. Department of Medicine, Georgetown University School of Medicine, 232 Building D, 4000 Reservoir Road NW, Washington, DC 20007.

E-mail address: verbalis@georgetown.edu (J.G. Verbalis).

doi:10.1016/j.ecl.2006.09.011

endo.theclinics.com

and brainstem cardiovascular centers [5]. Osmoreceptors located in the anterior hypothalamus stimulate AVP secretion in response to increased plasma osmolality and inhibit AVP secretion when decreased plasma osmolality is detected. Baroreceptors located in the carotid arteries and aortic arch also stimulate AVP secretion in response to decreases in mean arterial pressure or blood volume. AVP controls water permeability at the level of the nephron by binding to AVP V_2 receptors, causing aquaporin-2 (AQP2) water channel insertion into the luminal surface of collecting duct cells, thereby stimulating free water reabsorption and antidiuresis [6]. Chronically, AVP also increases the synthesis of AQP2 in principal cells of the collecting duct, resulting in enhanced water permeability and maximal antidiuresis [7].

Many different substances can stimulate AVP release, including acetylcholine, histamine, dopamine, prostaglandins, bradykinin, neuropeptide Y, and angiotensin II. Many others inhibit AVP release, including nitric oxide, atrial natriuretic peptide, and opioids [8–10]. Norepinephrine stimulates AVP release via α1-adrenoreceptors but also inhibits AVP release via α2-adrenoreceptors and β-adrenoreceptors [11,12]. Because AVP secretion is influenced by so many different factors, any one of which can predominate in a given clinical circumstance, dysregulated AVP secretion is often the cause of impaired water homeostasis in critical illness.

Hyponatremia

Hyponatremia is a common electrolyte abnormality that varies greatly in its clinical presentation. It has been estimated that approximately 1% of patients have acute symptomatic hyponatremia, 4% acute asymptomatic hyponatremia, 15% to 20% chronic symptomatic hyponatremia, and 75% to 80% chronic asymptomatic hyponatremia [13]. The incidence of hyponatremia (serum $[Na^+] \leq 134$ mmol/L) in the intensive care unit was prospectively found to be approximately 30% [14]. The in-hospital mortality rate for critical care patients with hyponatremia approaches 40%, and hyponatremia has been shown to be an independent predictor of mortality in the intensive care unit [15]. Hyponatremia is generally categorized based on serum tonicity as isotonic, hypotonic, or hypertonic. Although most instances of hyponatremia in critical illness are associated with hypotonicity, isotonic and hypertonic hyponatremia are also well documented and are discussed briefly first herein.

Isotonic hyponatremia

Isotonic hyponatremia is usually synonymous with so-called "pseudohyponatremia" and must be distinguished from true hypoosmolality. Plasma osmolality can be measured directly in the laboratory by osmometry or calculated based on the following formula:

$$\text{Posm (mOsm/kg } H_2O) = 2 \times \text{serum } [Na^+] \text{ (mmol/L)} \\ + \text{glucose (mg/dL)/18} \\ + \text{BUN (mg/dL)/2.8}$$

Normal serum is typically comprised of 93% water and 7% nonaqueous factors, including lipids and proteins [16]. Although the nonaqueous components do not affect serum tonicity, in states of marked hyperproteinemia or hyperlipidemia (typically, elevated chylomicrons or triglycerides), the nonaqueous proportion of serum is relatively increased with respect to the aqueous portion, artifactually decreasing the concentration of Na^+/L of serum although the concentration of Na^+/L of serum water is unchanged. Because isotonic hyponatremia does not cause movement of water between the intracellular fluid (ICF) and extracellular fluid (ECF) compartments, it is not a meaningful cause of disturbed body fluid homeostasis in the critical care setting but must be distinguished from more pathologic disorders.

Hypertonic hyponatremia

Hypertonic hyponatremia has also been termed *translocational hyponatremia* because the presence of osmotically active particles in the plasma induces an osmotic movement of water from the ICF to the ECF, decreasing serum [Na^+] even though serum osmolality remains elevated. Solutes such as glucose, mannitol, sorbitol, or radiocontrast agents all exert this effect. The generally accepted calculation to correct serum [Na^+] for hyperglycemia is a decrease in serum [Na^+] of 1.6 mmol/L for every 100 mg/dL increase in glucose concentration; however, some investigators have found a serum [Na^+] correction factor of 2.4 mmol/L to be more accurate, especially at higher plasma glucose concentrations (eg, $>$400 mg/dL) [17].

Hypotonic hyponatremia

Of most relevance in the critical care setting is hypotonic hyponatremia, a condition indicative of an excess of water relative to solute in the ECF. Hypotonic hyponatremia can occur as a result of solute *depletion*, a primary decrease in total body solute (often with secondary water retention), or solute *dilution*, a primary increase in total body water (often with secondary solute depletion) (Box 1) [4]. Hypotonic or hypoosmolar hyponatremia is generally subdivided according to the clinical ECF volume status. A recent retrospective analysis found the relative distributions of the types of hypotonic hyponatremia in the intensive care setting to be 24% hypervolemic, 26% hypovolemic, and 50% euvolemic [15].

Box 1. Pathogenesis of hypoosmolar disorders

*Solute depletion (primary decreases in total body solute plus secondary water retention)**

1. Renal solute loss
   - Diuretic use
   - Solute diuresis (glucose, mannitol)
   - Salt-wasting nephropathy
   - Mineralocorticoid deficiency
2. Nonrenal solute loss
   - Gastrointestinal (diarrhea, vomiting, pancreatitis, bowel obstruction)
   - Cutaneous (sweating, burns)
   - Blood loss

*Solute dilution (primary increases in total body water plus secondary solute depletion)**

1. Impaired renal free water excretion
   - A. Increased proximal nephron reabsorption
     - Congestive heart failure
     - Cirrhosis
     - Nephrotic syndrome
     - Hypothyroidism
   - B. Impaired distal nephron dilution
     - Syndrome of inappropriate antidiuretic hormone secretion (SIADH)
     - Glucocorticoid deficiency
2. Excess water intake
   - Primary polydipsia

* Virtually all disorders of solute depletion are accompanied by some degree of secondary retention of water by the kidneys in response to the resulting intravascular hypovolemia. This mechanism can lead to hypoosmolality even when the solute depletion occurs via hypotonic or isotonic body fluid losses. Disorders of water retention can cause hypoosmolality in the absence of any solute losses, but, often, some secondary solute losses occur in response to the resulting intravascular hypervolemia, which can further aggravate the dilutional hypoosmolality.

Hypovolemic hypoosmolar hyponatremia

Simultaneous water and sodium loss results in ECF volume depletion, with secondary AVP secretion and decreased free water excretion. Retention of water from ingested or infused fluids can then lead to the development of hyponatremia. Primary solute depletion can occur via renal or extrarenal sodium losses, each of which can have multiple etiologies.

Extrarenal solute losses

Vomiting, diarrhea, hemorrhage, and excessive sweating all cause extrarenal losses of sodium and potassium, and the fluid loss that accompanies the solute losses is a potent stimulus to AVP secretion. Hyponatremia in hypovolemic shock secondary to volume loss (from hemorrhage or gastrointestinal free water losses) or distributive shock (secondary to sepsis in which there is a relative hypovolemia from vasodilatation) is characterized by a urine sodium concentration (U_{Na}) generally less than 10 mmol/L, reflecting appropriate nephron function to maximize sodium reabsorption and to conserve body solute and ECF volume.

Renal solute losses

Diuretics, mineralocorticoid deficiency, and nephropathies are all important etiologies of renal sodium loss that can lead to the development of hypovolemic hyponatremia. In patients on diuretics, hypokalemia from kaliuresis can worsen hyponatremia by causing a net movement of sodium intracellularly. Thiazides are more commonly associated with severe hyponatremia than are loop diuretics such as furosemide [18]. Renal solute loss is characterized by high urine sodium excretion, typically $U_{Na} > 20$ mmol/L, despite the existence of degrees of volume depletion that would normally activate mechanisms causing renal sodium conservation.

Patients with mineralocorticoid deficiency from primary adrenal insufficiency, or Addison's disease, can present in the critical care setting with new onset adrenal insufficiency or following a period of inadequate steroid replacement and are typically profoundly volume depleted. Aldosterone secreted from the adrenal zona glomerulosa acts at the distal collecting duct to stimulate sodium reabsorption and hydrogen ion and potassium secretion. Conversely, aldosterone deficiency leads to excessive urinary sodium loss, intravascular volume depletion, and a decreased glomeruler filtration rate (GFR), which, in turn, stimulates baroreceptor-mediated AVP secretion and reduced water clearance with secondary water retention and hyponatremia [19].

A unique form of hyponatremia due to primary renal sodium losses sometimes seen in critically ill patients with neurologic lesions is cerebral salt wasting. This syndrome occurs following head injury or neurosurgical procedures. The initiating event is loss of sodium in the urine, which results in a decrease in intravascular volume leading to water retention and hyponatremia because of a hypovolemic stimulus to AVP secretion. Superficially, cerebral salt wasting resembles syndrome of inappropriate antidiuretic hormone secretion (SIADH); both are hyponatremic disorders often seen after head injury with relatively high urine sodium excretion rates and urine osmolality along with plasma AVP levels that are inappropriately high in relation to serum osmolality. In patients who have cerebral salt wasting, the increase in AVP is secondary to volume depletion, whereas a high AVP level is the primary etiologic event in patients with SIADH, who are euvolemic or have a modest increase in plasma volume from water retention. The relative distribution of cerebral salt wasting and SIADH among hyponatremic neurosurgery patients is unknown, and the etiology of cerebral salt wasting has not been definitively established. Abnormal sympathetic outflow to the kidney with a pressure natriuresis as well as abnormal secretion of atrial or brain natriuretic peptide have been proposed as potential causes [20,21]. Differentiation of cerebral salt wasting from SIADH hinges upon establishing that a period of urinary sodium loss and volume depletion preceded the development of hyponatremia. Because infusion of isotonic NaCl into a euvolemic patient with SIADH results in a rapid excretion of the salt and fluid load to maintain body fluid homeostasis, a high urine sodium concentration and urine flow rate alone do not establish that cerebral salt wasting is present. The patient's vital signs, weight, and input/output records should be reviewed carefully to determine what the patient's volume status and net fluid balance were just before and during the development of hyponatremia, and current physical findings and hemodynamic measures should also be taken into account [22].

In the critical care setting, depletional hyponatremia from decreased sodium ingestion rather than increased sodium loss can occur in patients on chronic enteral feedings because many tube feed preparations are relatively low in sodium content [23]. Elderly patients are at greater risk for hypovolemic hyponatremia from a variety of causes than are younger individuals [24].

Euvolemic hypoosmolar hyponatremia

Virtually any disease state causing hypoosmolality can present with what appears to be a normal hydration status based on the usual methods of ECF volume assessment. Clinical evaluation of volume status is not sensitive, whereas laboratory measures such as normal or low blood urea nitrogen (BUN) and uric acid concentrations and an elevated U_{Na} are useful correlates of normal ECF volume [4,25]. Many different disease states can present with euvolemic hyponatremia, and the largest subgroup of patients has presented with hypoosmolar hyponatremia in multiple studies over many years [1,15,26].

Syndrome of inappropriate antidiuretic hormone secretion

SIADH is the most common cause of euvolemic hyponatremia in critical illness. It is essential to recognize that hypoosmolality does not always imply that AVP secretion is inappropriate, especially in the hypovolemic patient. Diagnostic criteria for SIADH remain as defined in 1967 by Bartter and Schwartz (Box 2) [27]. First, ECF hypoosmolality must be present, and hyponatremia secondary to pseudohyponatremia or hyperglycemia must be excluded. Second, urinary osmolality must be greater than maximally dilute urine (ie, >100 mOsm/kg H_2O); however, urine osmolality must only be inappropriate at some plasma osmolality (ie, <275 mOsm/kg H_2O) and not for all levels of plasma osmolality, as is frequently found in patients with the *reset osmostat* variant of SIADH [28]. Third, clinical euvolemia must

Box 2. Criteria for the diagnosis of syndrome of inappropriate antidiuretic hormone secretion

Essential

1. Decreased effective osmolality of the extracellular fluid (P_{osm} <275 mOsm/kg H_2O)
2. Inappropriate urinary concentration (U_{osm} >100 mOsm/kg H_2O with normal renal function) at some level of hypoosmolality
3. Clinical euvolemia, as defined by the absence of signs of hypovolemia (orthostasis, tachycardia, decreased skin turgor, dry mucous membranes) or hypervolemia (subcutaneous edema, ascites)
4. Elevated urinary sodium excretion while on a normal salt and water intake
5. Absence of other potential causes of euvolemic hypoosmolality: hypothyroidism, hypocortisolism (Addison's disease or pituitary corticotropin [ACTH] insufficiency) and diuretic use

Supplemental

6. Abnormal water load test (inability to excrete at least 80% of a 20 mL/kg water load in 4 hours or failure to dilute U_{osm} to less than 100 mOsm/kg H_2O)
7. Plasma AVP level inappropriately elevated relative to plasma osmolality
8. No significant correction of plasma [Na^+] with volume expansion but improvement after fluid restriction

be present, because hypo- and hypervolemic states imply other etiologies of hyponatremia, as described elsewhere in this article. A patient with SIADH may experience hyper- or hypovolemia for other reasons, but a diagnosis of SIADH cannot be made until euvolemia is restored. An increased U_{Na} (> 30 mmol/L [25]) is the fourth essential criterion, but patients with SIADH can have low U_{Na} if hypovolemia or solute depletion is present. Although increased natriuresis is primarily a manifestation of free water retention [29], there may also be co-existing true sodium depletion secondarily [30]. SIADH is a diagnosis of exclusion and can only be made in the setting of normal renal, thyroid, and adrenal function. Because as many as 20% of patients who meet these criteria for SIADH do not have elevated AVP levels [31], some have proposed renaming this entity the syndrome of inappropriate antidiuresis (SIAD) [32].

It is always important to diagnose the underlying etiology of SIADH, because successful long-term correction of hyponatremia will also require treating the underlying disorder. The most common causes of SIADH in the critical care setting can be divided into five main categories: pulmonary disease, central nervous system disease, drug induced, tumors, and other etiologies (Box 3) [4]. Pulmonary infections common in the critical care setting, such as viral, bacterial, and tuberculous pneumonia, aspergillosis, and empyema can all cause hyponatremia, as can noninfectious pulmonary diseases such as asthma, atelectasis, pneumothorax, and acute respiratory failure. Some bacterial infections seem to be associated with a higher incidence of hyponatremia, particularly Legionella pneumonia [33,34]. Animal and human studies have demonstrated that hypoxia impairs free water diuresis via increased AVP secretion in the absence of decreased cardiac output, mean arterial pressure, or GFR [35]. Evidence suggests that hypercapnia also impairs free water excretion independent of the effect from hypoxia. In one prospective study of ventilated patients in the intensive care unit, plasma AVP levels were significantly elevated in hypercapneic patients ($PaCO_2$ >45 mmHg) in comparison with the nonhypercapneic state [36].

Glucocorticoid deficiency

Secondary adrenal insufficiency, or hypopituitarism, can also lead to hyponatremia but via a different mechanism than primary adrenal insufficiency. Secondary adrenal insufficiency causes a solute dilution via an increase in total body water rather than the solute depletion that characterizes primary adrenal insufficiency. The glucocorticoid deficiency that defines secondary adrenal insufficiency causes impaired free water clearance through AVP-dependent and AVP-independent mechanisms [37]. Because the main regulator of aldosterone secretion is the RAAS and not ACTH secretion by the pituitary, hyponatremia is not a result of renal salt wasting from mineralocorticoid deficiency in either secondary adrenal insufficiency or relative adrenal insufficiency in septic shock. Nevertheless, glucocorticoid deficiency can result in a clinical presentation almost identical to SIADH, because there is loss of hypoosmolar inhibition of osmoreceptor-mediated AVP release resulting in persistent nonosmotic AVP secretion [38]. This effect is further exacerbated in acute glucocorticoid deficiency by concomitant nausea, hypotension, and a decreased GFR that all further decrease free water clearance [39] and is particularly more marked in elderly patients [40]. With chronic glucocorticoid deficiency, impaired free water excretion also results from AVP-independent decreased cardiac output and renal perfusion, reducing volume delivery to the distal diluting tubules of the nephron [41].

Hypothyroidism

Hyponatremia can develop in hypothyroidism and in particular myxedematous states, although the mechanism by which hypothyroidism induces hyponatremia is not entirely understood. Patients with primary hypothyroidism have impaired free water excretion, which can be reversed by thyroid hormone replacement. It is well known that hypothyroidism is associated with low cardiac output, bradycardia, decreased cardiac contractility,

Box 3. Common etiologies of syndrome of inappropriate antidiuretic hormone secretion

Tumors

Pulmonary/mediastinal (bronchogenic carcinoma, mesothelioma, thymoma)

Nonchest (duodenal carcinoma, pancreatic carcinoma, ureteral/ prostate carcinoma, uterine carcinoma, nasopharyngeal carcinoma, leukemia)

Central nervous system disorders

Mass lesions (tumors, brain abscesses, subdural hematoma)

Inflammatory diseases (encephalitis, meningitis, systemic lupus, acute intermittent porphyria, multiple sclerosis)

Degenerative/demyelinative diseases (Guillan-Barré, spinal cord lesions)

Miscellaneous (subarachnoid hemorrhage, head trauma, acute psychosis, delirium tremens, pituitary stalk section, transphenoidal adenomectomy, hydrocephalus)

Drug induced

Stimulated AVP release (nicotine, phenothiazines, tricyclics)

Direct renal effects or potentiation of AVP antidiuretic effects (desmopressin [DDAVP], oxytocin, prostaglandin synthesis inhibitors)

Mixed or uncertain actions (angiotensin-converting enzyme [ACE] inhibitors, carbamazepine and oxcarbazepine, chlorpropamide, clofibrate, clozapine, cyclophosphamide, 3,4-methylenedioxymethamphetamine [Ecstasy], omeprazole, serotonin reuptake inhibitors, vincristine)

Pulmonary diseases

Infections (tuberculosis, acute bacterial and viral pneumonia, aspergillosis, empyema)

Mechanical/ventilatory (acute respiratory failure, chronic obstructive pulmonary disease, positive pressure ventilation)

Other

Acquired immunodeficiency syndrome and AIDS-related complex

Prolonged strenuous exercise (marathon, triathalon, ultramarathon, hot-weather hiking)

Senile atrophy

Idiopathic

and reduced ventricular filling [42–44]. Low cardiac output stimulates baroreceptor-mediated activation of AVP secretion. It has been postulated that AVP secretion is inappropriately high in severe hypothyroidism causing free water retention [45], but recent studies have demonstrated that hyponatremia is more likely to be mediated by AVP-independent mechanisms. In a series of patients with untreated myxedema due to primary hypothyroidism, all of whom underwent hypertonic saline infusion and a subpopulation who subsequently underwent water loading, there was a significantly lower basal plasma AVP level in the study group (0.5 ± 0.1 pmol/L) when compared with normal controls (2.5 ± 0.5 pmol/L). In addition, the subsequent rise in plasma AVP levels following hypertonic saline infusion was not exaggerated in any patients and was reported to be normal or even below normal in all patients. Plasma AVP was appropriately suppressed in the hyponatremic myxedema patients who demonstrated a degree of impaired urinary dilution during water loading, providing convincing evidence that decreased free water excretion in myxedema is not due to inappropriate plasma AVP elevation [46].

Severe hypothyroidism is also associated with decreased renal function and GFR. A study of patients with severe iatrogenic hypothyroidism demonstrated that approximately 90% had a significantly greater creatinine value in the hypothyroid as compared with the prior euthyroid state. Moreover, once thyroid hormone replacement was given and thyroid function normalized, creatinine values returned to their baseline euthyroid levels before the iatrogenically induced hypothyroid state [47]. Based on this combined evidence, the major cause of impaired water excretion in hypothyroidism appears to be an alteration in renal perfusion and GFR secondary to systemic effects of thyroid hormone deficiency on cardiac output and peripheral vascular resistance [48–50].

Hypervolemic hypoosmolar hyponatremia

In hypervolemic hyponatremia, there is an excess in total body water and total body sodium, resulting in clinically evident edema or ascites; however, in many cases, the increase in total body water is out of proportion to that of total body sodium, causing hyponatremia. Congestive heart failure, cirrhosis, and nephrotic syndrome all share this common pathophysiology, although the specific mechanisms vary among these different disease states.

Congestive heart failure

Although clearly a condition of total body ECF overload, the decreased cardiac output in congestive heart failure causes a perceived intra-arteriolar volume depletion, best described as a decrease in the effective arterial blood volume at the level of the carotid artery and the renal afferent arteriole baroreceptors [51,52]. Decreased renal perfusion activates the RAAS and the sympathetic nervous system, resulting in increased sodium reabsorption and secondary free water reabsorption [53]. Decreased renal perfusion and subsequent increased baroreceptor firing activate non-osmotic AVP secretion, resulting in increased free water reabsorption. The goal of these physiologic mechanisms is to restore normal renal perfusion in a perceived state of intra-arteriolar volume depletion, but the net effect is to further exacerbate hypervolemia and progressive hyponatremia in patients with congestive heart failure.

In a study of over 200 patients with severe congestive heart failure, those who were also hyponatremic were found to have a shorter median survival (164 versus 373 days). These patients were found to have elevated plasma renin activity, and there was a significant mortality benefit to treating this subgroup of patients with ACE inhibitors [54]. In addition, hyponatremia during the early phase of acute myocardial infarction has been found to predict long-term mortality independently of left ventricular ejection fraction and other accepted predictors of cardiac outcomes [55].

Cirrhosis

Once ascites develops as a sequelae of chronic liver disease, approximately 30% of affected patients will manifest hyponatremia (serum [Na^+] <130 mmol/L) [56]. Similar to the findings in congestive heart failure, there is impaired free water excretion in cirrhosis owing to non-osmotic release of AVP [57], but, in contrast to congestive heart failure, cirrhosis is characterized by a high cardiac output. Gastrointestinal endotoxin, which is less efficiently cleared due to portal-systemic shunting, stimulates nitric oxide production and vasodilatation [58]. Arterial dilatation, particularly in the splanchnic vasculature, leads to arterial underfilling and non-osmotic secretion of AVP [51,52]. Following disease progression with splanchnic vasodilatation, decreased mean arterial pressure and reduced renal perfusion can lead to the hepatorenal syndrome [59]. The increase in AVP secretion and water retention is proportional to the severity of cirrhosis, such that the extent of hyponatremia reflects hepatic disease progression with a serum [Na^+] less than 125 mmol/L, often indicative of end-stage disease [60]. In addition, the diuretic therapy that is commonly used to treat ascites often worsens hyponatremia by decreasing intravascular volume and renal perfusion, which increase AVP levels and further compromises the kidney's ability to excrete free water [61].

Advanced renal failure

Patients with mild-to-moderate renal dysfunction are generally able to excrete sufficient free water to maintain a normal serum [Na^+], whereas patients who have end-stage renal disease have impaired urinary dilution and free water excretion such that the minimum urine osmolality increases to 200 to 250 mOsm/kg H_2O, even though AVP secretion is appropriately suppressed. As a result, patients with advanced renal disease typically manifest hyponatremia owing to abnormal water retention.

Treatment of hyponatremia

The symptom severity of hyponatremia depends in large part upon the rapidity of the decrease in serum [Na^+]. Most patients are not symptomatic until the serum [Na^+] decreases to less than 125 mmol/L [62]. Symptoms are predominantly neurologic, including nausea, vomiting, headache, fatigue, irritability, and disorientation. Severe hyponatremia can progress to seizures, brainstem herniation, and death. The initial evaluation of patients in the critical care setting with hyponatremia includes a thorough history and physical examination, with particularly careful evaluation of ECF volume status including an assessment of orthostatic blood pressure and pulse. Initial laboratory evaluation should include serum electrolytes, glucose, an evaluation of renal function with BUN, creatinine, and uric acid, serum osmolality, and urine osmolality and sodium. Treatment of hyponatremia must strike a balance between the risks of the hyponatremia and the risks of correction. The magnitude of these risks depends on the degree of brain volume regulation that has transpired as a result of intracranial fluid and solute shifts [37]. The treatment of some hyponatremia-associated disease states involves treating the underlying etiology, such as steroids for adrenal insufficiency and thyroid hormone for hypothyroidism. In most cases, the appropriate treatment of hyponatremia relies on the identification of the underlying ECF volume status, the acuity with which the hyponatremia developed, and the severity of neurologic symptoms present (Fig. 1) [4].

Severe acute symptomatic hyponatremia

Acute hyponatremia (defined as <48 hours duration) with very low sodium values (<110–115 mmol/L) with seizures or coma is a medical emergency. The risk for neurologic complications is high, because cerebral edema can evolve quickly as a result of osmotic movement of water into the brain. In patients with severe acute hyponatremia, hypertonic (3%) NaCl should be infused at a rate to increase serum [Na^+] approximately 1 to 2 mmol/L/h until a less hyponatremic serum [Na^+] (ie, 125–130 mmol/L) has been achieved. In comatose or seizing patients, a faster rate of sodium correction of 3–5 mmol/L/h for a short period of time (ie, 1–2 hours) may be warranted to avoid imminent brainstem herniation [63].

In hypovolemic states, including the majority of patients with a U_{Na} less than 30 mmol/L, fluid resuscitation with isotonic NaCl with or without potassium is appropriate with a goal serum [Na^+] increase of 0.5 mmol/L/h. Accumulated evidence in experimental animals and humans confirms that a slower rate of serum [Na^+] correction minimizes the risk for central pontine myelinolysis [64]. The serum [Na^+] should be measured every 2 to 4 hours during acute corrections of hyponatremia to ensure that the increase in serum [Na^+] is proceeding at the desired rate. Young premenopausal women appear to be at greater risk for neurologic sequelae from hyponatremia, with 75% of cases of brain damage occurring in this subpopulation in some studies [65].

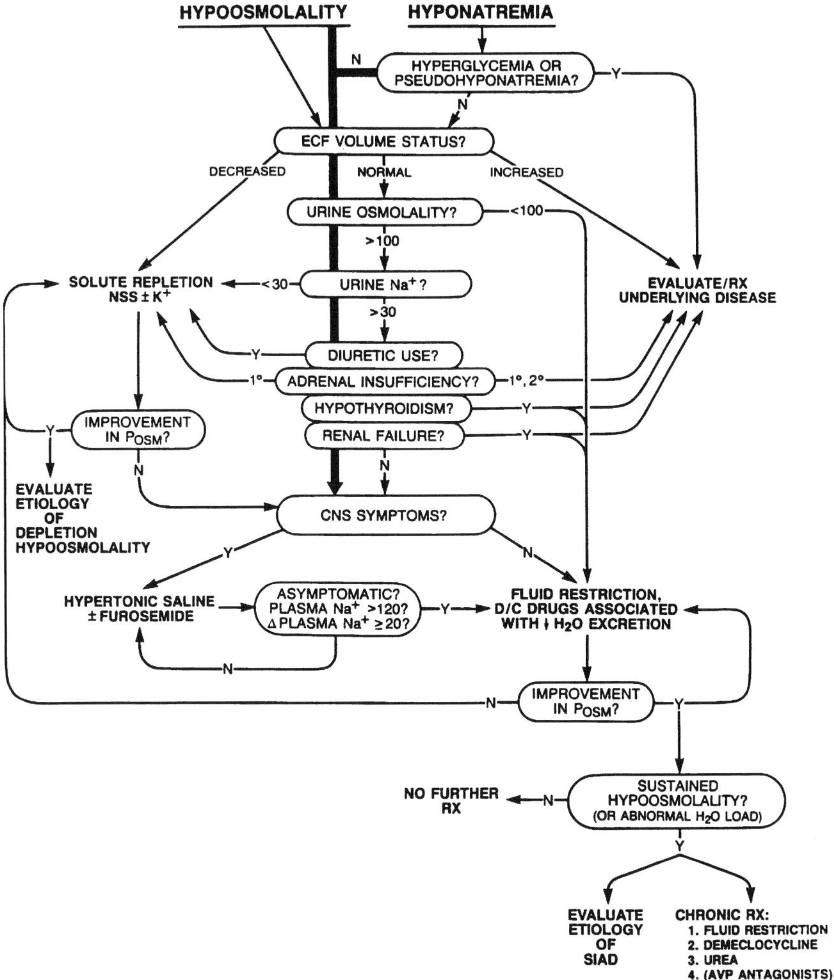

Fig. 1. Schematic summary of the evaluation of hypoosmolar patients. The dark arrow in the center emphasizes that the presence of central nervous system dysfunction due to hyponatremia should always be assessed immediately so that appropriate therapy can be started as soon as possible in symptomatic patients while the outlined diagnostic evaluation is proceeding. d/c, discontinue; ECF, extracellular fluid volume; N, no; NSS, normal (isotonic) saline; P_{osm}, plasma osmolality; Rx, treat; SIADH, syndrome of inappropriate antidiuretic hormone secretion; Y, yes; 1°, primary; 2°, secondary. The numbers referring to osmolality are in mOsm/kg H_2O; the numbers referring to Na^+ concentration are in mmol/L. (*Adapted from* Verbalis JG. SIADH and other hypoosmolar disorders. In: Schrier RW, editor. Diseases of the kidney and urinary tract. 7th edition. Philadelphia: Lippincott Williams & Wilkins; 2001. p. 2534; with permission.)

Treatment of hyponatremia in hypervolemic states includes free water restriction, diuresis with loop diuretics, and ACE inhibitors. Current clinical trials are underway investigating the use of AVP V_2 receptor antagonists for the treatment of euvolemic and hypervolemic hyponatremia.

Severe chronic symptomatic hyponatremia

In SIADH, fluid restriction is the mainstay of serum [Na^+] correction, with the goal of maintaining fluid intake 500 mL/d below urine output; however, this degree of fluid restriction is difficult to maintain in an intensive care setting where obligate fluid intakes for various therapies and parenteral nutrition often exceed this level. Furthermore, fluid restriction is not recommended to correct serum [Na^+] in hyponatremic patients with subarachnoid hemorrhage, because this patient subgroup has an increased risk for cerebral infarction that has been shown to be worsened by fluid restriction and lowered blood pressure [66].

Other current therapies for chronic hyponatremia include demeclocycline (600–1200 mg/d), furosemide (20–40 mg/d), NaCl tablets (3–18 g/d), and urea (30 g/d). Although these therapies are effective in some cases, in general they are suboptimal, and some patients, especially those with edema-forming states such as congestive heart failure and cirrhosis, are unable to tolerate the solute loads associated with many of these treatments. AVP receptor antagonists are a novel therapeutic class shown to be effective at preventing AVP-induced AQP2 membrane insertion in the renal collecting duct, causing the excretion of solute-free water, which has been termed *aquaresis* [67]. There are currently four nonpeptide agents in various stages of clinical trials, and the US Food and Drug Administration recently approved the use of conivaptan, the only combined AVP V1aR and V2R antagonist, for the treatment of euvolemic hyponatremia. Conivaptan is given as a 20-mg intravenous loading dose over 30 minutes followed by 20 to 40 mg as a continuous infusion over 24 hours for maximum of 4 days. Multiple studies have demonstrated that AVP V_2R receptor antagonists increase serum [Na^+] by inducing an aquaresis at a dose-dependent rate in patients with euvolemic and hypervolemic hyponatremia [68,69]. Clinical trials have documented that these agents are generally well tolerated and show great promise for the treatment of euvolemic and hypervolemic hyponatremia [68,69].

Hypernatremia

Similar to hyponatremia, hypernatremia can be induced by several illnesses in the critical care setting. Hypernatremia is generally categorized according to the causal factors involved: hypervolemic, hypodipsic, and increased free water losses (Box 4) [4].

Box 4. Pathogenesis of hyperosmolar disorders

Water depletion (decreases in total body water in excess of body solute)

1. Insufficient water intake
   - Unavailability of water
   - Hypodipsia (osmoreceptor dysfunction, age)
   - Neurologic deficits (cognitive dysfunction, motor impairments)
2. Hypotonic fluid loss*
   - A. Renal: diabetes insipidus
     - Insufficient AVP secretion (central diabetes insipidus, osmoreceptor dysfunction)
     - Insufficient AVP effect (nephrogenic diabetes insipidus)
   - B. Renal: other fluid loss
     - Osmotic diuresis (hyperglycemia, mannitol)
     - Diuretic drugs (furosemide, ethacrynic acid, thiazides)
     - Postobstructive diuresis
     - Diuretic phase of acute tubular necrosis
   - C. Nonrenal fluid loss
     - Gastrointestinal (vomiting, diarrhea, nasogastric suction)
     - Cutaneous (sweating, burns)
     - Pulmonary (hyperventilation)
     - Peritoneal dialysis

Solute excess (increases in total body solute in excess of body water)

1. Sodium
   - Excess [Na^+] administration (NaCl, $NaHCO_3$)
   - Sea water drowning
2. Other
   - Hyperalimentation (intravenous, parenteral)

* Most hypotonic fluid losses will not produce hyperosmolality unless insufficient free water is ingested or infused to replace the ongoing losses; therefore, these disorders also usually involve some component of insufficient water intake.

Hypervolemic hypernatremia

Hypervolemic hypernatremia can result from the infusion of hypertonic fluids (ie, $NaHCO_3$ or total parenteral nutrition) or from enteral feedings with inadequate free water administration.

Hypodipsic hypernatremia

Decreased water intake, or hypodipsia, probably represents the leading cause of hyperosmolality encountered in intensive care settings. This etiology is particularly prevalent among the elderly [70] or patients who have altered mental status who do not respond appropriately to physiologic stimuli that signal increased thirst.

Hypernatremia from increased water losses

A variety of diseases can cause increased free water losses in the critical care setting, including gastrointestinal water losses, intrinsic renal disease, hypercalcemia, hypokalemia, and solute diuresis, but the most common cause is hyperglycemia and glucosuria. Although these etiologies represent the most frequent causes of hypernatremia with critical illnesses, they must be differentiated from diabetes insipidus, which represents the quintessential clinical cause of hypernatremia. Generally, a urine osmolality less than 800 mOsm/kg H_2O in the setting of elevated serum osmolality is indicative of a renal concentrating defect. In the absence of glucosuria or other causes of osmotic diuresis, this generally reflects the presence of diabetes insipidus [4]. Diabetes insipidus is generally subdivided into central and nephrogenic disease.

Central diabetes insipidus

Central diabetes insipidus is caused by a deficiency of AVP secretion from the posterior pituitary but does not become fully manifest until more than 85% of the magnocellular AVP-secreting neurons are damaged [71]. Central diabetes insipidus is rare, with a prevalence of 1:25,000. Most cases (40% to 50%) are secondary to a hypothalamic lesion, such as a tumor, or infiltrative diseases such as sarcoidosis and histiocytosis. Approximately 20% to 30% of central diabetes insipidus is categorized as idiopathic, but most of these patients most likely have underlying autoimmune disease. Lymphocytic infundibuloneurohypophysitis is the foremost cause of spontaneous diabetes insipidus without prior head trauma or neurosurgery, potentially accounting for as many as 50% of all cases [72,73]. A small fraction of cases (5%) are genetic, often with a delayed onset. Sellar lesions and pituitary adenomas are not a common cause of diabetes insipidus, because, over time, the secretion of AVP from magnocellular neurons can shift to regions higher in the hypothalamus [5]. Because these lesions are typically slow growing, if a sellar lesion is detected in the setting of new-onset diabetes insipidus, this suggests the presence of a rapidly enlarging sellar mass such as metastatic disease. The absence of the posterior pituitary bright spot on saggital views of precontrast MR imaging can be useful to verify the presence of central diabetes insipidus with two important caveats: (1) there is an age-associated loss of the posterior pituitary bright spot in the absence of diabetes insipidus, and (2) the posterior pituitary bright spot may still be apparent in a patient with central diabetes insipidus secondary to the persistence of oxytocin, which is also stored in the posterior pituitary [5].

Nephrogenic diabetes insipidus

Nephrogenic diabetes insipidus is caused by end-organ resistance of the kidney to the antidiuretic effects of AVP. Whereas familial or hereditary nephrogenic diabetes insipidus is secondary to mutations of the AVP V_2 receptor or the AQP2 water channel, acquired nephrogenic diabetes insipidus is caused by hypercalcemia (serum [Ca^{++}] >13 mg/dL), hypokalemia (serum [K^+] <2.5 mmol/L), or medications such as lithium and demeclocycline. A plasma AVP level is useful to distinguish central diabetes insipidus from nephrogenic diabetes insipidus; however, to differentiate definitively nephrogenic diabetes insipidus from central diabetes insipidus and from normal individuals with primary polydipsia, performance of a water deprivation test is often necessary (Box 5) [4].

Treatment of hypernatremia

Treatment goals of hypernatremia include correcting the established water deficit and reducing ongoing excessive urine water losses. Patients in the intensive care setting are typically unable to drink in response to thirst, and progressive hypertonicity from untreated diabetes insipidus can be associated with grave consequences unless appropriately treated. The following formula is used to estimate the pre-existing water defecit [74]:

$$\begin{aligned}\text{Water deficit} = {} & 0.6 \times \text{premorbid weight} \\ & \times \left[1 - 140/\left(\text{serum}\left[Na^+\right]\ \text{mmol/L}\right)\right]\end{aligned}$$

This formula assumes that total body water is 60% of body weight, that no body solute is lost as hypertonicity developed, and that the premorbid serum [Na^+] is 140 mmol/L, but the formula does not take ongoing water losses into account. The serum [Na^+] should be lowered to approximately 330 mOsm/kg H_2O within the first 24 hours of correction to reduce the risk of exposure to the central nervous system of ongoing hypertonicity.

The treatment of central diabetes insipidus with DDAVP is an effective means of improving polyuria and hypernatremia. Initial doses in the acute setting are 1 to 2 μg (intravenous, intramuscular, or subcutaneous). If hypernatremia is present, free water should also be given in an effort to correct serum sodium, with 5% dextrose in water as the preferred intravenous replacement fluid. DDAVP is preferred over AVP, because the former has a longer duration of action, avoids the vasopressor effects of AVP at V_{1a} receptors, and is available in intranasal and oral preparations. Although some cases of nephrogenic diabetes insipidus respond to large doses of DDAVP, traditionally, nephrogenic diabetes insipidus is treated with sodium restriction and thiazide diuretics (any drug in this class may be used with equal

Box 5. Water deprivation test

Procedure

Initiation of the deprivation period depends on the severity of the diabetes insipidus. In routine cases, the patient should be given nothing by mouth after dinner. In cases with more severe polyuria and polydipsia, this may be too long a period without fluids, and the water deprivation should be begun early in the morning of the test (eg, 6 AM).

The test should be stopped when body weight decreases by 3%, the patient has orthostatic blood pressure changes, the urine osmolality reaches a plateau (ie, less than 10% change over three consecutive measurements), or the serum sodium is greater than 145 mmol/L.

Obtain a plasma AVP level at the end of the test when the plasma osmolality is elevated, preferably above 300 mOsm/kg H_2O.

If the serum sodium concentration is less than 146 mmol/L or the plasma osmolality is less than 300 mOsm/kg H_2O, infuse hypertonic saline (3% NaCl at a rate of 0.1 mL/kg/min for 1–2 h) to reach these endpoints.

Administer AVP (5 U) or DDAVP (1 μg) subcutaneously and continue following urine osmolality and volume for an additional 2 hours.

Interpretation

An unequivocal urine concentration after AVP/DDAVP (>50% increase) indicates neurogenic diabetes insipidus, and an unequivocal absence of urine concentration (<10%) strongly suggests nephrogenic diabetes insipidus or primary polydipsia.

Differentiating between nephrogenic diabetes insipidus and primary polydipsia as well as for cases in which the increase in urine osmolality after AVP administration is more equivocal (eg, 10% to 50%) is best done using the plasma AVP levels obtained at the end of the dehydration period or hypertonic saline infusion and the relation between plasma AVP levels and urine osmolality under basal conditions.

potential for benefit), which block sodium absorption and act to decrease renal diluting capacity and free water clearance. Prostaglandins increase renal blood flow and decrease medullary solute concentration, resulting in a small decrease in the interstitial gradient for water reabsorption. Drugs such as prostaglandin synthase inhibitors promote water reabsorption and impair urinary dilution, reducing free water clearance and urine output. These agents are helpful as adjunctive therapies in the treatment of nephrogenic diabetes insipidus.

Summary

Disorders of sodium and water metabolism are commonly encountered in the intensive care setting predominantly owing to the large number of varied disease states that can disrupt the balanced mechanisms that control the intake and output of water and solute. Disorders of body water homeostasis can be divided into hypoosmolar disorders, in which there is an excess of body water relative to body solute, and hyperosmolar disorders, in which there is a deficit of body water relative to body solute. Prompt identification and appropriate treatment of these disturbances are important to prevent the increased morbidity and mortality that accompany disorders of body fluid homeostasis in patients in critical care settings.

References

[1] Anderson RJ, Chung HM, Kluge R, et al. Hyponatremia: a prospective analysis of its epidemiology and the pathogenetic role of vasopressin. Ann Intern Med 1985;102:164–8.
[2] Subramanian S, Ziedalski TM. Oliguria, volume overload, Na^+ balance, and diuretics. Crit Care Clin 2005;21:291–303.
[3] Upadhyay A, Jaber BL, Madias NE. Incidence and prevalence of hyponatremia. Am J Med 2006;119:S30–5.
[4] Verbalis JG. Disorders of body water homeostasis. Best Pract Res Clin Endocrinol Metab 2003;17:471–503.
[5] Robinson AG, Verbalis JG. The posterior pituitary. In: Larsen PR, Kronenberg HM, Melmed S, et al, editors. Williams textbook of endocrinology. 10th edition. Philadelphia: WB Saunders; 2003. p. 281–329.
[6] Knepper MA. Molecular physiology of urinary concentrating mechanism: regulation of aquaporin water channels by vasopressin. Am J Physiol 1997;272:F3–12.
[7] Knepper MA. Long-term regulation of urinary concentrating capacity. Am J Physiol 1998; 275:F332–3.
[8] Baylis PH. Regulation of vasopressin secretion. Baillieres Clin Endocrinol Metab 1989;3: 313–30.
[9] Sklar AH, Schrier RW. Central nervous system mediators of vasopressin release. Physiol Rev 1983;63:1243–80.
[10] Sladek CD. Regulation of vasopressin release by neurotransmitters, neuropeptides and osmotic stimuli. Prog Brain Res 1983;60:71–90.
[11] Holmes CL, Patel BM, Russell JA, et al. Physiology of vasopressin relevant to management of septic shock. Chest 2001;120:989–1002.
[12] Leng G, Brown CH, Russell JA. Physiological pathways regulating the activity of magnocellular neurosecretory cells. Prog Neurobiol 1999;57:625–55.
[13] Boscoe A, Paramore C, Verbalis JG. Cost of illness of hyponatremia in the United States. Cost Eff Resour Alloc 2006;4:10.
[14] DeVita MV, Gardenswartz MH, Konecky A, et al. Incidence and etiology of hyponatremia in an intensive care unit. Clin Nephrol 1990;34:163–6.
[15] Bennani SL, Abouqal R, Zeggwagh AA, et al. Incidence, causes and prognostic factors of hyponatremia in intensive care. Rev Med Interne 2003;24:224–9.

[16] Fried LF, Palevsky PM. Hyponatremia and hypernatremia. Med Clin North Am 1997;81: 585–609.

[17] Hillier TA, Abbott RD, Barrett EJ. Hyponatremia: evaluating the correction factor for hyperglycemia. Am J Med 1999;106:399–403.

[18] Spital A. Diuretic-induced hyponatremia. Am J Nephrol 1999;19:447–52.

[19] Vachharajani TJ, Zaman F, Abreo KD. Hyponatremia in critically ill patients. J Intensive Care Med 2003;18:3–8.

[20] Damaraju SC, Rajshekhar V, Chandy MJ. Validation study of a central venous pressure-based protocol for the management of neurosurgical patients with hyponatremia and natriuresis. Neurosurgery 1997;40:312–6 [discussion: 316–7].

[21] Palmer BF. Hyponatraemia in a neurosurgical patient: syndrome of inappropriate antidiuretic hormone secretion versus cerebral salt wasting. Nephrol Dial Transplant 2000;15: 262–8.

[22] Palmer BF. Hyponatremia in patients with central nervous system disease: SIADH versus CSW. Trends Endocrinol Metab 2003;14:182–7.

[23] Rudman D, Racette D, Rudman IW, et al. Hyponatremia in tube-fed elderly men. J Chronic Dis 1986;39:73–80.

[24] Hodak SP, Verbalis JG. Abnormalities of water homeostasis in aging. Endocrinol Metab Clin North Am 2005;34:1031–46.

[25] Chung HM, Kluge R, Schrier RW, et al. Clinical assessment of extracellular fluid volume in hyponatremia. Am J Med 1987;83:905–8.

[26] Gross PA, Pehrisch H, Rascher W, et al. Pathogenesis of clinical hyponatremia: observations of vasopressin and fluid intake in 100 hyponatremic medical patients. Eur J Clin Invest 1987; 17:123–9.

[27] Bartter FC, Schwartz WB. The syndrome of inappropriate secretion of antidiuretic hormone. Am J Med 1967;42:790–806.

[28] Michelis MF, Fusco RD, Bragdon RW, et al. Reset of osmoreceptors in association with normovolemic hyponatremia. Am J Med Sci 1974;267:267–73.

[29] Leaf A, Bartter FC, Santos RF, et al. Evidence in man that urinary electrolyte loss induced by pitressin is a function of water retention. J Clin Invest 1953;32:868–78.

[30] Verbalis JG. Whole-body volume regulation and escape from antidiuresis. Am J Med 2006; 119:S21–9.

[31] Zerbe R, Stropes L, Robertson G. Vasopressin function in the syndrome of inappropriate antidiuresis. Annu Rev Med 1980;31:315–27.

[32] Robertson GL, Aycinena P, Zerbe RL. Neurogenic disorders of osmoregulation. Am J Med 1982;72:339–53.

[33] Sabria M, Campins M. Legionnaires' disease: update on epidemiology and management options. Am J Respir Med 2003;2:235–43.

[34] Sopena N, Sabria-Leal M, Pedro-Botet ML, et al. Comparative study of the clinical presentation of Legionella pneumonia and other community-acquired pneumonias. Chest 1998; 113:1195–200.

[35] Anderson RJ, Pluss RG, Berns AS, et al. Mechanism of effect of hypoxia on renal water excretion. J Clin Invest 1978;62:769–77.

[36] Leach RM, Forsling ML. The effect of changes in arterial PCO2 on neuroendocrine function in man. Exp Physiol 2004;89:287–92.

[37] Verbalis JG. SIADH and other hypoosmolar disorders. In: Schrier RW, editor. Diseases of the kidney and urinary tract. 7th edition. Philadelphia: Lippincott Williams & Wilkins; 2001. p. 2511–48.

[38] Oelkers W. Hyponatremia and inappropriate secretion of vasopressin (antidiuretic hormone) in patients with hypopituitarism. N Engl J Med 1989;321:492–6.

[39] Kamoi K, Tamura T, Tanaka K, et al. Hyponatremia and osmoregulation of thirst and vasopressin secretion in patients with adrenal insufficiency. J Clin Endocrinol Metab 1993;77: 1584–8.

[40] Yatagai T, Kusaka I, Nakamura T, et al. Close association of severe hyponatremia with exaggerated release of arginine vasopressin in elderly subjects with secondary adrenal insufficiency. Eur J Endocrinol 2003;148:221–6.
[41] Ishikawa S, Schrier RW. Effect of arginine vasopressin antagonist on renal water excretion in glucocorticoid and mineralocorticoid deficient rats. Kidney Int 1982;22:587–93.
[42] Crowley WF Jr, Ridgway EC, Bough EW, et al. Noninvasive evaluation of cardiac function in hypothyroidism: response to gradual thyroxine replacement. N Engl J Med 1977;296:1–6.
[43] Klein I, Ojamaa K. Thyroid hormone and the cardiovascular system. N Engl J Med 2001; 344:501–9.
[44] Wieshammer S, Keck FS, Waitzinger J, et al. Acute hypothyroidism slows the rate of left ventricular diastolic relaxation. Can J Physiol Pharmacol 1989;67:1007–10.
[45] Skowsky WR, Kikuchi TA. The role of vasopressin in the impaired water excretion of myxedema. Am J Med 1978;64:613–21.
[46] Iwasaki Y, Oiso Y, Yamauchi K, et al. Osmoregulation of plasma vasopressin in myxedema. J Clin Endocrinol Metab 1990;70:534–9.
[47] Kreisman SH, Hennessey JV. Consistent reversible elevations of serum creatinine levels in severe hypothyroidism. Arch Intern Med 1999;159:79–82.
[48] Derubertis FR Jr, Michelis MF, Bloom ME, et al. Impaired water excretion in myxedema. Am J Med 1971;51:41–53.
[49] Hanna FW, Scanlon MF. Hyponatraemia, hypothyroidism, and role of arginine-vasopressin. Lancet 1997;350:755–6.
[50] Schmitz PH, de Meijer PH, Meinders AE. Hyponatremia due to hypothyroidism: a pure renal mechanism. Neth J Med 2001;58:143–9.
[51] Schrier RW. Pathogenesis of sodium and water retention in high-output and low-output cardiac failure, nephrotic syndrome, cirrhosis, and pregnancy (1). N Engl J Med 1988;319: 1065–72.
[52] Schrier RW. Pathogenesis of sodium and water retention in high-output and low-output cardiac failure, nephrotic syndrome, cirrhosis, and pregnancy (2). N Engl J Med 1988;319: 1127–34.
[53] Oren RM. Hyponatremia in congestive heart failure. Am J Cardiol 2005;95:2B–7B.
[54] Lee WH, Packer M. Prognostic importance of serum sodium concentration and its modification by converting-enzyme inhibition in patients with severe chronic heart failure. Circulation 1986;73:257–67.
[55] Goldberg A, Hammerman H, Petcherski S, et al. Hyponatremia and long-term mortality in survivors of acute ST-elevation myocardial infarction. Arch Intern Med 2006;166: 781–6.
[56] Arroyo V, Rodes J, Gutierrez-Lizarraga MA, et al. Prognostic value of spontaneous hyponatremia in cirrhosis with ascites. Am J Dig Dis 1976;21:249–56.
[57] Bichet D, Szatalowicz V, Chaimovitz C, et al. Role of vasopressin in abnormal water excretion in cirrhotic patients. Ann Intern Med 1982;96:413–7.
[58] Guarner C, Soriano G, Tomas A, et al. Increased serum nitrite and nitrate levels in patients with cirrhosis: relationship to endotoxemia. Hepatology 1993;18:1139–43.
[59] Fernandez-Seara J, Prieto J, Quiroga J, et al. Systemic and regional hemodynamics in patients with liver cirrhosis and ascites with and without functional renal failure. Gastroenterology 1989;97:1304–12.
[60] Papadakis MA, Fraser CL, Arieff AI. Hyponatraemia in patients with cirrhosis. Q J Med 1990;76:675–88.
[61] Sherlock S, Senewiratne B, Scott A, et al. Complications of diuretic therapy in hepatic cirrhosis. Lancet 1966;1:1049–52.
[62] Arieff AI, Llach F, Massry SG. Neurological manifestations and morbidity of hyponatremia: correlation with brain water and electrolytes. Medicine 1976;55:121–9.
[63] Gross P, Reimann D, Neidel J, et al. The treatment of severe hyponatremia. Kidney Int Suppl 1998;64:S6–11.

[64] Sterns RH, Riggs JE, Schochet SS Jr. Osmotic demyelination syndrome following correction of hyponatremia. N Engl J Med 1986;314:1535–42.
[65] Ayus JC, Wheeler JM, Arieff AI. Postoperative hyponatremic encephalopathy in menstruant women. Ann Intern Med 1992;117:891–7.
[66] Wijdicks EF, Vermeulen M, Hijdra A, et al. Hyponatremia and cerebral infarction in patients with ruptured intracranial aneurysms: is fluid restriction harmful? Ann Neurol 1985; 17:137–40.
[67] Verbalis JG. Vasopressin V2 receptor antagonists. J Mol Endocrinol 2002;29:1–9.
[68] Greenberg A, Verbalis JG. Vasopressin receptor antagonists. Kidney Int 2006;69:2124–30.
[69] Palm C, Pistrosch F, Herbrig K, et al. Vasopressin antagonists as aquaretic agents for the treatment of hyponatremia. Am J Med 2006;119:S87–92.
[70] Phillips PA, Rolls BJ, Ledingham JG, et al. Reduced thirst after water deprivation in healthy elderly men. N Engl J Med 1984;311:753–9.
[71] Heinbecker P, White HL. Hypothalamico-hypophyseal system and its relation to water balance in the dog. Am J Physiol 1941;133:582–93.
[72] Huang CH, Chou KJ, Lee PT, et al. A case of lymphocytic hypophysitis with masked diabetes insipidus unveiled by glucocorticoid replacement. Am J Kidney Dis 2005;45:197–200.
[73] Imura H, Nakao K, Shimatsu A, et al. Lymphocytic infundibuloneurohypophysitis as a cause of central diabetes insipidus. N Engl J Med 1993;329:683–9.
[74] Robinson AG, Verbalis JG. Diabetes insipidus. Curr Ther Endocrinol Metab 1997;6:1–7.

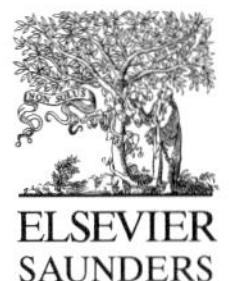

ELSEVIER
SAUNDERS

Endocrinol Metab Clin N Am
35 (2006) 895–913

ENDOCRINOLOGY
AND METABOLISM
CLINICS
OF NORTH AMERICA

Index

Note: Page numbers of article titles are in **boldface** type.

doi:10.1016/S0889-8529(06)00086-7

B

C

F

G

H

T

United States Postal Service

Statement of Ownership, Management, and Circulation

1. Publication Title: Endocrinology and Metabolism Clinics of North America
2. Publication Number: 0 0 0 - 2 7 5
3. Filing Date: 9/15/06
4. Issue Frequency: Mar, Jun, Sep, Dec
5. Number of Issues Published Annually: 4
6. Annual Subscription Price: $175.00
7. Complete Mailing Address of Known Office of Publication (*Not printer*) (*Street, city, county, state, and ZIP+4*)
   Elsevier, Inc.
   360 Park Avenue South
   New York, NY 10010-1710

   Contact Person: Sarah Carmichael
   Telephone: (215) 239-3681
8. Complete Mailing Address of Headquarters or General Business Office of Publisher (*Not printer*)
   Elsevier, Inc., 360 Park Avenue South, New York, NY 10010-1710
9. Full Names and Complete Mailing Addresses of Publisher, Editor, and Managing Editor (*Do not leave blank*)
   Publisher (*Name and complete mailing address*)
   John Schrefer, Elsevier, Inc., 1600 John F. Kennedy Blvd., Suite 1800, Philadelphia, PA 19103-2899
   Editor (*Name and complete mailing address*)
   Rachel Glover, Elsevier, Inc., 1600 John F. Kennedy Blvd., Suite 1800, Philadelphia, PA 19103-2899
   Managing Editor (*Name and complete mailing address*)
   Catherine Bewick, Elsevier, Inc., 1600 John F. Kennedy Blvd., Suite 1800, Philadelphia, PA 19103-2899
10. Owner (*Do not leave blank. If the publication is owned by a corporation, give the name and address of the corporation immediately followed by the names and addresses of all stockholders owning or holding 1 percent or more of the total amount of stock. If not owned by a corporation, give the names and addresses of the individual owners. If owned by a partnership or other unincorporated firm, give its name and address as well as those of each individual owner. If the publication is published by a nonprofit organization, give its name and address.*)

Full Name	Complete Mailing Address
Wholly owned subsidiary of	4520 East-West Highway
Reed/Elsevier, US Holdings	Bethesda, MD 20814

11. Known Bondholders, Mortgagees, and Other Security Holders Owning or Holding 1 Percent or More of Total Amount of Bonds, Mortgages, or Other Securities. If none, check box → None

Full Name	Complete Mailing Address
N/A	

12. Tax Status (*For completion by nonprofit organizations authorized to mail at nonprofit rates*) (*Check one*)
    The purpose, function, and nonprofit status of this organization and the exempt status for federal income tax purposes:
    Has Not Changed During Preceding 12 Months
    Has Changed During Preceding 12 Months (*Publisher must submit explanation of change with this statement*)

(*See Instructions on Reverse*)

PS Form **3526,** October 1999

13. Publication Title: Endocrinology and Metabolism Clinics of North America
14. Issue Date for Circulation Data Below: September 2006

15. Extent and Nature of Circulation			Average No. Copies Each Issue During Preceding 12 Months	No. Copies of Single Issue Published Nearest to Filing Date
a. Total Number of Copies (*Net press run*)			3550	3500
b. Paid and/or Requested Circulation	(1)	Paid/Requested Outside-County Mail Subscriptions Stated on Form 3541. (*Include advertiser's proof and exchange copies*)	1475	1333
	(2)	Paid In-County Subscriptions Stated on Form 3541 (*Include advertiser's proof and exchange copies*)		
	(3)	Sales Through Dealers and Carriers, Street Vendors, Counter Sales, and Other Non-USPS Paid Distribution	1056	1083
	(4)	Other Classes Mailed Through the USPS		
c. Total Paid and/or Requested Circulation [*Sum of 15b. (1), (2), (3), and (4)*] →			2531	2416
d. Free Distribution by Mail (*Samples, compliment-ary, and other free*)	(1)	Outside-County as Stated on Form 3541	126	117
	(2)	In-County as Stated on Form 3541		
	(3)	Other Classes Mailed Through the USPS		
e. Free Distribution Outside the Mail (*Carriers or other means*)				
f. Total Free Distribution (*Sum of 15d. and 15e.*) →			126	117
g. Total Distribution (*Sum of 15c. and 15f.*) →			2657	2533
h. Copies not Distributed			893	967
i. Total (*Sum of 15g. and h.*) →			3550	3500
j. Percent Paid and/or Requested Circulation (*15c. divided by 15g. times 100*)			95.26%	95.38%

16. Publication of Statement of Ownership
    Publication required. Will be printed in the **December 2006** issue of this publication. Publication not required
17. Signature and Title of Editor, Publisher, Business Manager, or Owner
    Joan Fanucci – Executive Director of Subscription Services
    Date: 9/15/06

I certify that all information furnished on this form is true and complete. I understand that anyone who furnishes false or misleading information on this form or who omits material or information requested on the form may be subject to criminal sanctions (including fines and imprisonment) and/or civil sanctions (including civil penalties).

Instructions to Publishers

1. Complete and file one copy of this form with your postmaster annually on or before October 1. Keep a copy of the completed form for your records.
2. In cases where the stockholder or security holder is a trustee, include in items 10 and 11 the name of the person or corporation for whom the trustee is acting. Also include the names and addresses of individuals who are stockholders who own or hold 1 percent or more of the total amount of bonds, mortgages, or other securities of the publishing corporation. In item 11, if none, check the box. Use blank sheets if more space is required.
3. Be sure to furnish all circulation information called for in item 15. Free circulation must be shown in items 15d, e, and f.
4. Item 15h., Copies not Distributed, must include (1) newsstand copies originally stated on Form 3541, and returned to the publisher, (2) estimated returns from news agents, and (3), copies for office use, leftovers, spoiled, and all other copies not distributed.
5. If the publication had Periodicals authorization as a general or requester publication, this Statement of Ownership, Management, and Circulation must be published; it must be printed in any issue in October or, if the publication is not published during October, the first issue printed after October.
6. In item 16, indicate the date of the issue in which this Statement of Ownership will be published.
7. Item 17 must be signed.
   Failure to file or publish a statement of ownership may lead to suspension of Periodicals authorization.

PS Form **3526,** October 1999 (*Reverse*)